Psychiatric Home Care

Anita W. Finkelman, MSN, RN
Visiting Assistant Professor
and
Interim Director of Continuing Education
University of Cincinnati College of Nursing
and Health
Cincinnati, Ohio

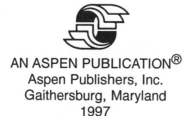

AN ASPEN PUBLICATION®
Aspen Publishers, Inc.
Gaithersburg, Maryland
1997

Library of Congress Cataloging-in-Publication Data

Finkelman, Anita Ward.
Psychiatric home care / Anita W. Finkelman.
p. cm.
Includes bibliographical references and index.
ISBN 0-8342-0928-4
1. Mentally ill—Home care. 2. Psychiatric nursing. 3. Home nursing. 4. Mentally ill—
Rehabilitation. 5. Mentally ill—Family relationships. I. Title.
RC439.5.F56   1997
362.2'4—dc21   96-48674
CIP

Orders: (800) 638-8437
Customer Service: (800) 234-1660

About Aspen Publishers • For more than 35 years, Aspen has been a leading professional
publisher in a variety of disciplines. Aspen's vast information resources are available in
both print and electronic formats. We are committed to providing the highest quality information available in the most appropriate format for our customers. Visit Aspen's Internet
site for more information resources, directories, articles, and a searchable version of Aspen's
full catalog, including the most recent publications: **http://www.aspenpub.com**
Aspen Publishers, Inc. • The hallmark of quality in publishing
Member of the worldwide Wolters Kluwer group.

Editorial Resources: Marsha Davies
Library of Congress Catalog Card Number: 96-48674
ISBN: 0-8342-0928-4
Printed in the United States of America
1 2 3 4 5

To my loving and caring husband, Fred, who has always supported my projects and writing, and to my daughters Shoshannah and Deborah, who have always believed in me.

Contents

Preface

With today's health care climate, it has become more and more critical to provide care in the community and to consider the cost-effectiveness of care. Home care is a treatment setting that offers many advantages to the psychiatric patient; however, the home is also a challenging place in which to provide care. Psychiatric home care is provided to patients with psychiatric diagnoses who may or may not have been hospitalized in the past, to medical patients who do not have a formal psychiatric diagnosis but do have major psychiatric symptoms, and to medical patients with psychological responses to their medical illnesses. These three categories of patients can be found in any home care program, even if the program does not offer formal psychiatric home care services. These patients have complex psychological and physical needs that require a high level of nursing care. The care provided must focus on psychiatric rehabilitation, using education of the patient, family, and/or significant other as a critical intervention. Home care is provided in the patient's real world, requiring staff to appreciate the daily problems that patient, family, and/or significant others encounter. Interventions must be realistic and flexible, and staff must relinquish control to the patient, family, and/or significant others.

Psychiatric Home Care may be used to assist in developing psychiatric home care services, to assist inexperienced psychiatric nurses to provide psychiatric home care, and to assist nursing education programs that include home care in their curricula. The book is divided into seven parts. Part I emphasizes the importance of developing a psychiatric treatment model that is used as a framework for the services provided. The chapters address patients with serious persistent mental illness, psychiatric rehabilitation and home care, the patient's family and significant others, the therapeutic relationship and communication, and psychoeducation. These topics represent the critical elements that should be considered as the treatment model is developed. Part II focuses on the administration of psychiatric home care services. Topics include administrative issues, the role of the psychiatric home care nurse, managed care, and case management. Part III describes the application of the nursing process in psychiatric home care. Topics include psychiatric assessment and diagnosis, and patient-centered, outcome-based care. Part IV emphasizes the importance of the biological component of mental illness and psychopharmacology related to the major psychiatric diagnostic categories. Topics include psychopharmacology in the 1990s, neuroscience, antianxiety medications, medications for obsessive-compulsive disorder, antimanic medications, antidepressant medications, antipsychotic medications, and anticholinergic medications. Part V provides an in-depth description of clinical problems in the home. Topics include anxiety disorders, depression, bipolar disorder, schizophrenia, dual diagnosis, neuropsychiatric complications of acquired immune deficiency syndrome (AIDS), and psychological care of the medically ill patient. Part VI focuses on the elderly patient in the home. Topics include principles of geropsychiatric home care treatment, and psychiatric disorders and neurological diseases in the elderly patient. Part VII discusses psychiatric emergencies in the home. Appendix A provides a glossary of psychiatric terms. The American Nurses Association standards of care for psychiatric-mental health nursing and home health nursing are found in Appendixes B and C.

Throughout the book, the emphasis is placed on the patient's responsibilities in the treatment process. I have struggled with the use of the term "patient" knowing that there is conflict in the nursing profession about the best term to use. In home health, both "patient" and "client" are used. This book was originally written using the term "client"; however, I never felt comfortable with it. As drafts were reread, I realized that I had to change back to the use of "patient." It was artificial for me to use "client" even though it has become preferred by many nurses. The belief is that the use of "client" implies that the "client" is in more control. I do not think the emphasis should be placed on the term we use to describe the person who needs and asks for health care but rather in our attitude toward that person, our recognition of the person as an individual who makes decisions about his or her health care after receiving advice from the health care provider and, in some cases, actual care. The reader will now find that "patient" has been used in this book. It is not done to offend anyone, but rather a decision that I made as an individual nurse. For those who are more comfortable with other terms, please substitute them, remembering where the emphasis must be placed rather than arguing about the "correct term." With the compassion and skill of home care staff, the psychiatric home care patient can often meet the goals of outcome-based treatment planning and learn self-management.

I

Development of a Psychiatric Treatment Model

1

Serious Persistent Mental Illness in the Home Care Patient

INTRODUCTION

Psychiatric home care has developed in response to a troubling time in psychiatric care. It has the potential of providing a creative change in health care for people with serious mental illness and for patients who have problems coping with medical illness. As home care agencies develop psychiatric services, they must consider the type of psychiatric treatment model that will be used as the framework for the care provided to patients and their families and/or significant others (SO). The first step in developing a psychiatric treatment model is to obtain an understanding of serious persistent mental illness and its effect on patients and their families/SOs. There are obstacles to developing home care services because of the "natural human tendency to move away from situations that are confusing and engender hopelessness. In home care, many of the mentally ill live in multi-problem situations, to which there is no easy answer."[1(pp.17–19)]

HOSPITALIZATION: EFFECTS ON THE PATIENT

The most common view of hospitalization is that it helps sick people. Psychiatric hospitalization, however, is more complex. According to Cohen, "The illness itself can be considered a traumatic experience, which is amplified by the iatrogenic trauma of psychiatric hospitalization."[2(p.80)] Caring for a patient in the home requires knowledge of his or her experience in other treatment settings. Hospitalization probably has occurred and, if not, it may occur at some time during home care. The continuum of psychiatric treatment includes hospitalization in both acute and long-term facilities and a variety of community settings such as partial hospitalization, outpatient therapy, halfway housing and treatment, crisis intervention clinics or emergency room visits, and psychiatric home care. Each of these affects the patient and his or her response to other treatment settings. It is clear that people with serious mental illness require treatment at different times in their lives and with different intensity. The health care system has not always met these needs. The quality of hospitalization can be highly variable, and the patient brings memories of past treatment into all treatment experiences. As Worley has observed, "The loss of self determination, autonomy, and freedom of action; the provision of all needs without the necessity of action on the part of the patient; and the regulation and standardization of life in institutions can lead to dependency, apathy, and the need to relearn the skills necessary to function in life outside of the institution."[3(p.22)] The patient who has been hospitalized has many needs, some of which may have resulted from hospitalization. Today, the length of stay has decreased considerably for most patients, with the average length of stay in 1994 at 15.2 days.[4] Even a short stay, however, places the patient in an environment in which decisions are made for him or her, a schedule is developed by staff, and structure is provided; even though the patient is encouraged to be as independent as possible, there are limits on independence in the hospital environment.

The shortened stays also means that the patient who is discharged is much sicker than in the past, with little time to adjust to medications. The adjustment that is needed from the hospital to the community is a major focus of psychiatric home care. A study that focused on postdischarge problems conducted a telephone follow-up of 127 patients with mixed diagnoses and an average length of stay of 14 days. Eight problem areas were identified.[5(p.25)]

1. *Medications:* forgetting to take, side effects, lack of funds to purchase, misuse, substitution
2. *Symptomatology:* actual occurrence, anxiety about occurrence
3. *Follow-up appointments:* forgetting, canceling, expressing feelings of lack of need, transportation problems
4. *Structuring time:* inability to transfer structure learned in hospital to home situation, frequent daily use of 10 to 12 hours of television to fill time; inability to think of alternative activities
5. *Sleeping:* inability to develop healthy sleeping patterns, inability to use or remember relaxation techniques taught during hospital stay
6. *Support groups:* lack of incentive or perceived value of support groups; difficulty with transportation to groups, inability to organize time
7. *Family/SO/patient relations:* discord with family/SOs, inability to work with feelings, inability to negotiate with family/SOs, resentment of family's/SO's vigilance
8. *Eating:* inability to follow food plan, inability to organize time for meal preparation, decrease in appetite, lack of sufficient intake, eating at inappropriate times

All of these problems can be addressed in home care, and each should be assessed for every patient admitted to home care.

STAFF

Besides confronting myths, as described in Exhibit 1–1, staff must recognize that, in the home setting, control shifts from the staff to the patient. Those who have worked in the hospital setting or any more structured setting may find it difficult to make the transition to the home care setting. Each home is an unfamiliar setting that usually includes contact with the patient's family and/or SOs. In most cases, this can be positive contact; however, there are some families/SOs with whom staff would prefer to have less contact. Collaboration and coordination among disciplines is more complex in the home. Staff in the hospital meet frequently to discuss patients and their care, but this is not possible in home care. Meetings are difficult to arrange; even telephone calls can be difficult due to schedule conflicts. Home care staff work alone most of the time and lack the support that hospital staff provide one another, especially during times of stress. Coping with suicidal behavior, escalating behavior, and acting out is more complex in the home because safety is a critical issue. There is also less staff support, less structure, and fewer physical restraint resources. Staff may feel this burden and fear patient behavior.

The home care nurse carries much more responsibility than the hospital nurse; however, this can have its advantages. Nurses can be more creative in the home setting, and the situation usually demands it. For many nurses, this can be a positive experience. Staff can actually see how the patient lives, the daily problems, and interactions with family/SOs—all in the patient's real world. The psychiatric nurse may be confused about the nursing role in the home, one that does have different components than the hospital nurse and clearly is different from nonpsychiatric home care nursing. The psychiatric patient is more disorganized than the medical patient, requiring less technical and procedure-oriented care. Such a patient may lead the home care nurse with limited psychiatric experience to ask, "What is there left to do?"

THE PATIENT IN HOME CARE

The patient in the home is in an environment that focuses on past and present conflicts with family/SOs and provides less structure and more isolation than the patient may need. The hospital does provide an environment in which contact with family/SOs is less intense, and a structure that alleviates anxiety for many patients. The hospitalized patient has more contact with others, even though it

Exhibit 1–1 Myths and Facts about Mental Illness

Myth: A person who has been mentally ill can never be normal.
Fact: Often mental illness is temporary, lasting only a short time. Many people will not get sick again. Some people do have illness that continues throughout their lives.

Myth: Persons with mental illness are unpredictable.
Fact: During active illness the person may be unpredictable but, after recovery, the person will probably be predictable with consistent behavior.

Myth: Mentally ill persons are dangerous.
Fact: Only a very small number of mentally ill persons are dangerous, trying to hurt themselves or others.

Myth: Recovered mental patients could become dangerous suddenly and go beserk.
Fact: Few patients go beserk. After discharge, it is more likely that a person might become depressed rather than suddenly dangerous.

Myth: You cannot talk to someone who has been mentally ill.
Fact: You can talk with patients who have been mentally ill. It is only patients who are very confused or severely depressed who might not be able to talk, and this is usually for only a short time. Some communication is always possible.

Myth: A former mental patient makes a bad employee.
Fact: Most former patients have no problems working. Those who do may need to find a more flexible job or a less stressful one.

Myth: Mental retardation is a form of mental illness.
Fact: These are not the same.

Myth: A person usually stays in the hospital for months or even a year.
Fact: Most patients stay in the hospital for several days to a week or two.

Myth: Mental illness can happen with the rich and the poor.
Fact: This is true. Mental illness has nothing to do with income.

Myth: If you are different from others, you are mentally ill.
Fact: Saying someone is "different" does not mean that the person is mentally ill.

Myth: A readmission to a hospital means treatment has failed.
Fact: Some patients need help periodically. For them, any time spent outside the hospital is a success.

continues

Exhibit 1–1 continued

> *Myth:* There have been no great changes in treatment for mental illness in the last 50 years.
> *Fact:* There have been major changes, such as the use of medications.
>
> *Myth:* Most patients with mental illness need to be hospitalized.
> *Fact:* Most patients are treated outside the hospital as outpatients.
>
> *Source:* Adapted from *The 14 Worst Myths About Recovered Mental Patients*, DHHS Publication No. (ADM) 88-1391, © 1988, U.S. Government Printing Office.

may be forced upon the patient. Allowing the patient to return home may communicate to the patient that he or she is cured; and consequently, the patient may wonder why further treatment, such as home care, is required. Understanding how the patient interprets the hospital discharge and the need for home care is a critical first step in the home care admission assessment. In addition, negative hospital experiences may lead the patient to be wary of any type of treatment or staff. Patients who have never experienced psychiatric home care may be very confused about staff roles, especially if physical care is also provided by the same nurse. Psychiatric nurses in the hospital do not usually provide physical care.

The patient, however, may experience many benefits from home care. The natural setting of the home puts the patient in control, requiring independence rather than dependence, and there is less of a stigma associated with home care. More staff time may be available for actual patient care, because in the hospital setting staff are very busy and interruptions are common. Because the nurse actually sees the home and observes interactions in the home setting, the nurse's understanding of the patient's needs often is more realistic and facilitates more realistic interventions.

Today, if it is appropriate, patients can be discharged sooner from the hospital to another treatment program that can meet their needs. Home care is less costly than hospital care for the patient, and yet it is a treatment service whose intensity can be adapted. With a better assessment of the patient and the problems, home care may be used to prevent unnecessary hospitalizations. Patients with complex psychiatric and physical problems can receive care from the same source, and this reduces the patient's stress. All psychiatric patients need education about their illnesses, treatment, and skills. Teaching patients in their homes is more comfortable for them. Patients can be more independent and apply their learning in their real world. They do not have to wait to try to apply information received in the hospital, which may or may not be realistic or helpful, after discharge from the hospital. It is hoped that learning in the patient's home will result in increased patient compliance and self-management.

THE FAMILY AND/OR SIGNIFICANT OTHERS

Many families/SOs fear that, because there is a lack of treatment choices for psychiatric patients, the home will become the treatment setting by default and the family/SOs will serve as the treatment staff. They fear that the decision will not be made because the home setting is the best place for the patient, but because it is the only place. If this is true, then psychiatric home care will have limited success in meeting the needs of patients and families/SOs. It must be recognized that there are families/SOs who are reluctant to participate in care, unable to participate in care, burned out from past experiences, or even destructive to the care. Listening to the family/SO's view of home care is very important. The patient's symptoms and problems may only fuel unhealthy conflict with the family/SOs, particularly if they do not receive help in coping with the conflicts that arise from daily living with an ill family member. The family/SOs may also be confused about the role of the nurse and other home care staff and unsure how to get help from the nurse. In the hospital they may have had limited or negative experiences with the nursing staff. They may want the structure and control to be in the nurse's hands and not in the patient's. They may fear certain behaviors and worry about their safety and the safety of the patient in the home. For many families/SOs, home care may offer new choices for them. There is less stigma than with hospitalization. Staff may have the opportunity to listen to family/SOs and to develop a better understanding of their needs and problems. The family/SOs will have time with the ill family member in a more natural setting and will have the opportunity to maintain more natural relationships but with support from a professional. In addition, home care is less costly. This can be very important if the family/SOs have used much of their financial resources or if insurance coverage is limited. According to Hatfield, "Families of the mentally ill, like other consumers of goods and services in our society, want the power of informed choice. They want safe, efficacious, cost-effective help. They want increased control over their own lives. Making informed choices in the arena of mental health, however, presents nearly insurmountable difficulties because there is such a confusing diversity of theory and practice."[6(p.11)]

Given these disadvantages and advantages, what can be gained from providing psychiatric care in the home? The nurse will see the patient in the patient's natural setting coping with daily problems and interacting with people who are important. The nurse will become involved in this environment, its relationships, and communications processes, and the nurse can problem solve in the patient's environment. Psychiatric home care can be stressful for all; however, there are many positive aspects for the staff, the patient, and the family/SOs. To use the home to the advantage of the patient, the nurse needs to understand the illness and its effect on the patient's daily life.

STRESS-VULNERABILITY-COPING-COMPETENCE

"Mental illness is one of those catastrophic events that strikes infrequently, but when it does, it has devastating consequences for patients and families."[7(p.19)] There is a need to understand mental illness, to understand the relationship between the biological and the behavioral-affective-social aspects of the illness as a catastrophic event. Parts IV and V of this book include information about the biological aspect of mental illness and its implications for treatment. The history of psychiatry does not suffer from the lack of theories about mental illness, its process, and etiology. In fact, this history has led to much conflict about identifying the correct theory. Today it is important to describe an approach that includes the new biological information, as psychiatric professionals consider many important questions: What is the relationship between the biological and the behavioral-affective-social aspects of the illness? Is there a relationship? Do we throw out one aspect for the other? As psychiatric professionals consider these questions, nursing has tried to focus on the biopsychosocial with efforts to view all aspects of each patient. Nursing has not always been successful, because it is a complex approach.

The following basic beliefs about the importance of the biological information in psychiatric care have been identified by Andreasen:[8(pp.29–33)]

- The major psychiatric illnesses are diseases, just as the medical illnesses diabetes, heart disease, and cancer are diseases.
- These diseases are caused principally by biological factors, and most of these factors reside in the brain.
- Clinical evaluation of patients involves careful history-taking, observing the course of symptoms over time, physical examination, and sometimes laboratory tests.
- Serious or severe mental illnesses include depression, inappropriate elevations in mood or mania, schizophrenia, severe anxiety disorders, and illnesses leading to senility or the dementias.
- The treatment of these diseases emphasizes the use of "somatic therapies." It also recognizes the importance of social and economic functioning.
- Mental illnesses are not due to "bad habits" or weakness of will.
- Mental illnesses are not caused by bad parenting or bad "spousing."

- The somatic therapies are very effective methods for treating many mental illnesses.

Frequently, patients and families/SOs want to discuss these issues and particularly their feelings about them. In this discussion, the home care nurse should share information about facts and myths of mental illness and its treatment.

In addition to the biological factors, other factors are important to patient functioning. Liberman has developed the stress-vulnerability-coping-competence approach as a model of mental illness that incorporates the biological and psychosocial factors. The model explains the onset, course, and outcomes of symptoms and social functioning as a complex interaction among biological, environmental, and behavioral factors.[9] Figure 1–1 illustrates this model and describes the factors that affect psychiatric disability.

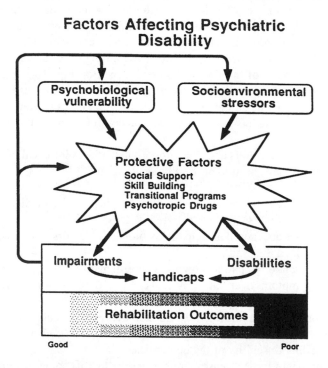

Figure 1–1 Factors Affecting Psychiatric Disability. *Source:* Reprinted with permission from R. Liberman, ed. "The Practice of Psychiatric Rehabilitation: Historical, Conceptual, and Research Base," *Schizophrenia Bulletin*, Vol. 12, No. 4, p. 547, © 1986, American Psychiatric Press.

The first component of the model is the biological process. Psychobiological vulnerability factors put the person at risk and are "relatively enduring pathological abnormalities present before, during, and after symptomatic episodes."[10(p.12)] The second component consists of socioenvironmental stressors, those transient or environmental experiences or events that occur and require some adaptation.[11] The third component of the model consists of the protective factors that "determine whether a given level of vulnerability to mental disorder leads to manifest symptomatology under a given current level of stress."[12(p.12)] The goal is to decrease the effects of stress and decrease the chance of relapse—to find equilibrium between the patient's psychobiological vulnerability, the socioenvironmental stressors, and the patient's personal coping and competence. As indicated in the figure, typical protective factors are social support, skill building, transitional programs, psychotropic drugs, and case management.

Applying this model to care of the patient in the home requires an appreciation of the interactive nature of the illness between the biological deviations and the socioenvironmental stressors, the risk of exacerbation or relapse of illness, and the importance of protective factors or methods for preventing or lessening symptomatology. The nurse must assess the patient's biological condition and potential and present stressors and then develop interventions to support the protective factors. Liberman identifies the following three principles that can guide the nurse:[13(p.26)]:

1. the optimism that desirable change is possible, given the harnessing of principles of human learning to the needs of the patient
2. the belief that motivation for change can come from special arrangements of the patient's rehabilitation and natural environments as well as from within the patient
3. the confidence that building from the patient's assets and interests, including supportive treatment and family environments, even small improvements can lead to significant functional changes in and uplifting of the patient's quality of life

Nurses who work in home care are uniquely prepared to apply the stress-vulnerability-coping-competence model to help the psychiatric home care patient. Coping and adaptation are important components of all nursing care. According to Hatfield, "The theory of coping and adaptation starts with the assumption that all living systems strive to maintain themselves in their environment, to overcome obstacles, and to achieve autonomy and self-determination . . . usually to master conditions of threat, harm, or challenge when the usual strategies are insufficient."[14(p.20)] Potential modifiers of stress are the action of medications and the patient's problem solving, coping capacity, and the social environment.

EXPERIENCING SERIOUS PERSISTENT MENTAL ILLNESS: DEMORALIZATION

Viewing persons with mental illness as having chronic illness is no longer acceptable. As early as 1978, Talbott commented that the term *chronic* stigmatizes the person, implying hopelessness and progressive deterioration.[15] This viewpoint has only become stronger over the years, particularly by some organizations such as the National Alliance for the Mentally Ill (NAMI). The more acceptable term is *serious persistent mental illness*, which includes any person with bipolar disorder, schizophrenia, major depression, or any mental illness that persists over time. Liberman has identified three measurements to use in describing serious mental illness: (1) diagnosis; (2) disability as measured by social and vocational level of function; and (3) duration of symptoms, disability, and hospitalization episodes. According to Mechanic:

> The problems of integrating mental health care into health care are complicated by the orientation of the general health sector toward acute care, and in this sense, serious mental illness shares common problems with many other chronic disabling diseases. Such conditions typically disrupt the ability to perform ordinary role activities, undermining patients' everyday functioning, confidence, and self esteem. Effective care requires not only dealing with medical manifestation but also helping individuals to maintain the skills and supports necessary to counteract negative consequences and providing assistive strategies and devices that facilitate coping.[16(p.895)]

Most patients who are admitted to a psychiatric home care program have serious persistent mental illness. They are experiencing demoralization as a result of their illness and its effect on their lives. According to Mosher and Burti, "Low self-esteem and a lack of self-confidence, competence, and a sense of efficacy define the demoralized person."[17(pp.77–78)] One parent described her adult son's mental illness in the following way: "Stuart not only appeared to lose his ability to concentrate, he also acted as though he was intimidated by his friends. This was really puzzling because Stuart was an easygoing fellow who had had very relaxed, long-term relationships with his buddies. He had been the kind of child who loved to play and was always in a good humor."[18(p.84)] It is impossible to understand fully the patient's experience of mental illness or how the patient experiences the demoralization, but it is important to attempt to understand it as much as is possible. This understanding will help staff provide care that focuses on what the patient needs rather than what the staff think the patient needs. This effort to understand requires connecting symptoms to behavior, as behavior has meaning for the patient.

Hatfield has described some of the elements of mental illness that help staff, families, and SOs to develop a better understanding of the illness experience.[19]

- *Altered perceptions:* The patient's senses are heightened or decreased, usually with increased acuteness. Visual and auditory experiences are increased, usually more intense or louder. Misperceptions or distortions may occur. The patient may become focused on one or two thoughts or perceptions. Particularly important to all aspects of nursing care are the difficulty the patient may have in synthesizing incoming stimuli and difficulty filtering out irrelevant stimuli. This can interfere with interpersonal relationships, problem solving, and teaching the patient.
- *Attention deficits:* The patient's attention and concentration can be inadequate. Distractions can easily interfere with concentration. If the patient has hallucinations, they will affect attention. The patient may have difficulty deciding what is important.
- *Cognitive confusion:* Cognitive confusion may result in disorientation, thought blocking, loosening of associations, and a confused attitude. The patient may think concretely with little or no ability to think abstractly. Logical thinking may be impaired. These difficulties directly affect the patient's ability to problem solve and cope with stress.
- *Changes in emotions:* The most common changes in emotions are exaggerated feelings and inappropriate emotions. Exaggerated feelings can be anywhere on a continuum of too much or too little (for example, from a patient who is extremely psychotic to a patient who is so depressed that movement is difficult). Inappropriate emotions can be identified when the patient responds to a situation in a manner that would not be expected, such as laughing at a sad situation.

These experiences all affect the patient's sense of self, resulting in a feeling of loss, emptiness, and loneliness. Not all patients experience all of these deficits, as there are individual differences as well as diagnostic differences. More specific descriptions related to the experience of mental illness will be discussed in Part V.

Demoralization is usually the experience of most patients who are referred to psychiatric home care. The focus of psychiatric home care is on "remoralization." This is the helping process "in which patients are given opportunities to develop options, solve problems, overcome obstacles, and accomplish goals."[20(p.78)] According to Godschalx, "The impact upon life experiences is of greater concern to people with schizophrenia than are the symptoms of the illness."[21(p.29)] This is also true for patients with other diagnoses. The tendency is to focus on the symptoms without seeing what the symptoms are doing to the patient's life. By focusing on the patient's life experiences, it will be easier for staff to ask, "What works for the patient?"

The Patient and Grieving

Patients with a mental illness experience many losses during the course of their illness. If they are newly diagnosed with a mental illness, they may just be beginning to experience losses. Hospitalization has its own potential losses for the patient, including loss of freedom, choice, self-care, independence, contact with important persons, job, school, and hope for the future. Individual patients experience these losses with a different intensity, and treatment can help the individual cope with the loss and even recover some of the losses. After hospitalization, the patient experiences more losses, particularly related to self-concept, self-esteem, and the view that others have of the patient. As the patient adjusts to the illness, grieving takes place. The illness may have exacerbations and relapses that renew grieving for the patient. For many patients, it is very difficult to accept that they may never be the same or may never achieve a goal that they thought was important in the past. The patient can develop positive self-esteem and a different self-concept that incorporates the need for treatment and any limitations from the illness. The patient can again achieve important goals, but they may need to be modified. Nursing care in the home assists the patient as the grieving process is experienced, focusing on a positive resolution.

Relapse: Effects on Patient, Family/Significant Others, and Staff

The long-term nature of mental illness indicates that relapse will occur for most patients (for example, depression returns or the patient becomes psychotic again). This exacerbates demoralization, and it is painful for the patient and the family/SOs. Relapse disrupts progress, which makes everyone involved feel that they are taking one step forward and two steps back. The nurse may also feel hopelessness due to the relapses; however, if the nurse allows these feelings to negatively affect the patient's care it will be detrimental for all. Relapses must be viewed as opportunities to learn more about the illness and its effects on the patient, and then everyone must work toward moving forward. The nurse identifies with the patient positive aspects of hospitalization (e.g., shorter treatment than last time, a chance for the patient to focus on a specific problem, or an opportunity to try a new medication). Helping the patient and the family/SOs to frame the hospitalization in a positive way facilitates progress.

SUMMARY

Providing home care services for the patient with serious persistent mental illness is complex and demanding. According to Keating and Kelman, "It is the caring nature of the nurse that generates trust and collaboration in the care of the ill patient and maintenance of health of other family members. The nurse's genuine concern and care for these patient systems is the foundation for building a trusting relationship, contractual agreements, delivery of care, patient and family compliance with medical orders, participation in the nursing prescription, and the eventual consumption of self-care."[22(p.77)] Treatment in the home is very different from treatment in the hospital—for the patient, family/SOs, and the staff. This transition from treatment in the hospital to the home is not easy, but it can be very positive in the long run. It requires an understanding of the illness and its effects on daily life, as well as an understanding of the care of the psychiatric patient in the home. One approach, psychiatric rehabilitation, can be very helpful for the patient and family/SOs and can be applied by nursing staff in the home.

NOTES

1. M. Walsh, "The Challenge of Mental Health Home Care," *Caring* 5, no. 7 (1986): 17–19.
2. L. Cohen, "Psychiatric Hospitalization as an Experience of Trauma," *Archives of Psychiatric Nursing* 8, no. 2 (1994): 78–81.
3. N. Worley, "Independent Living for the Chronically Mentally Ill," *Journal for Psychosocial Nursing* 27, no. 9 (1989): 18–23.
4. "NAPHS Survey Finds Member Facilities Treating More Patients; Inpatient Care Continues to Drop," *Psychiatric Services* 46, no. 10 (1995): 1088.
5. J. McIntosh and N. Worley, "Beyond Discharge: Telephone Follow-Up and Aftercare," *Journal of Psychosocial Nursing* 32, no. 10 (1994): 21–27.
6. A. Hatfield, *Family Education in Mental Illness* (New York: Guilford Press, 1990), 11.
7. Hatfield, *Family Education in Mental Illness*, 19.
8. N. Andreasen, *The Broken Brain: The Biological Revolution in Psychiatry* (New York: Harper & Row, 1984), 29–33.
9. R. Liberman, "Social Factors in Schizophrenia," in *American Psychiatric Association Annual Review*, Vol. 1, ed. L. Grinspoon (Washington, DC: American Psychiatric Press, Inc., 1982), 12.
10. R. Liberman, "Coping with Chronic Mental Disorders: A Framework for Hope," in *Psychiatric Rehabilitation of Chronic Mental Patients*, ed. R. Liberman (Washington, DC: American Psychiatric Press, Inc., 1988), 1–28.
11. Liberman, "Coping with Chronic Mental Disorders," 12.
12. Liberman, "Coping with Chronic Mental Disorders," 12.
13. Liberman, "Coping with Chronic Mental Disorders," 26.

14. Hatfield, *Family Education in Mental Illness*, 20.

15. J. Talbott, *The Chronic Mental Patient: Problems, Solutions, and Recommendations for a Public Policy* (Washington, DC: American Psychiatric Association, 1978), 57.

16. D. Mechanic, "Integrating Mental Health into a General Health Care System," *Hospital and Community Psychiatry* 45, no. 9 (1994): 893–897.

17. L. Mosher and L. Burti, *Community Mental Health: Principles and Practice* (New York: W.W. Norton & Company, 1989), 77–78.

18. P. Backlar, *The Family Face of Schizophrenia* (New York: G.P. Putnam's Sons, 1994), 84.

19. Hatfield, *Family Education in Mental Illness*, 83–93.

20. Mosher, *Community Mental Health: Principles and Practice*, 78.

21. S. Godschalx, "Experiencing Life with a Psychiatric Disability," in *Chronic Mental Illness: Coping Strategies*, ed. J. Maurin (Thorofare, NJ: SLACK, Inc., 1989), 3–29.

22. S. Keating and G. Kelman, *Home Health Care Nursing: Concepts and Practice* (Philadelphia: J.B. Lippincott Co., 1988), 77.

SUGGESTED READING

Bachrach, L. 1995. Recurring themes and a tribute. *Psychiatric Services* 46, no. 6: 553–554, 557.

Brince, J. 1986. The psychiatric patient: Hospital care—home care. *Caring* 5, no. 7: 13–16.

Mechanic, D. 1994. Integrating mental health into a general health care system. *Hospital and Community Psychiatry* 45, no. 9: 893–897.

O'Conner, F. 1994. A vulnerability-stress framework for evaluating clinical interventions in schizophrenia. *Image* 26, no. 3: 231–237.

Reif, L., and K. Martin. 1996. *Nurses and consumers: Partners in assuring quality care in the home.* Washington, DC: American Nurses Association.

Walsh, M. 1986. The challenge of mental health home care. *Caring* 5, no. 7: 17–19.

CHAPTER

2

Psychiatric Rehabilitation: Application in Psychiatric Home Care

INTRODUCTION

Psychiatric rehabilitation may seem to be an unusual place to begin a discussion of psychiatric home care; however, it includes the critical elements that must be considered as a home care agency and individual nurses begin to develop and apply a treatment model to the clinical situation—the care of the seriously mentally ill patient in the home. Psychiatric rehabilitation activities are very similar to psychiatric nursing activities. In addition, psychiatric rehabilitation is an approach that can respond to many important patient needs. According to Munich and Lang, "It addresses difficulties in three domains of patients' lives: clinical status, functional status, and quality of life."[1(p.661)]

DEMORALIZATION

Most psychiatric patients in the home experience demoralization or feelings of low self-esteem, low self-confidence, and problems with competence. Demoralization results from the patient's illness, past psychiatric treatment, and the lack of or limited acceptance of mental illness from the community. The illness limits the patient's ability to cope and may prevent the patient from learning important communication and social skills. The symptoms may interfere with the patient's ability to develop options to solve a problem. Those who offer help need to consider normalization or help the patient to identify options that are most nearly normal.[2] Treatment does not always help the patient, and hospitalization is not always supportive. Frequently a patient's memories from past treatment affect acceptance of and compliance with future treatment. The community has not been accepting of mental illness. Stigma and shame are common experiences for both the patient and family/significant others (SOs). According to Backlar, "Shame is a powerful and destructive force. Subtly it can underlie the diverse and persistent dilemmas which abound for the families of people with mental illness."[3(p.15)] A parent of an adult child who has a mental illness stated, "Sometimes I say that I am not ashamed of this happening—of my son being mentally ill—that I am not embarrassed by it, but I have found in the past that this is not really true. At one time or another I have had feelings of shame and anger. I like to think that I don't have a problem with it but when I'm really honest I have to admit that there is always a little residual embarrassment, a kind of tightness that makes me feel that I must both explain and hold myself back."[4(p.83)]

Prevention of further damage from the illness, its treatment, and the community is difficult to achieve. Successful prevention requires comprehensive, coordinated services. Psychiatric home care is one of these important services. Treatment that blends psychiatric treatment and rehabilitation is based on the following assumptions.[5(pp.551–554)]

- Major mental illness is a real disease with an underlying biological component.
- The expression of mental illness is determined by the interaction of underlying vulnerability (genetic and biological factors), personal attributes (psychodevelopmental factors), and environmental characteristics (family and sociocultural factors).
- Persons with severe mental illness have an underlying biological vulnerability that is likely to be always present. Recovery, not cure, is possible.
- Appropriate assessment is important. Both functional and syndromal diagnoses must be carefully made. (*Functional diagnoses* identify skills and abilities. *Syndromal diagnoses* predict course and stages of recovery indicating psychophysiological vulnerabilities and help identify somatic treatments.)
- The illness label must be separated from the person with the illness.
- The types of treatment or rehabilitation interventions that are most appropriate change as the phase of the illness and the developmental needs of the person change.
- Patients who are capable of making decisions about their treatment, rehabilitation, and lifestyle have the right to do so.
- People who lack decision-making capacity have a right to the treatment they need. Such people may require involuntary treatment for significant periods of time.
- Patients have the right to live as independently as their capabilities allow.
- Treatment and rehabilitation should be tailored to the individual patient.
- To consider the patient's many needs, the expertise of each staff member on the multidisciplinary team needs to be used appropriately.
- Treatment and rehabilitation must occur concurrently.

- Treatment and rehabilitation are professional endeavors, and professional boundaries must be maintained.
- Treatment of major mental illness must be as active and aggressive as necessary.
- Treatment and rehabilitation must ensure that each patient's basic needs, including the need for a supportive and safe environment in which to live, are met.
- Individuals cannot be treated or rehabilitated without the participation of family members and significant others in evaluation, treatment, education, and support.
- All treatment and rehabilitation are collaborative.
- Treatment and rehabilitation teams must use the findings of sound research.

The psychiatric home care nurse applies nursing interventions that incorporate psychiatric rehabilitation to assist the patient who is demoralized. According to Mosher and Burti, "The helping process can be viewed as one of remoralization, in which patients are given opportunities to develop options, solve problems, overcome obstacles, and accomplish goals."[6(p.78)] Nurses as well as other health care professionals often provide care that encourages dependency rather than independency. Mosher and Burti recommend that community mental health, which includes psychiatric home care, should preserve and enhance the patient's personal power and control.[7(pp.106–107)] The nurse cannot give the patient power. It is often easier for nurses to do for the patient rather than help the patient do for himself or herself. The home care nurse should ask the patient, "What do you want?" and "How can I help you get it?" Strategies the nurse can use to preserve and enhance the patient's personal power and control include the following:[8]

- Provide information.
- Help identify options.
- Encourage role playing and practicing scenarios.
- Exercise advocacy.
- Keep the patient involved in the process.
- Serve as a facilitator.
- Demystify medical issues.
- Limit direct action as much as possible.
- Involve a network of resources.
- Encourage patient responsibility.

The patient and the nurse agree upon goals and strategies that help the patient to feel more positive and more successful or "remoralized." This requires working on concrete problems and building from one success to another. A critical point with remoralization, however, is patient power. The more the patient is actively engaged in the process, the more the patient will gain.

Working with home care patients may place the nurse in a position of trying to be all things for the patient. This is never successful. According to Mosher and Burti, "Overenthusiastic intrusion into all aspects of patients' lives will leave them expectant, dependent, and ultimately disillusioned when this month's savior proves to be no more reliable than last's. . . . There is no magical relief from pain and suffering. You need to 'be with' and 'do with' patients, while expecting them to learn better how to help themselves. You may also experience disappointment about your patients' perceived failures."[9(p.377)] Ultimately, the nurse must remember that the patient's life is his or her own, not the nurse's. This is not always easy to accomplish as the nurse becomes more and more involved in the patient's daily problems with limited support from other staff to discuss the appropriate level of involvement. When it is discussed, other staff members rarely have the opportunity to interact with the patient and lack firsthand experience with the patient. For this reason, it is very important to frequently ask: "What does the patient want?"

DEFINITION OF PSYCHIATRIC REHABILITATION

The concept of psychiatric or psychosocial rehabilitation has been developing over the past 45 years, and it has had many definitions. Liberman states that psychiatric rehabilitation emphasizes "strategies to help people cope with the environment rather than succumb to it, health induction rather than symptom reduction, and improvement of the person's ability to do something in a specific environment, even in the presence of residual disability."[10(p.4)] The International Association of Psychosocial Rehabilitation Services defines psychiatric/psychosocial rehabilitation as "the process of facilitating an individual's restoration or habitation to an optimal level of independent functioning in the community."[11(p.vii)] Bachrach defines it as "a therapeutic approach to the care of mentally ill individuals that encourages each patient to develop his or her fullest capacities through learning procedures and environmental supports."[12(p.1456)] Sartorius's definition emphasizes the quality of life: "Rehabilitation means restoring or creating a life of acceptable quality for people who suffer from a mental illness or who have impaired mental capacity that causes a certain level of disability."[13(p.1180)] Another definition is offered by a nurse: "an approach to mental health care that focuses on interpersonal relationships, social roles and interactions, and activities of daily living as well as the treatment of symptoms of mental illness."[14(p.24)] This is the definition that will be used in this book. Exhibit 2–1 highlights key concepts from these definitions.

Exhibit 2–1 Psychiatric Rehabilitation: Key Concepts

- strategies to cope
- health as opposed to illness
- improvement
- facilitation
- independent function in the community
- development of fullest capacity
- learning
- environmental supports
- quality of life
- interpersonal relationships
- social roles
- activities of daily living
- treatment of symptoms

Rehabilitation begins as soon as an acute episode is stabilized. Disabled persons need skills and environmental supports to fulfill the demands of living. Psychiatric rehabilitation focuses on any of the following:

- communication skills
- problem solving
- affect identification
- needs recognition
- social relatedness
- self-care
- family/SO relationships
- interpersonal relationships
- coping skills
- psychoeducation
- case management
- psychotropic medications
- housing
- vocational skills and support
- leisure and recreational activities
- nutrition
- exercise
- general health

All of these areas may be included in nursing care. The individual patient must participate actively in the process as clinical status, functional status, and quality of life are discussed and improved, and the patient must commit to working toward a solution. The level of commitment varies, depending on the individual patient. Psychiatric rehabilitation involves assessment, training, and modification of living environments with specific goals or outcomes.

PSYCHIATRIC REHABILITATION PRINCIPLES AND CONCEPTS

Psychiatric rehabilitation principles have been identified from the literature to provide a framework for the development of psychiatric rehabilitation that meets patients' needs. These principles are found in Exhibit 2–2. Other principles that are important to psychiatric rehabilitation include the following:

- Improvement should focus on the quality of life as perceived by the patient and family/SOs.
- As outcomes are identified, the patient's strengths are emphasized.
- The nurse must keep in mind the patient's perception rather than the nurse's perception.
- The nurse does not do *for* the patient but *with* the patient, recognizing that there are individual differences among patients and that each patient changes over time.

These principles emphasize the importance of flexibility. Rigidity will lead to problems for the psychiatric patient in the home as well as for the family/SOs and the nurse.

Bachrach has identified seven important concepts related to psychiatric rehabilitation that can be incorporated into psychiatric home care.[15(pp.18–19)]

1. Individualization or to enable the patient to develop to the fullest extent of his or her capabilities
2. Environmental factors are changed to meet the patient's needs or the patient's capabilities are adapted to the environment.
3. Hope is restored supporting the patient's functional capacity and self-esteem.
4. Optimistic work goals are set.
5. Social and recreational life is supported, and social skills developed.
6. Active involvement in care is required of each patient.
7. Continuity of care is critical to the ongoing process.

These seven psychiatric rehabilitation concepts are important in nursing practice as well as in psychiatric home care. If these principles are not incorporated into nursing practice, the patient has little chance of success in home care. Nurs-

Exhibit 2–2 Principles of Psychosocial Rehabilitation

- All people have an underused capacity that should be developed.
- All people can be equipped with skills (social, vocational, educational, interpersonal).
- People have the right and responsibility for self-determination.
- Services should be provided in as normalized an environment as possible.
- Assessment of needs and care should be differential (i.e., based on the unique needs, abilities, deficiencies, and environment of each patient).
- Maximum commitment is required from staff members.
- Care is provided in an intimate environment without professional authoritative shields and barriers.
- Early intervention is preferable.
- Environmental agencies and forces are recruited to assist in the provision of service.
- Attempts are made to modify the environment in terms of attitudes, rights, services, and behavior (social change).
- All patients are welcome for as long as they want to be served (with the exception of specific, short-term, high-demand programs).
- Work and vocational rehabilitation are central to the rehabilitation process.
- Emphasis is on social rather than a medical model of care.
- Emphasis is on the patient's strengths rather than on pathologies.
- Emphasis is on the here and now rather than on problems from the past.

Source: Reprinted with permission from R. Cann et al., "Perceptions of Consumers, Practitioners, and Experts Regarding Psychosocial Rehabilitation Principles," *Psychosocial Rehabilitation Journal*, Vol. 16, No. 1, p. 97, © 1992, International Association of Psychosocial Rehabilitation.

ing strongly supports patient strengths, patient participation, individualized care, and the importance of the environment for the patient. The nursing process emphasizes continuity throughout all stages of care. The principles and concepts of psychiatric rehabilitation are so similar to psychiatric nursing principles and concepts that it is difficult to distinguish them.

CRITICAL TERMINOLOGY[16–22]

Critical terminology related to psychiatric rehabilitation should be understood by home care staff as psychiatric rehabilitation principles and activities are incorporated into nursing care.

- *pathology*—lesions or abnormalities in the central nervous system caused by agents or processes responsible for the etiology and maintenance of the biobehavioral disorder
- *impairment*—any loss or abnormality of psychological, physiological, or anatomical structure or function (resulting from underling pathology)
- *disability*—any restriction or lack of ability (resulting from an impairment) to perform an activity in the manner or within the range considered normal for a human being
- *handicap*—a disadvantage for a given individual (resulting from an impairment or a disability) that limits or prevents the fulfillment of a role that is normal (depending on age, sex, social, and cultural factors) for that individual
- *social support*—the interpersonal transactions involving the expression of positive affect of one person to another, the affirmation of another's view or behaviors, and/or the provision of aid to another, either materially or symbolically
- *psychosocial protective factors*—factors that buffer the impact of stressors and thereby reduce the probability of relapse
- *coping*—processes that may confer protection from relapse in major mental disorders when an individual with a given biological vulnerability is confronted with environmental stressors
- *self-efficacy*—the belief or conviction that one can successfully execute the behaviors required to produce a desired outcome; thought to be a precursor or at least a concomitant of the striving behavior itself
- *self-care*—the practice of activities that individuals initiate and perform in their own behalf in maintaining life, health, and well-being
- *self-determination*—the ability to decide for one's self to engage in acts necessary for self-care in day-to-day living (*Self-help* is a similar term, in which the patient is encouraged to develop problem-solving strategies him- or herself with help from staff. The staff are not the experts but intervene to prevent destructive actions. Self-help might be described as mutual help.)
- *contextualization*—keeping the patients in as close contact with their usual surroundings, both geographical and interpersonal, as possible
- *functional status*—level of the patient's ability to perform independently activities related to self-care, social relations, occupational functioning, and use of leisure time
- *illness trajectory*—the course of the illness or chronic condition, which depends on the individual, the interventions utilized, and unpredictable events that occur during the course of the illness
- *activities of daily living*—self-care activities (such as eating, personal hygiene, dressing, recreational activities, and socialization) that are performed

daily by healthy individuals as part of independent living; during periods of illness, individuals may not be able to perform some or all of these self-care activities

- *social skills*—the coping process by which social competence is achieved; the skills (verbal and nonverbal communication, internal feelings, attitudes, and perceptions of the interpersonal context) mediate successful outcomes of social interactions that are reflected in the achievement of the individual's goals and the favorable impression made on others

For additional terms related to psychiatric home care, see the glossary in Appendix A.

PSYCHIATRIC TREATMENT, THE REHABILITATION PROCESS, AND THE NURSING PROCESS

The psychiatric rehabilitation process is not different from the nursing process and, thus, it is easy for nursing staff to apply to their practice. Initially, parts of the psychiatric rehabilitation process may seem unfamiliar; however, on closer view they are similar processes. According to the American Nurses Association (ANA), psychiatric nursing practice is "characterized by interventions that promote and foster health, assess dysfunction, assist patients to regain or improve their coping abilities, and prevent further disabilities."[23(p.12)] A review of the ANA *Standards of Psychiatric-Mental Health Clinical Nursing Practice* found in Appendix B supports the similarities between rehabilitation and nursing. The standards also identify the importance of the home visit "as an effective method of responding to the mental health needs of an individual or a family."[24(p.14)] Nursing has always been more practically oriented and tries to help patients and their families/SOs cope with illness and its effects on daily living. The emphasis has been health based or on a realistic assessment of assets and limitations. Because helping patients to function and repairing deficits have always been part of nursing care, nurses can easily apply psychiatric rehabilitation interventions that have the same goals.

If it is accepted that psychiatric rehabilitation can easily be applied to psychiatric nursing, the next logical question is its relationship to psychiatric home care. Can psychiatric rehabilitation only be applied in a hospital setting or some type of structured community program? Because of the short length of hospitalization and the inadequacy of hospitalization to assist patients with problem solving, coping skills, social skills, and psychoeducation, patients need other resources. Patients who are discharged with limited preparation to deal with environmental stressors soon need more intensive care. In addition, these patients are unprepared to use after-care resources (e.g., a patient may be so frightened that he or she cannot leave home to go to an outpatient clinic; a patient may not know how to solve simple problems when out of the house, such as missing the bus or not enough having change for the bus; a patient may become angry and not know how to control this feeling in public situations). The list is endless and, for those patients who are homebound because of their illness, help must be given in the home until they are able to obtain it elsewhere. The goal is always normalization. Providing treatment in the setting that is most normal for the patient is critical for achieving this goal. The home is a stopping-off point to the clinic, private practitioner, or a community program. By using psychiatric rehabilitation principles and interventions as well as nursing interventions, psychiatric nursing may provide the bridge to help the patient make the transition from the home to normalized life.

The Psychiatric Rehabilitation Process

The psychiatric rehabilitation process correlates with the nursing process. It includes three steps: assessment, planning, and monitoring. Figure 2–1 provides a flowchart of the application of this approach to treatment. The approach focuses on how "assessment and treatment interlock in a continuing fashion over time."[25(p.66)] The steps depicted in this figure are very familiar to nurses. The ANA *Standards for Home Health Nursing Practice* state that "the nurse, guided by the care plan, intervenes to provide comfort, to restore, improve, and promote health, to prevent complications and sequelae of illness, and to effect rehabilitation"[26(p.11)] (see Appendix C). Combining the two approaches of nursing and psychiatric rehabilitation facilitates care that is more appropriate to the needs of the psychiatric home care patient.

Assessment

The psychiatric rehabilitation assessment includes an assessment of symptoms, functional abilities, and resources. These are also included in the nursing assessment. The patient's behavioral assets and deficits are assessed. As with nursing, strengths as well as limitations are emphasized. Kuehnel and Liberman recommend that the functional assessment include the following:[27(p.60)]

- stressors that may overwhelm the individual's coping skills and competencies in social and instrumental roles, leading to an exacerbation or relapse of symptoms
- the presence or absence of premorbid and current coping skills and competencies that may serve as buffers against stress

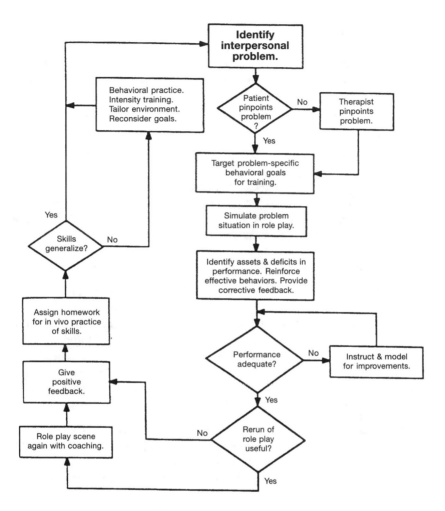

Figure 2–1 Flowchart: Basic Skills Training. *Source:* Reprinted with permission from R. Liberman, *Psychiatric Rehabilitation of Chronic Mental Patients*, p. 167, © 1988, American Psychiatric Press.

- the reasons for deficits in an individual's coping and problem-solving skills, such as disuse, reinforcement of the sick role, or loss of motivation

This assessment, just as with the nursing assessment, provides direction for setting goals, measuring outcomes, and monitoring progress. For both types of assessments, the patient's participation is critical.

Rehabilitation Plan

As is true of the nursing assessment, the rehabilitation assessment does not occur in a sequentially linear fashion but rather in an overlapping one. This means that the plan will change and that flexibility is important. Applying this to nursing is not difficult. Suggested steps for the psychiatric rehabilitation plan are as follows:[28]

- Set specific goals/outcomes (short-term goals oriented toward the here and now and long-term goals).
- Prioritize skills to be acquired and resources to be mobilized.
- Establish timelines to help the patient, family/SOs, and nurse realize that progress is expected, does occur, and has definite value and satisfaction; recognize that flexibility is required.
- Ensure coordination between all agencies, professionals, and support groups.
- Identify responsibilities.

As is true in nursing, ongoing monitoring is the most important step in the psychiatric rehabilitation process. Outcomes should be measured for the patient and the nurse to appreciate progress and to determine the next direction to be taken. Assessments and plans are useless if results are not monitored. Typically, psychiatric rehabilitation plans contain interventions that focus on social skills and psychoeducation. Social skills include affective, cognitive, and motor functioning. As the plan is developed, the required skills for social interactions are considered. These may include, for example:[29]

- accurate social perception or reception of the relevant characteristics of an interpersonal situation (an awareness of the other person's feelings and aims and one's rights and responsibilities)
- cognitive ability to process or translate social perceptions into alternate courses of action and to decide upon the best alternative
- ability to implement or send the chosen alternative response back to the other person using appropriate verbal and nonverbal behaviors

SUMMARY

The practice of psychiatric rehabilitation has been evolving since the early nineteenth century, and there has been increased interest in this area since the 1980s. Some professionals are concerned that psychiatric rehabilitation may be oversold and that the term *recovery* may be misused. According to Lamb, however, "Whatever positions are taken on these issues, we do have consensus about what is perhaps the most important issue: that psychiatric rehabilitation is effective and that it should be made available to every person with long-term severe mental illness."[30(p.1019)] Home care is a setting and treatment modality in which psychiatric rehabilitation, even though modified in many cases, can be provided.

NOTES

1. R. Munich and E. Lang, "The Boundaries of Psychiatric Rehabilitation," *Hospital and Community Psychiatry* 44, no. 7 (1993): 661–665.

2. L. Mosher and L. Burti, *Community Mental Health: Principles and Practice* (New York: W.W. Norton & Company, 1989), 107.

3. P. Backlar, *The Family Face of Schizophrenia* (New York: G.P. Putnam's Sons, 1994), 15.

4. Backlar, *The Family Face of Schizophrenia*, 83.

5. M. Munetz et al., "An Integrative Ideology to Guide Community-Based Multidisciplinary Care of Severely Mentally Ill Patients," *Hospital and Community Psychiatry* 44, no. 6 (1993): 551–555.

6. Mosher and Burti, *Community Mental Health*, 78.

7. Mosher and Burti, *Community Mental Health*, 106–107.

8. Mosher and Burti, *Community Mental Health*, 106–107.

9. Mosher and Burti, *Community Mental Health*, 377.

10. R. Liberman, "Coping with Chronic Mental Disorders: A Framework for Hope," in *Psychiatric Rehabilitation of Chronic Mental Patients*, ed. R. Liberman (Washington, DC: American Psychiatric Press, Inc., 1988), 1–28.

11. International Association of Psychosocial Rehabilitation Services, *A National Directory: Organizations Providing Psychosocial Rehabilitation and Related Community Support Services in the United States* (Columbia, MD: 1990).

12. L. Bachrach, "Psychosocial Rehabilitation and Psychiatry in the Long-Term Patient," *American Journal of Psychiatry* 149, no. 11 (1992): 1455–1463.

13. N. Sartorius, "Rehabilitation and Quality of Life," *Hospital and Community Psychiatry* 43, no. 12 (1992): 1180–1181.

14. M. Boyd, "Rehabilitation into Psychiatric Nursing Practice," *Issues in Mental Health Nursing* 15, no. 1 (1994): 13–26.

15. Bachrach, "Psychosocial Rehabilitation," 18–19.

16. W. Anthony and R. Liberman, ed., "The Practice of Psychiatric Rehabilitation: Historical, Conceptual, and Research Base," *Schizophrenia Bulletin* 12, no. 4 (1986): 631–647, at 631–634.

17. Liberman, "Coping with Chronic Mental Disorders," 12–13.

18. R. Kahn, "Aging and Social Support," in *Aging from Birth to Death: Interdisciplinary Perspectives*, ed. M. Riley (Boulder, CO: Westview, 1979), 77–91, at 77.

19. D. Orem, *Nursing: Concepts of Practice* (New York: McGraw-Hill, 1980), 35.

20. Mosher and Burti, *Community Mental Health*, 82, 105.

21. American Nurses Association, *A Statement on Psychiatric-Mental Health Clinical Nursing Practice and Standards of Psychiatric-Mental Health Clinical Nursing Practice* (Washington, DC: American Nurses Publishing, 1994), 1–47, at 42–43.

22. R. Liberman, "Social Skills Training," in *Psychosocial Rehabilitation of Chronic Mental Patients*, ed. R. Liberman (Washington, DC: American Psychiatric Press, Inc., 1988), 148–198, at 149–150.

23. American Nurses Association, *A Statement on Psychiatric-Mental Health Clinical Nursing Practice and Standards of Psychiatric-Mental Health Clinical Nursing Practice*, 12.

24. American Nurses Association, *A Statement on Psychiatric-Mental Health Clinical Nursing Practice and Standards of Psychiatric-Mental Health Clinical Nursing Practice*, 14.

25. T. Kuehnel and R. Liberman, "Functional Assessment," in *Psychiatric Rehabilitation of Chronic Mental Patients*, ed. R. Liberman (Washington, DC: American Psychiatric Press, Inc., 1988), 59–116.

26. American Nurses Association, *Standards of Home Health Nursing Practice* (Washington, DC: 1986), 11.

27. Kuehnel and Liberman, "Functional Assessment," 60.

28. Kuehnel and Liberman, "Functional Assessment," 110.

29. Liberman, "Social Skills Training," 150.

30. H. Lamb, "A Century and a Half of Psychiatric Rehabilitation in the United States," *Hospital and Community Psychiatry* 45, no. 10 (1994): 1015–1020.

SUGGESTED READING

Abraham, I. et al. 1992. Integrating the bio into the biopsychosocial: Understanding and treating biological phenomena in psychiatric-mental health nursing. *Archives of Psychiatric Nursing* 6, no. 5: 296–305.

Anthony, W. et al. 1990. *Psychiatric rehabilitation.* Boston: University Center for Psychiatric Rehabilitation.

Anthony, W., and L. Spaniol, eds. 1994. *Readings in psychiatric rehabilitation.* Boston: Boston University Center for Psychiatric Rehabilitation.

Cohen, M. et al. 1986. *Psychiatric rehabilitation trainer packages: Functional assessment.* Boston: Boston University Center for Psychiatric Rehabilitation.

Deegan, P. 1985. Recovery: The lived experience of rehabilitation. *Psychosocial Rehabilitation Journal* 11, no. 4: 11–19.

Krauss, J., and A. Slavinsky. 1982. *The chronically ill psychiatric patient and the community.* Boston: Blackwell Scientific Publications.

Lamb, H. 1994. A century and a half of psychiatric rehabilitation in the United States. *Hospital and Community Psychiatry* 45, no. 10: 1015–1019.

Moller, M., and M. Murphy. 1996. Relapse prevention to reduce hospitalization. *Current Approaches to Psychoses: Diagnosis and Management* 5, no. 1: 14–16.

Munetz, M. et al. 1993. An integrative ideology to guide community-based multidisciplinary care of severely mentally ill patients. *Hospital and Community Psychiatry* 44, no. 6: 551–555.

Munich, R., and E. Lang. 1993. The boundaries of psychiatric rehabilitation. *Hospital and Community Psychiatry* 44, no. 7: 661–665.

Postrado, L., and A. Lehman. 1995. Quality of life and clinical predictors of rehospitalization of persons with severe mental illness. *Hospital and Community Psychiatry* 46, no. 11: 1161–1165.

Unzicker, R. 1989. On my own: A personal journey through madness and re-emergence. *Psychosocial Rehabilitation Journal* 13, no. 1: 71–77.

3

The Patient's Family and Significant Others

INTRODUCTION

Families and the mental health system have had a long and often negative relationship. The use of terms such as *psychotic-level, pathogenic, dysfunctional, multiproblem,* and *disorganized* family only remind the family of negative experiences. Families may have been told that their relative's behavior is due to parents' marital problems, family communication style, family underinvolvement or overinvolvement; in other instances, the ill family member is viewed as misbehaving instead of mentally ill. More recently, the emphasis has been on high expressed emotion, which places the family into one of two categories: high expressed emotion or overinvolved, hostile, critical family, which is seen as bad, and low expressed emotion, warm, understanding, tolerant family, which is seen as good. These past experiences and the attitudes cited in Exhibit 3–1 have led families to be distrustful of health care professionals. According to Taylor, "There surely is a need to enlighten many of us (nurses) about the efficacy of empowering consumers and their families. Far too many of us, including me, were educated in an era when those with a mental illness were seen as objects to be cared for and their families were viewed as impediments to the achievement of that task. That orientation, no matter how well-intentioned, has made it difficult for some of us to wholeheartedly embrace the notion that patients and their significant others have something valuable to contribute to the treatment regimen."[1(p.289)]

Families and significant others (SOs) do need help in determining what role they will play in the support and care of their relative, but not by means of intensive probing of their own dynamics. It is with this new role that home care staff can help the family/SOs and thus improve the daily life of the patient, who may be an adult child or an elderly parent.

Exhibit 3–1 Attitudes of Family/Significant Others toward Mental Health Professionals

---

- blame of families for onset and course of mental disorders
- focus on pathology and deficits
- lack of empathy for stressors and disappointments experienced by families/SOs
- lack of respect for efforts put forth by families/SOs with the mentally ill relative
- inadequate information on mental illness
- unwillingness to educate families
- inadequate assistance in the daily management of the mentally ill relative
- insufficient family/SO participation in the treatment and after-care process
- tendency for rebuff, isolation, or dissociation
- insufficient emotional support

Source: Reprinted with permission from S. Kazarian and D. Vanderheyden, "Family Education of Relatives of People with Psychiatric Disability: A Review," *Psychosocial Rehabilitation Journal*, Vol. 15, No. 3, p. 68, © 1992, International Association of Psychiatric Rehabilitation.

MENTAL ILLNESS: A CATASTROPHIC EVENT

Understanding stress-coping-adaptation will help the home care staff to assist the patient and the family/SOs cope with the illness and learn to manage it. Coping is the effort a person makes to deal with situations of threat, harm, or challenge. When a person cannot adapt, the results often are strong feelings and confusion. Regardless of whether the illness occurs slowly or acutely, it can have disastrous effects on the family. According to Peternelj-Taylor and Hartley, "Increasingly, evidence suggests that families of psychiatric patients tend to experience significant levels of continuing or chronic strain, a concept referred to as objective and subjective family burden.[2(p.25)] *Objective burden* consists of concrete problems, such as adverse effects on the household, financial problems, role changes, crises and problems with community resources, difficulties in finding treatment resources, and disruption of personal lives. *Subjective burden* consists of the effects of the concern and worry about the ill family member, which usually result in excessive stress and problems leading to anxiety, grief, depression, and health problems.

The onset of mental illness produces a crisis. The family's usual problem-solving strategies do not work; however, the illness experience requires rapid adjustment. As a consequence, psychological stress is expected and should not be pathological. Mental illness requires family members to modify identity, image, and roles within the family. Cognitive functioning for family members may be greatly reduced. Families/SOs at this time are described as "being in distress." They often have the following characteristics:[3(p.21)]

- narrow, fixed spans of attention
- sense of urgency that "something must be done"
- alienated and alone
- profound sense of loss of identity
- drastically reduced capacity to make decisions
- unsatisfactory performance of usual social roles

The family's response to the crisis will depend on the family configuration, socioeconomic level, culture, family traditions and values, community attitudes and resources, social supports and networks, age and health of the caregivers, personality characteristics, and relationships between the patient and caregivers. The home care nurse should identify when the family is in crisis by assessing the family for shock, denial, helplessness, and grieving. The nurse helps to provide objective reality about the illness; however, it is critical that the nurse consider how the family/SOs interpret the illness. They may experience as individuals and as a family a threat to self-esteem and integrity, anxiety, threat of loss or deprivation, and depression. The best way for home care staff to emphasize and to increase their understanding of the family's/SO's experience is to imagine what it would be like to have a child or an adult child with a serious mental illness. Families have dreams for their children. What are they? What if they are taken away? What is the emotional impact of mental illness on the family?

The Grieving Process

Parents who have a child who develops a serious mental illness experience the same grief that parents experience if their child dies, regardless of the age. Their reactions are not usually seen as grief by society or by health care professionals; rather, these reactions are often seen as evidence of pathology. How can this grief possibly be the same grief that is felt at the death of a child? Parents who lose a child feel as if a part of themselves has been cut away. Serious mental illness in a child results in the same feeling.

There is no required way to experience grief; however, some aspects are similar for most people. Kubler-Ross developed one of the first theories about the grieving process that helped health care professionals begin to focus on grief and provide care for those who are grieving.[4] However, other ideas about the process have since been developed. More recently, Rando described the mourning process in three phases,[5] and MacGregor has applied these to families who experience mental illness.[6]

1. *Avoidance phase.* In the early phase of grief, the family experiences numbness and shock, disorientation, sleeplessness, poor memory, loss of desire for food, and unpredictable emotional swings. Some family members may worry that they may be going crazy. Denial is important at this time.

2. *Confrontation phase.* During this phase, family members experience very intense emotions, anger, sadness, fear, anxiety, guilt, longing, and depression. They become obsessed with reviewing the circumstances of the death and try to find some meaning in the child's suffering. Inability to protect the child not only brings on guilt but also lowers self-esteem. This is even worse when the illness cannot be easily understood, such as serious mental illness in a child or adult child. Parents are angered by their helplessness and are very vulnerable and oversensitive to responses from others. They find that the safest target for this anger is the self, in the form of guilt or depression, or anger toward the spouse. Because both parents are grieving, it is difficult for them to help each other, and this can lead to serious mutual problems. Grieving methods may be different for each spouse, which can cause additional problems. Grief also changes people. It is important to help parents understand all of their losses and help them recognize each other's grief.

3. *Reestablishment phase.* During this phase, parents—even though changed—are able to move on or develop equilibrium. There will be reminders at birthdays, anniversaries, special holidays, etc., and the loss never disappears. Families experiencing loved ones with mental illness will have greater problems during this phase, because for most parents there can be no real conclusion or equilibrium. Watching a child or adult child change his or her personality, cognition, and functioning levels causes deep feelings and begins a "lifetime of losses." The onset of mental illness may occur at the time when the child is at the "brink of young adulthood" or is a young adult. Family members see their child's loss of independence, friendships, hopes, careers, education, role in the family, marriage and children, joy and pleasure, talents and competence, and the future. The number of such losses experienced and their depth will vary, but at the horrifying time of diagnosis these losses loom over all family experiences. Internally, parents personally feel loss of self-esteem and competence, their dreams, control, pleasure in their child's success, and positive sense of family past. They are now filled with questions such as: What went wrong? Did I do something wrong? Externally, they experience financial loss, problems with living arrangements, time lost from work to care for the adult child, changes in friendships and social life, and loss of freedom or independence.

Grieving parents whose child dies have societal support (e.g., funeral, mourning rituals, etc.). Those who have lost a child through mental illness do not have this support. A family member has described mental illness as the "no casserole illness." Friends and neighbors do not rally around as they might for a medical illness. Most people would not even acknowledge that the family grieves. If family members are not allowed to grieve for their losses, their grief may become chronic, and their ability to cope will lessen. Not only do they have no rituals that offer support, but also they must deal with stigma and shame. Parents may deny their losses as they hold on to hope for complete recovery with no long-term damage. At the same time, their child is still alive, and it requires energy to support the adult child; treatment, housing, and other catering responsibilities are ever present and demanding. If they ask professionals for help with their feelings of loss, often these feelings get turned into pathology. They might be told that strongly expressed emotions are harmful to their child. They feel alone in their grief and lack understanding about what they are grieving for and that it is normal. If, however, they search for information about the illness and its treatment, this can help them increase their self-esteem and competence, and decrease feelings of helplessness, fear, anger, and guilt. The home care nurse can help with their search for information and let parents know that this is a positive step. Parents need to know that grieving is normal and appropriate and that home care staff will help them cope with it.

As the family/SOs experience the illness of a loved one, they need to confront many threats to their daily living.[7]

- *Threat of loss and deprivation.* Mental illness causes the patient to lose temporarily or permanently many of his or her personality characteristics. The cyclic nature of the illness makes these losses more difficult to experience. The nurse probably never knew the patient when he or she was healthy; however, the family/SOs knew the healthy family member, which makes their loss worse. It is very difficult when the ill family member pushes the family away and isolates himself or herself. The family feels a loss in the family group. The patient may also be aware of what is lost personally and by others. This grieving reaction is an important one for families/SOs and the patient. Grieving may lead to feelings such as anxiety, depression, sorrow, dejection, fear, agitation, panic, anger, denial, shock, numbness, relief, and resentment. The family/SOs may dwell on the past when things were better or remember presumed mistakes. They may also experience physical reactions due to intense grief (e.g., shortness of breath, loss of appetite, loss of sleep, or uncontrolled crying). In addition, the family/SOs will be deprived of sleep, vacations, relaxation time, and personal time.

- *Threat to self-esteem and self-worth.* When helping families/SOs, it is important to maintain their self-esteem. According to Hatfield, "The sacrifices that parents make over a long period of child rearing ordinarily have their rewards by having upstanding competent adult children to point to with pride. What happens, then, to the self-image of parents whose children have severe mental illnesses and who may never fulfill the role of the 'successful parent'?"[8(p.28)] Embarrassment, shame, guilt and blame, and stigma are common family/SO reactions.
- *Threat to integrity and optimism.* The experience of having an ill family member makes the family realize how vulnerable they are, and they feel weakened. If they had an optimistic viewpoint prior to the illness, it, too, will be challenged.
- *Threat to security.* To feel secure in an environment, a person must feel physically safe, able to predict events, and able to exert some control over life events. This sense of security is lost with illness, and the resulting insecurity leads to anxiety and tension. Dangerousness, usually reflecting poor impulse control, may be directed at the family/SO and is often due to jealousy, hypersensitivity to criticism, perceived obstruction of desires, carelessness with cigarettes or with cooking, unwillingness to seek medical and dental care, and susceptibility to attack by others in the community. Worries about homelessness and wandering are common in families who experience serious mental illness. In some homes, family members may fear physical assault by the ill family member. Family members may themselves lose control due to the tension of living with an ill family member or for personal reasons. With this unpredictability, the family/SO must stay on guard. Will the patient get better or worse? When will it happen? How will the patient be able to manage? How will it happen? How long will the relapse last? Will the patient be in worse condition when he or she recovers from the next relapse? These questions can be overwhelming. Older parents may worry about what will happen when they die. The National Alliance for the Mentally Ill (NAMI) has developed some resources to help family members with this issue. Cost of treatment will become more and more of a concern. Some families/SOs may be willing to sell everything, to give away other siblings' college funds, etc., just to find the treatment that will cure the patient. The family carries much of the responsibility, but they feel that they have little power to influence the illness itself, its treatment, or its costs. They must struggle with the dilemma of making decisions for the patient who is an adult. This lack of power is related to a lack of information. Families who do not understand mental illness and their choices may be led into the wrong decisions or feel uncomfortable challenging the mental health system and its professionals.

Siblings

Often the focus of health care providers is on the patient and the patient's parents; however, the patient's siblings experience many of the same feelings as the parents. In addition, siblings may experience strong feelings of jealousy due to the attention given to the ill family member. The financial burden that the family carries may directly affect the sibling (e.g., the sibling is denied material items and is affected by stress the family experiences over the lack of funds). Siblings need support and education about the illness and the treatment. They may hold their feelings inside due to concerns about upsetting their brother or sister and parents. In the long run, this may affect their own health. Changes in roles and relationships need to be openly discussed. Parents need guidance about providing time for others in the family. Participating in a sibling support group might decrease stress at home by providing a safe place for the sibling to express conflicted feelings. The home care nurse should be assertive about including siblings in planning and education and allowing time for siblings to discuss their personal concerns.

FAMILY/SIGNIFICANT OTHERS

Family/SOs become the major caregivers when an ill family member lives at home. The caregivers may be parents caring for an adult child, adult children caring for an elderly parent, or a spouse caring for a spouse. All of these situations present problems and daily stress for the caregivers. Role changes will be inevitable, and past problems may complicate the caregiving relationship. Both the caregiver and the patient may be very uncomfortable with the required changes in their relationship, even though these changes are necessary to maintain a stable home environment. How do family members/SOs try to maintain a stable environment and yet meet the changing needs of an ill family member and live with the impairments caused by the illness? Family members who are forced to be caregivers and are unprepared for the job must learn behavioral management techniques to cope with the following challenges and problems:[9]

- *Difficulty in self-regulation.* The patient may exhibit excesses in smoking, eating, and sleeping and behaviors such as refusal to bathe, too much bathing, excessive spending, refusal to spend money, or problems with dress. Problems managing medications can influence all other problems for the patient and the family/SOs.
- *Conflict between dependence and independence.* How much protection and support to give to the ill family member is a common concern for the family/ SO. The patient may not be able to solve problems; however, when the family

tries to do it for the patient, the patient may become angry and feel that the family is controlling. It is often very difficult to find the right balance.

- *Persistent avoidance of threatening situations.* The patient may spend a lot of time avoiding ordinary life situations, considering them too threatening. In addition, the patient may be very sensitive to threats to self-esteem, anticipate failure and rejection, and be unable to cope well with anxiety. Family/SO communication may be inadequate, and everyone may avoid trying to communicate their true feelings to one another, fearing the reactions.

- *Social isolation.* The ill family member is frequently lonely; however, it may not be very rewarding to be around the ill family member. This feeling may be difficult for the family/SOs to verbalize. Fears about what others will think about the patient's behaviors and illness may make the patient less likely to try social interactions. The family/SOs may be embarrassed about the patient's behavior in public.

- *Self-destructive and risk-taking behaviors.* The patient may exhibit self-destructive and risk-taking behaviors (e.g., excessive or limited eating, smoking, carelessness with fire, failure to treat injuries and illnesses, susceptibility to drug and alcohol abuse, and suicidal behaviors). The family may feel that they can resolve all of the patient's problems and save the patient. Home care staff may also feel this way. Everyone must accept that this cannot be done. The patient needs to take some responsibility.

- *Exploitive and provocative behavior.* The ill member may become exploitive and provocative due to a need to have some control. This behavior can be very disturbing to family life, so much so that it becomes the focus. In this way, the patient will feel in control; however, this behavior is not healthy for the patient or for the family.

- *Hostile and abusive behavior.* Some families live in a continual state of anxiety, wondering when the next angry outburst will occur. In some situations, setting limits may lead to anger; however, this does not mean that limits should not be set. The family/SOs need to consider if the threatening behavior is due to uncontrollable impulses or if the patient is able to control the behavior. According to Hatfield, "We believe that most mentally ill people have it within their power to modify their actions and develop behaviors conducive to living with others. Families can learn to enforce basic limits so that their safety, privacy, and comfort are maintained."[10(p.41)]

- *Invasion of privacy.* The patient has little ability to delay gratification and, as a consequence, may not recognize other family members' need for privacy. Time for privacy for all family members is important.

- *Use of poor judgment.* Poor judgment affects decision making and can lead to poor relationships, money problems, legal problems, and destruction of property. All of these increase the family's problems.

- *Problems with the mental health system.* The patient and the family/SOs may have a history of many problems accessing and using the mental health system. Typically their problems relate to confidentiality, legal issues, patient rights versus patient needs, inadequate communication and collaboration, access to services, and inadequate services.

Home care staff need to develop a partnership with the patient's family as well as with the patient. As staff work with the family/SOs, they should do the following:[11]

- Clarify mutual goals or outcomes.
- Learn rehabilitation/educational approaches.
- Avoid forcing the family to fit staff's model.
- Acknowledge limitations.
- Use teamwork.
- Identify family/SO strengths.
- Respond to intense feelings.
- Encourage family/SO enrichment or time devoted to themselves.
- Learn about psychiatric illness and medications.
- Provide practical advice.
- Learn about community resources.
- Meet with local support groups.
- Acknowledge diverse beliefs.
- Develop staff supports.

Exhibit 3–2 describes guidelines to help patients and families/SOs communicate with health care professionals. These guidelines help decrease the gap between health care professionals and the family/SOs and prevent some problems from developing between the staff and the family/SOs.

Reintegration of the Family Unit

The home care agency "occupies a unique position in that it can potentially produce maximum change with the least expenditure of time and resources."[12(p.40)] The home environment can be more easily assessed when staff visit it. Home care staff can observe family interactions in their natural environment. Due to the nature of the immediate needs of the patient and the family/SOs, staff are in a better position to have their advice taken. The reintegration of the family unit must first begin with a family assessment that provides information about the family's needs, particularly in the areas of education about the patient's illness, treatment, and behavioral family management skills.

Exhibit 3–2 Family Guidelines for Communicating with Professionals

---

- Effective assertiveness requires reasonable expectations. Before you can be assertive, be clear about what you can reasonably expect from someone else.
- In establishing realistic expectations, you need to understand that communicating with families about mental health issues is complex for the professional. The therapist (or any other health care professional) is guided by many factors: his/her training, theoretical model, employment setting, personality, financial considerations, caseload demands, as well as ethical codes and rules.
- Additional constraints on communication include client rights, client availability, and level of functioning.
- Families want to be heard. They want support for their struggle with mental illness, and they want to be a part of the treatment team. Families do not want to be blamed or made to feel guilty; they do not want unclear jargon or professional terminology; they do not want controlling or judgmental attitudes from the mental health professional.
- If individual family members need help, they should get it. Dealing with a family member's mental illness is very difficult. It can be unpredictable, frightening, expensive, tragic, long-term, and very stressful.
- The ability to explain what you want and why you want it is helpful. You might discuss your thoughts with someone else in advance to get feedback on the appropriateness of your question. Write down your thoughts in advance to be sure you are asking what you intend. If more than one family member will be in attendance, decide on one spokesperson.
- Look for areas of agreement and build on those. Remember that association with your relative's health care professionals is different than developing a therapeutic relationship. If this is a new relationship, give it a chance to develop.

Source: Adapted with permission from "Guidelines for Communicating with Professionals," *Alliance for the Mentally Ill of MD, Inc., Newsletter,* Vol. 11, No. 2, p. 6, © 1993, Alliance for the Mentally Ill of MD.

The Return Home

Ideally, when the ill family member is hospitalized, discharge planning begins on admission to the hospital. The family/SOs should be involved. As soon as it is determined that the patient will be discharged to the family's home, hospital staff, the patient, and the family/SOs should begin to prepare for discharge to the home. If home care will be used, home care staff should be included in the planning. The family/SOs as well as the patient may not be happy about the discharge decision. Home care staff should recognize this reaction and allow time for family to express feelings openly. Hospital and home care staff can begin to make plans that minimize anticipated problems during the first days at home. The following are often considered in the planning:[13]

- Consider ways to handle initial problems that may occur because the mentally ill individual may behave inappropriately in one or more of the following ways:
  1. continue to behave like an inpatient (e.g., passivity)
  2. selfishly want his or her way
  3. show little respect for the welfare of others
  4. physically or verbally abuse other persons
  5. act out sexually
  6. disregard the effects of the actions on the activities of others
  7. disrespect the privacy of other family members
  8. deviate from the routines of sleeping, eating, taking medication, or exercising
  9. refuse to or otherwise be unable to bathe, dress, and tend to personal grooming needs; do little of anything that is required of an individual in a family unit
- Anticipate the initial response, reactions, and possible biases of family members outside the immediate family, friends, neighbors, and other social or work contacts.
  1. Plan to let people know that the ill relative is coming home. What, when, and how will you tell others about your ill relative? Whom will you tell, and under what circumstances will you tell them?
  2. Let close friends know what is happening. Denying or covering up or hiding the relative will only make matters worse.
  3. Encourage family members/SOs and others to learn about mental illness, and stress the fact that mental illness is an organic disease of the brain, much the same as cancer or diabetes is a disease of other parts of the body. The more that family members/SOs accept the illness, the more it will encourage society to accept it as any other disease.
  4. It is important that family members/SOs, as well as the ill person, have time to themselves. Be sure to consider this in your planning. Family members may need help finding respite care or they may have help from other family members.
- Plan ways to get life back on track. As with other illnesses, family members tend to overprotect the mentally ill person. The relative needs to recover from being hospitalized. The more quickly things are "normalized," the better.
- Set goals to rehabilitate the ill family member, as well as the entire family. Whenever possible, a short visit at home before discharge may decrease some anxiety and help to identify some potential problems. Insurance coverage is

decreasing for this type of visit, and when the visits do occur, hospital staff must be very clear about outcomes and document carefully.

Clearly, what has been described about planning before hospital discharge does not happen for many patients. With shorter lengths of stay, fewer hospital staff, and less time for inpatient patient education and planning with the patient and the family/SOs, many patients are referred to home care with minimal or no planning for the return home. On the first visit, home care staff often find a patient and family/SOs in turmoil and stress. They have no idea how to cope. The home care nurse must then conduct the assessment as well as do crisis resolution for problems that have already occurred since discharge.

FAMILY ASSESSMENT

The home care nurse needs to be very careful in assessing the family and to avoid identifying families as the cause of mental illness. The focus of the assessment is not on family psychopathology but rather on the nature of family assets and limitations. The overall goal for the family/SOs is to help them better manage the patient at home with the least amount of disruption to the family. Elements of the family assessment include the following:

- past history with the patient at home
- reactions to patient's past treatments
- motivation to help the patient
- involvement in the patient's life in the past, and present needs for involvement
- family power structure
- family communication methods
- family problem-solving methods
- family perceptions of the development of the mental illness
- knowledge and understanding of the illness and its treatments
- conflicts and irritability
- family time budget
- management of household tasks and responsibilities
- subjective attitudes expressed by each member of the family about one another
- privacy
- temperature of the family emotional climate
- use of alcohol/drugs by family members
- family assets and deficits

- family members' expected outcomes for the patient
- financial status

Gerace suggests some important questions about the family for the home care nurse to consider during assessment. "Are their responses realistic? Can they allow the patient to be unique or to have privacy? Can they allow participation in family activities at the patient's own pace? Are they able to set limits when necessary and to seek professional help when needed? Are they using some of the self-help agencies and groups that are available in the community?"[14(p.12)]

Methods for assessing the family are varied. The most common method is the database or formal interview. Much information can also be gained by observation and informal interviews. Providing opportunities for the family/SOs to interact with the patient can provide valuable data. To gain a better understanding of how the family members/SOs perceive problems, ask each family member/SO to describe something that happened during the past week that was a source of tension or distress. Then discuss whether the descriptions and feelings are shared by all.[15] The family/SOs might also be asked to spend five minutes resolving a problem together while the nurse observes the process. Questions to consider during the exercise include the following:[16]

- Who takes the lead?
- How clearly is the problem presented?
- Are the alternatives realistic?
- How do they determine the alternative selected?
- What is the role of the patient in this process?
- What is the emotional climate during the process?

Home care staff should remember that the family is coping with the problems as best they can, given their present resources and capabilities. Home care staff then need to enhance the family's capabilities. There are no easy answers for accomplishing this, because each family and situation is different. The family will have to make decisions, to solve problems, and to take actions, and few know what to expect with mental illness.

There are two ways to view family/SO adjustment—focusing on individual family members/SOs or on the family as a unit. The family as a unit is very important for the patient. There will be changes in roles, family routines and schedules, social activities, and how individual family members get their needs met. Success will depend not only on the family's response to the illness, but also on the family's response to other life stresses it experiences. Interdependent roles in the family mean that change in one member's role will affect all others. Much will depend upon the past role of the ill family member (e.g., mother/wife, brother/

sister, son/daughter, father/husband). There will be a drain in energy as new roles are taken on. Some family members may be resentful of time required for the ill member. As changes within the family occur, what is important is "a fair and equitable division of tasks and a fair allocation of resources within the family unit."[17(p.44)] Family members may find that they have less to give friends and yet may need friends more. Some social isolation may be inevitable, but this is not evidence of family pathology.

INTERVENTIONS WITH FAMILY/SIGNIFICANT OTHERS

Behavioral family management is highly structured, relatively brief treatment requiring an active, directive nurse. It requires the identification of desired outcomes and the development of a plan to work on specific tasks with the patient and, if required, the family/SOs. The overall goal is to develop a positive and supportive home environment and to support all who live in the environment by providing the family/SOs with behavioral management skills. Education is the major method used. Because education does not presume "pathology" or "dysfunction," it is a more acceptable approach for most families. Education should turn the patient and family/SOs into real "experts." When symptoms are discussed, the nurse asks each family member to give his or her own perspective of specific symptoms. Some patients are surprised that anyone is interested in how they feel. Practicing skills and discussing feelings and problems with the help of home care staff will help the family reintegrate as a unit. To do this, family members/SOs need to listen to each other first, and this requires initiating positive statements and suggestions, acknowledging positive actions of others, making positive requests of others, practicing active listening and empathic responsiveness, and expressing negative feelings constructively.[18]

There are many interventions that can be used by the family/SOs to create a more supportive home environment. Home care staff must help the family/SOs identify those that might be helpful for their family and the ill family member.[19-20]

- Increase a sense of coherence. The two major interventions that help the patient have a sense of coherence are medications and a predictable, stable environment. The patient needs definite expectations and few decisions. Daily routine with established times for meals, bedtime, and daily tasks, as well as a weekly schedule with particular events assigned to certain days provide structure in the home. The decisions that the patient makes should be carefully assessed. As the patient improves, the patient is given more decision-making responsibility. Each family needs to determine what is most important to their family functioning; however, family members will need to compromise.

- Provide continuity of experience. Patients often appear rigid and inflexible and respond to change poorly due to the stress experienced with changes. They may view each experience as new, as if they have no past experiences from which they have learned. Time is also a problem, but nagging the patient about time is not helpful. The patient needs specific help with planning, such as knowing how much lead time is required, using clocks and calendars, and anticipating events. Some patients enjoy hearing about their past from family, and others do not because it reminds them of their incomplete memories, their confusion, or their pain over their loss of happier times.

- Strive for predictability of events. Predictability is very important to the patient. Consistency must be considered at all times, as inconsistency increases anxiety. Helping the patient anticipate what an experience will be like will help decrease anxiety about unpredictability. Due to the unpredictability of the illness, the family/SOs will need to learn to live one day at a time. Some days will be better than others, and flexibility is important.

- Bring demand and capability into balance. The patient may have great difficulty coping with the ordinary requirements of daily life. Significant "demand-capability imbalance" produces high levels of stress. Home care staff should help the patient and teach the family/SOs how to help the patient by using the following guidelines:[21]

    1. Due to cognitive overload, confusion, and inability to focus, the patient will have times when stimulation should be decreased. Too many people, activities, and tension may increase the patient's problems with sorting out stimuli and responding properly. The patient may then feel more incompetent and more tension.

    2. Language should be simple and direct. Present simple ideas one at a time, with careful observation to determine if the patient understands.

    3. Staff expectations about family communication need to be realistic, as change takes time and practice.

    4. When assessing the patient's tolerance, the meaning of events to the patient is important.

    5. Hovering over the patient is not helpful; limit family/SO face-to-face contact with the patient when the patient is experiencing excessive anxiety.

    6. Home care staff and the family/SOs must remember that it is the patient's view of stress, not the family's or the nurse's, that is important.

    7. Some patients react to stress by withdrawing and becoming preoccupied; becoming agitated and angry; or experiencing sleeping problems,

fatigue, etc. The patient needs to learn other methods for coping with overwhelming situations.

8. Understimulation can also be unhealthy for the patient, increasing isolation and reducing self-esteem.

9. If expectations exceed patient capability, everyone will experience increased stress. With shortened lengths of stay in the hospital, the patient who comes home with only some symptoms decreased continues to experience major problems. "After the initial stabilization, a period of inactivity, lethargy, and excessive sleep is common."[22(p.115)] The patient may have too high expectations. During the initial home visit, the approach is to delay commenting on unrealistic expectations. This does not mean that the staff and family/SOs must be permissive of any and all behavior. The patient must have some responsibilities and soon discuss expectations with staff. If not, the patient may begin to believe that he or she is more disabled.

10. Help the patient to develop an acceptable identity. "The chronically ill person must be helped to give up a role of being 'sick' for that of being 'different.' . . . a new meaning and a new way of life must be found."[23(p.117)] This can be a very frightening time for the patient. At some point the patient needs to acknowledge the losses, because grieving is required for adaptation. The patient may have a period of sadness, tearfulness, lack of motivation, and possibly suicidal ideation, or the patient may use avoidance rather than learning about the illness and management of the illness.

11. Provide a supportive environment. The characteristics of a supportive environment include continuity and predictability, adequate structure, limited amount and intensity of stimulation, clear and calm communication, appropriate expectations, and encouragement and positive feedback.[24]

12. Plan for holidays and special family events. Holidays and special family events are supposed to be happy times, but for most families they are also stressful times. This is particularly true for a family member who is already vulnerable to stress and is having problems with too many activities at one time, too intense sights and sounds, new experiences that occur quickly, too much noise, too many people, and too many things to remember. With a confused and chaotic inner world, the patient needs a calm outer world. What can be done to help?[25]

     −Plan what will be occurring and identify what might be difficult for the ill family member.

     −Recognize that it will not be like it was in the past.

−Try to keep the ill relative's schedule as normal as possible; he or she needs the structure and continuity.

−Assess the amount of stimulation the ill family member can tolerate and allow him or her personal space.

−Talk with your family member about expectations and schedules.

−Expectations should be reasonable.

−If time is a problem for the ill family member, plan for extra time.

−Give the ill member a special task, if he or she is up to it, so that the patient feels included.

−If the situation becomes confusing, remain calm and talk clearly and simply with the ill family member.

−Remember that memories may arise from past experiences for all who are participating.

−Family members/SOs need to give themselves extra time and try to keep their own stress at a minimum.

EXPECTED OUTCOMES

Monitoring the process of care and rehabilitation is very important, but expected outcomes must be clearly identified first. Without outcomes, it is difficult to determine progress. The patient must participate in the development of outcomes. Family/SO involvement is also helpful. Desired outcomes must be reasonable and as attainable as possible. It is best to develop them step by step. They should be written. As progress is monitored with the patient and family/SO, changes in treatment may be required. Positive feedback should be given during every evaluation session, and these sessions should be frequent. Staff should document these sessions, indicating how the patient and family/SO participated. Examples of some methods of obtaining data to assist in monitoring outcomes are homework assignments, behavioral progress records, symptom monitoring logs, and rating scales.

SUMMARY

Before home care staff can really help someone with serious mental illness and the family/SOs, staff members must understand the personal side of mental illness. The patient's description is not the experience itself, but it helps to understand the patient's experience of the illness and the struggle that families/SOs experience daily.

NOTES

1. C. Taylor, "Consumers and Their Families," *Archives of Psychiatric Nursing* 8, no. 5 (1994): 289–290.

2. C. Peternelj-Taylor and V. Hartley, "Living with Mental Illness: Professional/Family Collaboration," *Journal of Psychosocial Nursing* 31, no. 3 (1993): 23–28.

3. H. Hansell, *The Person-In-Distress: On the Biosocial Dynamics of Adaptation* (New York: Human Sciences Press, 1976), 21.

4. E. Kubler-Ross, *On Death and Dying* (New York: The MacMillan Company, 1969).

5. T. Rando, "The Unique Issues and Impact of the Death of a Child," in *Parental Loss of a Child*, ed. T. Rando (Champaign, IL: Research Press, 1986), 5–44.

6. P. MacGregor, "Grief: The Unrecognized Parental Response to Mental Illness in a Child," *Social Work* 39, no. 2 (1994): 161–163.

7. A. Hatfield, *Family Education in Mental Illness* (New York: Guilford Press, 1990), 29–35.

8. Hatfield, *Family Education in Mental Illness*, 28.

9. Hatfield, *Family Education in Mental Illness*, 38–41.

10. Hatfield, *Family Education in Mental Illness*, 41.

11. L. Spaniol et al., "How Professionals Can Share Power with Families: Practical Approaches to Working with Families of the Mentally Ill," *Psychosocial Rehabilitation Journal* 8, no. 2 (1984): 77–84.

12. D. Dunn and C. Galloway, "Mental Health of the Caregiver: Increasing Caregiver Effectiveness," *Caring* 5, no. 7 (1986): 37–42.

13. A. Esser and S. Lacey, *Mental Illness: A Homecare Guide* (New York: John Wiley & Sons, 1989), 95.

14. L. Gerace, "Nursing Assessment in Psychiatric Home Health Care," *Journal of Home Health Care Practice* 2, no. 3 (1990): 9–15.

15. R. Liberman, "Behavioral Family Management," in *Psychiatric Rehabilitation of Chronic Mental Patients*, ed. R. Liberman (Washington, DC: American Psychiatric Press, Inc., 1988), 197–244, at 225.

16. Liberman, "Behavioral Family Management," 226.

17. Hatfield, *Family Education in Mental Illness*, 44.

18. Liberman, "Behavioral Family Management," 231.

19. Hatfield, *Family Education in Mental Illness*, 110–118.

20. H. Lefley, "Aging Patients as Caregivers of Mentally Ill Adult Children: An Emerging Social Problem," *Hospital and Community Psychiatry* 38, no. 10 (1987): 1063–1070.

21. Hatfield, *Family Education in Mental Illness*, 110–118.

22. Hatfield, *Family Education in Mental Illness*, 115.

23. Hatfield, *Family Education in Mental Illness*, 117.

24. Hatfield, *Family Education in Mental Illness*, 119.

25. A. Hatfield, "Thoughts on Coping with the Holidays," *AMI of Maryland, Inc., Newsletter* 8, no. 3 (1990): 4.

SUGGESTED READING

Backlar, P. 1994. *The family face of schizophrenia.* New York: G.P. Putnam's Sons.

Basolo-Kunzer, M. 1994. Caring for families of psychiatric patients. *Nursing Clinics of North America* 29, no. 1: 73–79.

Biegel, D. et al. 1995. A comparative analysis of family caregivers' perceived relationships with mental health professionals. *Psychiatric Services* 46, no. 5: 477–482.

Chesla, C. 1989. Parents' illness models of schizophrenia. *Archives of Psychiatric Nursing* 3, no. 4: 218–225.

Dunn, C., and C. Galloway. 1986. Mental health of the caregiver: Increasing caregiver effectiveness. *Caring* 5, no. 7: 37–42.

Eakes, G. 1995. Chronic sorrow: The lived experience of parents of chronically mentally ill individuals. *Archives of Psychiatric Nursing* 9, no. 2: 77–84.

Esser, A., and S. Lacey. 1989. *Mental illness: A homecare guide.* New York: John Wiley & Sons.

Gamble, G., and K. Midence. 1994. Schizophrenia family work: Mental health nurses delivering an innovative service. *Journal of Psychosocial Nursing* 32, no. 10: 13–16.

Gerace, L. 1990. Nursing assessment in psychiatric home health care. *Journal of Home Health Care Practice* 2, no. 3: 9–15.

Hatfield, A. 1987. The expressed emotion theory: Why families object. *Hospital and Community Psychiatry* 38, no. 4: 341.

Hull, M. 1993. Coping strategies of family caregivers in hospice home care. *Caring* 12, no. 2: 78–88.

Kanter, J. 1984. *Coping strategies for relatives of the mentally ill.* Arlington, VA: National Alliance for the Mentally Ill.

Kazarian, S., and D. Vanderheyden. 1992. Family education of relatives of people with psychiatric disability: A review. *Psychosocial Rehabilitation Journal* 15, no. 3: 67–84.

Lefley, H. 1987. Aging parents as caregivers of mentally ill adult children: An emerging social problem. *Hospital and Community Psychiatry* 38, no. 10: 1063–1070.

MacGregor, P. 1994. Grief: The unrecognized parental response to mental illness in a child. *Social Work* 39, no. 2: 160–166.

Manderino, M., and V. Bzdek. 1989. Social-skill building with chronic clients. In *Chronic mental illness: Coping strategies,* ed. J. Maurin, 187–195. Thorofare, NJ: SLACK, Inc.

Mason, S. et al. 1990. Patients' and caregivers' adaptation to improvement in schizophrenia. *Hospital and Community Psychiatry* 41, no. 5: 541–544.

Najarian, S. 1995. Family experience with positive client response to Clozapine. *Archives of Psychiatric Nursing* 9, no. 1: 11–21.

Parker, B. 1993. Living with mental illness: The family as caregiver. *Journal of Psychosocial Nursing* 31, no. 3: 19–21.

Pearson, M. 1993. The nurse, the elderly caregiver, and stress. *Caring* 12, no. 1: 14–17.

Peternelj-Taylor, C., and V. Hartley. 1993. Living with mental illness: Professional/family collaboration. *Journal of Psychosocial Nursing* 31, no. 3: 23–28.

Ragaisis, K. 1994. Critical incident stress debriefing: A family nursing intervention. *Archives of Psychiatric Nursing* 8, no. 1: 38–43.

Schiff, H. 1977. *The Bereaved Parent.* New York: Penguin Books USA, Inc.

Spaniol, L. et al. 1984. How professionals can share power with families: Practical approaches to working with families of the mentally ill. *Psychosocial Rehabilitation Journal* 8, no. 2: 77–84.

Stone, R. 1991. Familial obligations: Issues for the 1990s. *Generations* 15, no. 3: 47–50.

Surpin, R., and F. Grumm. 1990. Building the home care triangle: Clients and families, paraprofessionals, and agencies. *Caring* 9, no. 4: 6–10, 12–15.

CHAPTER

4

The Therapeutic Relationship and Communication

INTRODUCTION

The relationship that the patient and the family/significant others (SOs) develop with home care staff is a critical component of the home care treatment for the psychiatric patient. For the patient who refuses to leave the home to see other psychiatric treatment providers, the home care staff is the only person-to-person contact that the patient has with a psychiatric treatment provider. Home care staff interactions with the patient will affect patient progress. Patients need to learn how to cope with their feelings, understand how they relate to others, improve relationships, and improve their communication with others. Patients are assisted in accomplishing these goals by relating to staff and others.

This patient-staff-family interaction occurs in the home, which is a different environment for most nurses. Bowers describes this environment: "The nurse enters an alien world, the private world of the patient, which is hidden from public view. As the patient opens the door to welcome the nurse in, the nurse passes into foreign territory, a land which is unknown and uncharted to him, full of strangeness. By allowing the nurse access, the patient allows the nurse a transient sojourn in that foreign land, and in effect shows a willingness for the nurse to abide for a while and see, touch and feel the nature of the private domain."[1(p.70)] Home care staff will find that their professional boundaries will be challenged as they develop a staff-patient relationship and cope with the issues of self-disclosure, gifts and hospitality, and maintaining a therapeutic distance.[2]

THE STAFF-PATIENT RELATIONSHIP

The therapeutic relationship helps the patient cope with problems and learn new skills, but a therapeutic relationship in the patient's home has different char-

51

acteristics than one experienced in other settings. The patient is in charge in the home, and home care staff need to use more persuasion and negotiation.[3] Personal space and territoriality are important issues. The home care nurse experiences a more intimate understanding of living with a chronic illness. Socialization is part of the home visit, but it cannot consume all of the visit. According to Stulginsky, "Home health nurses are invited into homes. It is not a place they own. They are guests. Entrance is granted, not assumed, as is the case in hospitals. To gain entrance, nurses need to establish trust and rapport quickly."[4(p.405)] There is less concentrated time with the patient than in the hospital, and thus rapport must occur quickly in order to develop a working relationship. One way to do this is by validating the illness. Patients "need to sense that someone hears how illness affects their life and is willing to react to it."[5(p.477)]

As patients repeat behaviors that have caused them problems, home care staff use these opportunities to teach patients new behaviors. Everything that is done with a patient is part of the staff-patient relationship. Patients need time to interact with others, times that are supportive and positive. The therapeutic or helping relationship is one in which a home care staff member tries to help the patient cope, adapt, learn, and grow. The staff member accepts the patient as a person and respects the patient's rights. Trust is an important part of the relationship. This includes honesty when expressing feelings to the patient, but it does not mean that all staff feelings about the patient should be expressed. Trust means that the patient feels that staff will not intentionally hurt him or her but will try to help. It also means that staff can be relied upon. Most psychiatric patients have problems related to trust. Trusting a staff member may be difficult for the patient due to past experiences with others.

Home care patients have many different problems and past experiences. Some of these may be difficult for staff to understand and/or accept (e.g., abortion, divorce, different religious beliefs, substance abuse, history of experiencing or participating in abuse, homosexuality, acquired immune deficiency syndrome [AIDS], suicide, and violence of all types). Some patients are people that the home care staff would not associate with outside work because of their histories or problems; however, staff must care for them as home care patients and provide a place where they can be accepted. Staff do not have to agree with patients; however, they should not challenge patients. Staff listen and help to teach patients new ways to cope with their feelings and problems.

Phases of the Relationship

The phases of the staff-patient relationship are preorientation, orientation, working, and termination. The depth of any of these phases depends upon the amount of time the patient is in home care, the patient, the staff member, the amount of contact the staff member has with the patient, the patient's problems, and the home environment. The patient's past relationships with health care providers is a critical factor. If that history has been negative, it can affect the relationship and its development. During the preorientation and orientation phases, home care staff should assess the patient's history. The *preorientation phase* focuses on the initial contact between the home care nurse and the referral source, initial admission data, and—when possible and appropriate—a meeting with the referral source and the patient. Such a meeting might occur when the patient is in the hospital, and the home care nurse visits the treatment team in the hospital to develop plans for the patient. The *orientation phase* is the "getting to know one another" phase. The admission assessment is completed, and the treatment plan is initiated. The patient becomes involved in identifying problems and treatment outcomes. Other home care staff who will work with the patient in the home are introduced and begin to provide care. The *working phase* focuses on meeting the patient's needs. It is a time for clarification of perceptions and expectations between the staff and the patient. As the patient and staff work together to resolve problems, they experience increased intensity and commitment in the relationship. The patient begins to see staff as people who can help; however, there will be testing and fluctuating dependency and independency. The final phase is *termination*. In most cases, the home care staff will have an estimate of when the patient will be discharged based on the patient's problems and the patient's insurance coverage. Preparing for termination begins on admission. It must be an integral part of the treatment plan. For some patients, the termination phase can be a very difficult time; symptoms may get worse or reoccur, and the patient may regress. The patient may feel anxious, fearful, and angry. Home care staff must provide time to discuss the patient's concerns and problem solve to alleviate stress. The patient and the patient's family/SOs will need frequent reinforcement to emphasize that they will be able to cope. Resources that they can use after home care is completed are discussed prior to discharge.

As the staff-patient relationship develops, its intensity may lead to problematic reactions for the staff and consequently for the delivery of home care. These reactions include rescue fantasies, overidentification with the patient, fear of responsibility, and fear of aggression. *Rescue fantasies* are more common in caring for psychiatric patients than in caring for patients with medical problems. There is a desire to cure, to solve all of the patient's problems. This approach will fail and bring with it feelings of staff guilt. *Overidentification* can occur if the patient is feeling something that the staff member has felt. If it affects the interventions taken, it can be very problematic. There must be a clear separation between staff and patients, both in behavior and feelings. *Fear of responsibility* is not new to nursing; however, providing psychiatric care in the home increases the feeling of responsibility and, for those who have less psychiatric experience, helping the patient cope with complex problems may increase this fear. *Fear of aggression* is a concern with psychiatric patients, but sometimes it is exaggerated. Staff need to assess the patient's potential for aggression carefully and plan interventions; however, fear can prevent the implementation of appropriate care. For all four of these potential problems, staff supervisors can help to provide a place to openly discuss these concerns and determine ways to resolve them.

Guidelines for Staff-Patient Relationships

Guidelines for staff-patient relationships include the following:

- Confidentiality is very important. Staff should not talk about patients after work outside the work setting. If the patient wants to read his or her medical record, the home care agency's policy should be followed.
- Privacy is part of a relationship. Patients have times when they need privacy, and this is fine as long as the patient is safe. The family/SOs may need help in understanding the patient's need for privacy, just as the patient may need help understanding the family/SOs' needs for privacy. Staff should not share details of their private lives with patients. Patients really do not want to hear about staff problems. Often patients ask about staff as a strategy to avoid talking about themselves. Staff may say that they are married, have children, are divorced, etc., but staff should quickly turn the conversation back to the patient. Staff home telephone numbers and addresses should not be shared. The patient should contact staff through the agency.
- Staff anxiety will affect the patient. When staff anxiety is interfering with work, staff members should try to understand why it is occurring and, if possible, correct the causes. Discussing problems with the supervisor may be helpful. All staff members will need support at some time. Knowing when to ask for help is very important for staff and for the patients. Getting support from and giving support to other staff members is an important part of working as a team. Staff who are aware of the needs of one another will work better with one another and better with patients.
- Staff cannot solve all patient problems. Patient problems need to be left at work. Staff relaxation is very important in decreasing staff stress. Psychiatric patients are not easy to care for and drain staff of energy. This causes problems for staff who cannot take a break from their work.
- Fear can be dangerous for staff and for patients. If staff are afraid of a patient, most patients recognize this fear. If staff experience fear, they should

take actions to reduce this fear. Staff can talk with another staff member about the fear and try to understand it. Often identifying why it is occurring can help to understand the patient better and reduce fear.

- Staff may notice that they work better with some patients than with others (e.g., a staff member may work better with a depressed patient rather than a patient with schizophrenia). This is not unusual, but it is important is to understand it. Staff cannot always pick their patient assignments, but if staff know that they have a particular reaction, they can be alert for it. A negative reaction towards the patient will interfere with the patient's care.

- Sharing information is a part of all of the care provided in the home. Staff need to know what is going on with the patient. Sharing information includes what is observed and heard. This information is shared in reports, documentation, team meetings, supervisory visits, and telephone conversations.

- Consistency is very important for the psychiatric patient. It means that the staff members agree on an approach or intervention with a patient, and all follow it. It can also mean that individual staff members are consistent with a patient. It is confusing to patients when staff say one thing and then turn around and contradict it at another time. There will be times when changes are necessary, but it is helpful to explain this to the patient.

- Patients can respond to touch in positive and negative ways. Touching a patient is not recommended when a patient is first admitted and frightened. Being touched by a stranger may not be comforting and may be seen as an attack. For some patients, even a handshake may be difficult. When in doubt, do not touch a patient. Staff can show support and caring by their tone of voice and by simply listening to the patient. Patients who have a history of abuse or rape may be especially sensitive to touch and react negatively to it.

- The boundary between staff and the patient may be more blurred in the home. Keeping the home visit from becoming a social visit can be difficult, particularly with patients who do not require hands-on nursing care. Structuring the visit and using psychiatric rehabilitation methods will help clarify the purpose of the visit. When the patient asks personal questions about staff, the staff member should give a simple response and then change the conversation back to the patient.

Potential Problems

All staff-patient relationships will encounter problems. Some problems are more important than others. Exhibit 4–1 describes danger signals that indicate serious problems in a staff-patient relationship that should be corrected.

Exhibit 4–1 Danger Signals in Staff-Patient Relationships

- You do not accept that the patient has problems and is in need of treatment. (Thinking that the patient is only "as normal as everyone else" will deny the patient care.)
- You feel that you are the only one who understands the patient. You feel that other home care staff are too critical of the patient or that other staff are jealous of your relationship with the patient. (You need to ask for direct feedback from other staff and learn new ways to work with the patient. If this situation is not relieved, staff-staff communication and teamwork will break down, and this will affect the patient's treatment.)
- You are guarded and defensive when other home care staff question your interaction or relationship with the patient. You play the "yes, but . . ." game, or you say "this situation is different." (You can make mistakes like everyone else. It is important to accept this and accept advice.)
- Your patient talks freely with you—especially in light, superficial conversation and perhaps even with sexual overtones—but remains silent and defensive or avoids other home care staff when they visit. (You may be reinforcing the patient's problems. The patient needs to learn how to deal with problems rather than avoid them. Talking with you only about unimportant topics and avoiding other staff is not helpful for the patient.)
- You keep secrets with the patient; certain information is not documented or reported. (This is destructive to treatment.)
- Often you make excuses about why other home care staff or the patient's physician do not need to know the secret information. (This is called *rationalizing*. You separate yourself from the treatment team and make yourself the "treatment team.")
- You report only negative aspects of patient behavior. (Your perception of the patient and observations are influenced by negative feelings toward the patient.)
- You view the client as "your" patient. (You listen less and less to what others say about the patient and become less objective.)
- You receive gifts, cards, letters, or personal telephone calls from the patient. (These actions indicate that the patient views your relationship as a personal relationship.)

THE COMMUNICATION PROCESS

Communication is part of everything that is done in psychiatric home care. It is critical to the patient's care, staff-patient relationships, and staff-family/SO relationships. Communication also includes staff-staff communication, which is an important part of home care. Documentation or written communication is important as well, as it provides information that is shared with others.

Communication is a two-way process used to convey a message or idea between two or more people. It includes the spoken word and nonverbal methods of communicating thoughts, attitudes, and feelings. The communication process contains five components:

1. *Sender*—the person who sends the message (This is more than just the words; it includes the nonverbal signals and everything that makes up the person.)
2. *Message*—what is actually said, including nonverbal signals, the sender's attitude toward himself or herself, the message, and the receiver
3. *Receiver*—the person to whom the message is sent
4. *Feedback*—the message the receiver sends to the sender in response to the sender's message
5. *Context*—the setting in which the communication is taking place

Figure 4–1 describes the relationship among these components of the communication process.

Nonverbal communication includes communication that is not the spoken word. It can be a deliberate or unintentional way of communicating, but it is critical to all communication. Examples of nonverbal communication are gestures, facial expressions, bodily movements, tone of voice, volume of speech, posture, gait, physical appearance including hygiene and dress, written word, decorations in a person's room, etc. Interpreting nonverbal communication can be difficult. Asking the other person to define nonverbal messages verbally is the most reliable method, but it is not always possible to do.

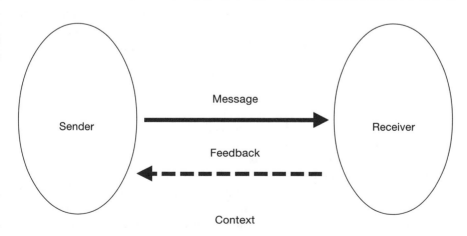

Figure 4–1 The Communication Process

Nonverbal communication can be constructive or destructive. Home care staff need to be aware of their own feelings, as this will help them better understand their own nonverbal communication. Observing the patient's nonverbal messages and comparing them to what the patient is saying is very important (e.g., when the patient is saying she is happy, but her facial expression appears sad). Describing for the patient what has been heard and what has been seen can be helpful and encourages the patient to assess behavior and feelings as a part of communication.

Clear communication includes respect for attitudes and values. Home care staff may not agree with the patient, but they need to respect the patient's right to have feelings. Staff should not criticize patient's values, nor should they force their own values onto the patient. Trust and respect for the patient are important. Staff members' interest in what the patient is saying communicates to the patient that staff care and view the patient as a human being. It is also important that patients do not make staff into perfect people who can solve all problems. Sometimes this may mean that staff need to admit that they do not have a solution to a problem or admit to an error.

Issues that may arise with some home care patients may be difficult for home care staff; however, the patient continues to require care. Examples of these include the following:

- *Homosexuality.* How do home care staff feel about a patient who has AIDS or who tests positive for human immunodeficiency virus (HIV), who says that he or she will not change sexual behaviors? Arguing with the patient may lead to decreased communication. Staff must provide information and guidance but must keep their own personal reactions to themselves. Homosexuality may not be an acceptable lifestyle to a staff member, but the patient must be respected. The patient needs help in understanding the positive and negative results of behavior. Staff cannot force a change in behavior on the patient.
- *Abortion.* A patient may have a history of an abortion, and staff may personally disagree with abortion. However, staff cannot discuss this personal viewpoint with the patient. The abortion decision is the patient's decision. Staff provide opportunities for the patient to talk about her feelings, to solve problems, and to learn ways to cope.
- *Sexual abuse, child abuse, or physical abuse of other adults.* Abusive behavior can be quite disturbing to staff, particularly to staff with children. Helping such a patient requires a separation of the staff member's personal negative feelings from the work. The patient is in a therapeutic relationship that allows for appropriate expression of feelings and problem solving.

PATIENT INTERVIEW

It is important to learn from each interview; however, not everything staff learn can be applied to every patient interview. Each interview is different. Home care staff may worry about the right words to say. There are no magic formulas or words. It is not unusual to fear that the wrong words will damage the patient; however, it does not work that way. Three professionals could interview the same patient differently. Styles vary as do people. Staff cannot be given a script and told exactly what to say. It would not be real for the patient or for staff. Staff can be given suggestions about what they might say; but in a conversation, staff and the patient will be affected by feelings, the situation, the environment, the staff member's past relationship with the patient, the patient's past relationships, staff member's past relationships with others, communication skills of staff and the patient, and timing. Controlling any of these is very difficult.

Interviewing Problems

Interviewing the patient who is experiencing acute symptoms may be very difficult. The home care nurse must determine if continuing the interview is in the best interest of the patient. The information gained will be sketchy at best and may not be accurate. Family/SOs may be used as alternative data sources until the patient is more able to participate. If the patient is agitated, a break in the interview may make it possible to continue the discussion after the patient has regained control. A change of topic or type of questions may also decrease the patient's agitation. If the patient is suspicious, the interview may only increase the suspiciousness. The patient should always be given an explanation about the need for the information and how it will be used. An open discussion about confidentiality may help. Patients who are delusional or hallucinating should not be challenged about these symptoms, which are real to the patient. In addition, problems with conceptual disorganization such as blocking, circumstantiality, flight of ideas, and loosening of associations make it very difficult to interview the patient. When these symptoms occur, staff should repeat questions, define terms, rephrase and refocus, and assess illogical and irrelevant comments. For such patients, questions that are closed ended may be more successful. Structure is important and helps the patient.

Communication Techniques

There are many therapeutic communication techniques. Some of the techniques that might be used by home care staff with the patient and family/SOs include the following:

- *Listening.* Listening focuses on hearing as much as possible in a message from the patient. This includes identifying the nonverbal communication and understanding its relationship to the verbal communication.
- *Questioning.* A question should be clear and understandable. After the question is asked, staff need to stop and listen for the response.
  1. Ask one question at a time.
  2. Open-ended versus closed-ended questions is an important consideration. An open-ended question allows the patient to give as much information as he or she wants to give (e.g., "How did you feel about your discussion with your father about your argument?"). Closed questions limit the patient to a specific answer (e.g., "Did you talk with your father about your argument?").
  3. Double questions can be problematic. These are either-or questions, asking the patient to choose from two options (e.g., "Did you watch TV last night or go to bed?"). Maybe the patient did not do either of these and is confused as to how to answer the question.
  4. The use of "why" often sends the message that staff consider the topic to be "bad" or that an action should not be done (e.g., instead of saying, "Why didn't you follow your plan for the day?" it is better to say "You usually follow your plan for the day. What was going on with you today that kept you from following it?")
- *Seeking clarification.* Staff ask the patient for more information to make the message clearer (e.g., "I'm not sure that I understand").
- *Restating.* Staff repeat what they think the patient has communicated to them. In doing this, staff are asking the patient if they heard the message correctly (e.g., "Let me repeat what you have said to make sure I understand").
- *Silence.* Silence can be used in a positive way. It allows time for thought, and time to just be together. Silence can be helpful during times of intense emotions to provide a break. Because it may take longer for the elderly patient to communicate, this patient may need silent times. If the staff member is unsure what to say, sometimes silence can be helpful to bridge this gap. According to King: "Silence gives the patient time to ponder thoughts, feelings and decisions. Silence provides time to formulate questions about new strategies for care. Silence may provide a clue to either party that information is not new or meaningful."[6(p.65)]
- *Focusing.* Staff help the patient talk about one topic or problem in more depth.
- *Summarizing.* Staff tell the patient what they think are the main ideas that have been discussed. This usually is done at the end of a discussion, and then staff ask the patient to evaluate the discussion.

- *Giving broad openings.* This technique provides the patient with the chance to choose the topic (e.g., "Is there something you would like to talk about today?" or "Where would you like to begin?").
- *Offering general leads.* This technique encourages the patient to continue to talk (e.g., "Tell me more about it" or "And then what happened?").
- *Making observations.* When staff make observations, they verbalize or put into words what they are seeing or observing (e.g., "You seem sad today" or "Are you uncomfortable when we discuss your progress?").
- *Encouraging comparison.* The staff member encourages the patient to make comparisons and to identify whether an experience, feeling, or problem is similar to or different from another (e.g., "How was this family discussion like your last one?" or "Have you had a similar problem with another person before?").
- *Giving information.* Giving information is probably the most frequent technique used. It is sharing facts with the patient. It is a very basic level of communication that must be used; however, it can be abused if other techniques are not used.

Communication Problems

All staff-patient communication will encounter some problems, and all staff use nontherapeutic techniques at times. The home care staff need to be alert to potential problems and use of nontherapeutic techniques, prevent them when possible, and intervene early when they occur. The following are some examples of these problems.

- Arguing with a patient over basic values does not help the patient problem solve. Some patients ask for staff opinion; however, the focus should be on the patient's reactions and options. Staff should focus the conversation on the patient, away from the staff.
- Simply knowing certain facts about the patient can interfere with the patient-staff relationship, even though the patient never speaks about them. Such examples may be the patient who has abused his or her children or the patient who has had an abortion. If staff have feelings about these issues that interfere with communication, they need to recognize this communication problem and discuss it with their supervisor or professional colleagues to resolve the conflict so that the patient can receive care.
- Abusive behavior from the patient is not appropriate patient behavior. Staff do not have to tolerate verbal or physical abuse. They must set limits with the patient. When discussing this with the patient, staff should focus on the

patient's behavior rather than staff behavior. Staff set limits because they respect the patient and themselves.

- Silence is difficult to handle. An initial staff reaction to silence is to feel that something has been done wrong or that the patient does not like the staff member. "What did I do wrong to get the patient to clam up?" Silence is seen as a negative experience, a bad thing; however, staff and the patient need to learn to be comfortable with silence. There are many possible reasons for silence:
  1. The patient may need to sort out thoughts and feelings.
  2. They patient may require a break from conversation.
  3. The situation may be confusing to the patient, or the patient may be confused as to what to say or do next.
  4. The patient may not be ready to reveal anything or may be showing resistance.
  5. The patient may refuse to accept questioning from staff.
  6. Short pauses may mean that the patient is searching for more thoughts and feelings to express.

  There may be a connection between the silence and what was said before the silence began. Staff, however, may not ever learn the reason for the silence. Sometimes the patient will explain the silence. With some patients, staff can comment on the silence and see if the patient provides some clues about the silence (e.g., "You are very quiet now"). The patient should not be told he or she is silent. During silence, observe the patient's nonverbal signals (e.g., gestures, facial expressions, posture, hand movements, etc.). Staff should also be concerned with their own nonverbal signals. Are staff communicating to the patient that they are confused, angry, bored, or restless? Staff should learn how to sit through some silence with patients. It is helpful if staff can remember times when they were silent. What were the reasons for it? What expectations did the staff member have at those times? What helped the staff, and what did not help during the silence?

Listening, Empathizing, and Questioning

Listening is more than merely hearing verbal sounds. It is hearing the whole picture, getting the message. It is hard work to listen to someone. If the listener's mind is wandering to other subjects, he or she cannot really listen. A good listener is interested in what is being said and shows this interest through posture, attention, and other nonverbal clues. Staff hear the way things are said (e.g. tone, expressions, gestures). What is not said? What is hinted at? What is perhaps being held back? "Why didn't I see that?" may be a question staff ask themselves some days. There will be days and times when a staff member's listening skills are not as good as other days. Many factors can interfere with listening, such as the staff member's mood, personal problems, fatigue, health, busy workday, worry about the next home visit, the topic of conversation, what is happening in the home environment, and personal reactions to the patient and/or the patient's problems. Listening skills can be improved by

- decreasing distractions
- listening to the content rather than to the way the patient is communicating
- listening to all of the communication before answering
- keeping an open mind even if content is very emotional
- listening for themes

Empathy is feeling yourself into or participating in the inner world of another person while remaining yourself. Staff need to try to see the world through the patient's eyes. Empathy is understanding *with* a person, not *about* a person. It is, however, important to remember that the staff member is a separate person from the patient.

Questioning is probably the most frequently used communication method with patients. Problems that may occur with questioning are

- asking too many questions
- asking confusing questions
- asking questions that interrupt the patient
- asking more than one question at a time
- only asking questions that have "yes" or "no" answers

The patient may begin to feel like an object who answers questions when asked and otherwise keeps quiet, an object with information that is the only reason staff members are interested in the patient. For some patients, this may communicate to them that the staff member is the authority. The patient agrees to this, expecting staff to come up with a solution—a solution that staff often do not have. The patient may wonder, "What are staff good for?" and feel that staff should be able to put information together and come up with the magic answer. Staff have failed the patient, just like everyone else has. These feelings may need to be discussed with the patient by saying: "I don't have the answer for you. I will help you look at your feelings, behavior, and the facts about the situation. Then we can work on choices you might have." Bombarding the patient with questions is not helpful. One question after another only puts the patient in the position of answering, giving little chance for the patient to choose the topic. The patient may begin to feel that there is one correct answer, but he or she cannot come up with it.

When a patient answers questions like a robot with no feelings, this indicates that the patient has communication problems, there are problems with the staff-patient relationship, or the environment is not helpful. It may be that too many questions are being asked. Questioning the patient is often the way staff deal with their own anxiety. Staff do not know what to say, so they ask a question. If staff begin to ask too many questions, they should evaluate their own anxiety as it is probably high.

More Communication Problems

- Anger toward the patient is not an uncommon problem. Staff may need time to get away from the patient to release anger appropriately rather than to lose control with the patient. After a patient exhibits behavior that arouses anger, it should be discussed with the patient. What happened? What was the patient feeling? What did the patient think was going on with staff? If possible, staff and the patient should identify other choices that the patient had as an alternative to inappropriate behavior. A similar intervention can be used when a patient has a conflict with family/SOs. Staff need to help the patient and family/SOs look at what is going on between them. Patients may not understand what they are doing to stimulate another person to respond negatively. Staff and family/SOs need to let the patient know that they consider the patient responsible for his or her own actions, thoughts, and feelings.
- If staff are overly concerned about what they will say next, they have difficulty listening, and this affects communication. When staff feel themselves jumping ahead of what the patient is saying, they need to listen more and respond to what the patient is saying and the patient's feelings.
- Staff should not tell the patient what to think or feel. Respecting the patient's thoughts and feelings does not mean agreeing with all of them. It does not mean thinking or feeling the same way as the patient or having the same values. The patient has as much right to his or her ideas, feelings, and values as staff do, and staff want to do everything possible to understand the patient's ideas, feelings, and values.
- Time limits should not be ignored. For some discussions with patients, it is important to identify the time limit before the discussion begins. If the patient initiates a conversation shortly before a visit is to end, staff need to tell the patient that time is limited. Depending on the subject matter, staff may (1) suggest continuing the conversation at the next visit, specifying when that visit will be; (2) telephone the patient to complete the discussion; or (3) if it is an emergency (such as admission of suicidal feelings), extend the visit. If the patient routinely does this, staff should discuss the behavior with the patient to determine why the patient waits until the end of a visit to begin a discussion. Patients can be very sensitive to staff behavior, but they need to learn about limits.

- If staff are not really listening to the patient and are eager to get to the end point, they may jump to conclusions. Staff then assume they know what the patient is communicating, and often they are incorrect.
- Changing the subject is a way to avoid a subject that makes a person feel uncomfortable. Either the patient or staff may do this in a conversation. If staff do it, the patient may think that staff do not want to talk about what interests the patient. If the patient changes the subject, staff need to assess this behavior and perhaps comment about it. The patient's changing the subject may indicate that the subject is a difficult one. Is it a subject the patient never talks about? Is it a subject that is important? Is there enough privacy for the patient?
- Lack of staff consistency occurs when staff change what they have said in the past. It is confusing to the patient if staff tell the patient to do one thing and then change their instructions without an explanation. For patients who use manipulation, this only exacerbates their problems and manipulative behavior. A treatment plan that is communicated to all home care staff who work with the patient can help prevent inconsistency if staff follow it.
- Lack of trust is a serious problem in a relationship, and it will affect communication. The receiver in the communication process needs to believe that the sender means what he or she is saying. Honesty, consistency, clear communication, and involvement of the patient in all aspects of the treatment planning will increase trust between the patient and home care staff.
- Failure to use reality testing will make it difficult to understand the message from the patient. Is what the patient discussing real? If a patient is hallucinating, staff may not understand the message from the patient. Clarification may be necessary, but it must be nonconfrontational.
- When staff talk about themselves rather than the patient, the patient feels unimportant. It is easy for staff to begin to talk about personal information when the patient discusses personal problems, but it must be avoided.
- When staff members talk too much, this gives the patient little time to talk. Staff should give the patient enough time to make statements and discuss thoughts before staff begin talk.
- If the staff ignore the patient's feelings, they will experience incomplete communication. Feelings are a critical part of communication. Staff need to identify feelings and help the patient express them.
- Use of pronouns such as *he, she, it, they,* and *them* may be confusing to the patient and to staff. If staff do not understand the patient, staff should ask for an explanation. Staff should also avoid using these pronouns unless they make their meaning clear to the patient.
- Ignoring nonverbal communication will decrease the meaning of a message. Nonverbal communication is critical to communication. Staff need to be aware

of their own nonverbal signals to the patient and of the patient's nonverbal signals. What are the nonverbal signals communicating? Is the message the same as the verbal communication? If it is different, staff may want to comment on this to the patient.

- It is not always helpful to reassure the patient. Reassuring occurs when staff say such things as, "Everything will be all right." Such a statement is false and not helpful, and staff should not promise this to a patient.

Solution-Focused Interviewing[7]

Brief, solution-focused approaches tend to mobilize hope, use existing support systems, and support patient strength. Several authors have identified the following suggestions as solution-oriented questions. These questions increase the patient's involvement in identifying goals for solution.

- *presession change questions*
    1. Many times in between the call for an appointment and the first session, people notice that things already seem different. What have you noticed about your situation?
    2. What changes have you already noticed since your discharge from the hospital?
- *miracle questions:* Suppose one night there is a miracle while you are sleeping, and the problems that led you to get treatment are solved. Because you were sleeping, you don't know that a miracle has happened. What do you suppose you will notice is different the next morning that will tell you that there has been a miracle? Who will be the first person to notice the next day that something is different about you after the miracle? What will be different between you and your (mother, father, wife, husband, etc.)?
- *exception questions*
    1. Are there times now that some of this miracle happens even just a little bit?
    2. Tell me about those times when this problem does not occur? How do you get this to happen?
- *scaling questions*
    1. On a scale of 1 to 10, where 10 is the problem solved and 1 is the worst it has ever been, where are you today?
    2. On a scale of 1 to 10, with 10 being that you have every confidence this problem can be solved and 1 being no confidence at all, where would you put yourself today?
    3. What would it take for you to go (e.g.) from a 3 to a 3.5 or 4?

- *coping questions*
  1. How have you prevented things from getting worse?
  2. How did you manage to get yourself up this morning?
  3. What keeps you going?

STAFF COMMUNICATION WITH FAMILY/SIGNIFICANT OTHERS

All of the information discussed pertaining to staff-patient communication is applicable to staff communication with family/SOs. The staff will be communicating with family/SOs when they are very vulnerable; however, the situation is different from communicating with them during an inpatient experience. According to Stulginsky, "On their own turf, families feel freer to question advice, do things their own way, establish their own time schedule, and set their own priorities. Sometimes what they decide is opposite to what is advised."[8(p.405)] Chapter 3 discusses families/SOs in more depth.

TELEPHONE COMMUNICATION

The telephone is a very important communication method in home care. Home care staff use it to communicate with the home care agency, other staff, other health care resources, the patient's physician, and the patient/family/SOs. Clear communication on the telephone is important. For calls where there might be questions later about what was said, the staff should keep notes. Telephone calls that should be documented, such as calls to the physician or to the patient, need to be documented in a timely manner and should include all of the relevant information.

STAFF-STAFF COMMUNICATION

Communication among staff members is a critical part of home care and, with more complex patient problems, its importance increases. Staff need to communicate about the patients, working relationships with one another, and staff planning and scheduling. Verbal and written communication is used. Communication is affected by the organization of the home care agency or service; its standards, policies, and procedures; and the communication system. Time is always a problem, and finding the best time to communicate with staff, referral sources, physicians, etc., can be difficult. For some contacts, it may be helpful to set up a specific time for one-to-one meetings or telephone calls. Preparing for these contacts will make them more productive and efficient. Developing a rapport is also critical to the success of long-term staff relationships and communication. Patient care will benefit from positive staff relationships.

DOCUMENTATION

According to Erickson, "Documentation serves as a primary measure of clinical practice and reimbursement eligibility and as a tool of professional accountability and quality assurance."[9(p.22)] Documentation is a part of communication about, with, and for the patient. For the psychiatric patient, information that is documented must be specific and behaviorally focused. It is easy to document that staff are helping the patient ventilate about his or her anxiety or talk about anxiety; however, for reimbursement and for others to understand, it is important to describe specific interventions and their results (e.g., the patient was taught the symptoms of anxiety and asked to identify those that apply to him; the patient was taught relaxation techniques and was able to do them; the patient reported using the relaxation techniques and experiencing a decrease in anxiety so that he was able to participate in the family meal). Documentation must be as specific as possible and applicable to the individual patient.

SUMMARY

The therapeutic relationship is rarely easy to develop, particularly due to time pressures and intermittent home care visits. Each staff member must develop his or her own style in working with patients and their families/SOs. Communication is an integral part of every relationship. Being in the position of developing a relationship and communicating with a home care patient whose major problems relate to relationships and communications puts the staff in a challenging position; however, it can be done with most psychiatric patients and their families/SOs.

NOTES

1. L. Bowers, "Ethnomethodology II: A Study of the Community Psychiatric Nurse in the Patient's Home," *International Journal of Nursing* 29, no. 1 (1992): 69–79.
2. M. Stulginsky, "Nurses' Home Health Experience: Part II: The Unique Demands of Home Visits," *Nursing & Health Care* 14, no. 9 (1993): 476–485, at 482.
3. Bowers, "Ethnomethodology II: A Study of the Community Psychiatric Nurse in the Patient's Home," 69.
4. M. Stulginsky, "Nurses' Home Health Experience: Part I: The Practice Setting," *Nursing & Health Care* 14, no. 8 (1993): 402–407, at 405.

5. Stulginsky, "Nurses' Home Health Experience: Part II: The Unique Demands of Home Visits," 477.

6. K. King, "Using Therapeutic Silence in Home Healthcare Nursing," *Home Healthcare Nurse* 13, no. 1 (1995): 65–68, at 65.

7. D. Webster et al., "Introducing Solution-Focused Approaches to Staff in Inpatient Psychiatric Settings," *Archives of Psychiatric Nursing* 8, no. 4 (1994): 254–261, at 254–255, 258.

8. Stulginsky, "Nurses' Home Health Experience: Part I: The Practice Setting," 405.

9. G. Erickson, "Multidisciplinary Documentation for Home Care," *Caring* 11, no. 1 (1992): 22–26.

SUGGESTED READING

Boling, P., and J. Keenan. 1992. Communication between nurses and physicians in home care. *Caring* 11, no. 5: 26–29.

Bowers, L. 1992. Ethnomethodology II: A study of the community psychiatric nurse in the patient's home. *International Journal of Nursing Studies* 29, no. 1: 69–79.

Braverman, B. 1990. Eliciting assessment data from the patient who is difficult to interview. *Nursing Clinics of North America* 25, no. 4: 743–750.

Carey, R. 1989. How values affect the mutual goal setting process with multiproblem families. *Journal of Community Health Nursing* 1, no. 3: 207–215.

King, K. 1995. Using therapeutic silence in home healthcare nursing. *Home Healthcare Nurse* 13, no. 1: 65–68.

Morrison, J. 1993. *The first interview.* New York: Guilford Press.

Pruitt, R. et al. 1987. Mastering distractions that mar home visits. *Nursing & Health Care* 8, no. 6: 345–347.

Shea, S. 1988. *Psychiatric interviewing: The art of understanding.* Philadelphia: W.B. Saunders Company.

Stulginsky, M. 1993. Nurses' home health experience: Part I: The practice setting. *Nursing & Health Care* 14, no. 8: 402–407.

Stulginsky, M. 1993. Nurses' home health experience: Part II: The unique demands of home visits. *Nursing & Health Care* 14, no. 9: 476–485.

5

Psychoeducation in the Home

INTRODUCTION

Patient and family/significant other (SO) education is a critical component of psychiatric home care. Every visit to the home is an opportunity to teach new skills to improve self-management. This learning process must be collaborative. The home care nurse should discuss collaborative learning with the patient and the family/SOs at the initial visit. Patient education is an intervention defined as "planning, implementation, and evaluation of a teaching program designed to address a patient's particular needs."[1(p.483)] It must be included in every patient's home care plan and documented in the patient's record. The American Nurses Association (ANA) recommends that "education should be offered in a manner in which the patient is fully informed regarding care, and assumes ownership, gives consent, and uses the knowledge to direct the process of psychopharmacology. Patients and significant others need to know about the disorder, its symptoms, and psychopharmacologic treatments, as well as concurrent and alternative treatment modalities."[2(p.33)]

THE LEARNING PROCESS

The learning process can be described in the same way as the nursing process. It requires assessment, outcome identification, development of specific interventions or teaching methods and strategies, implementation, and evaluation of learning. Three principles are important in the process.[3]

1. Effective teaching results in learning.
2. Patient teaching is concerned with helping people acquire the knowledge, attitudes, skills, and behaviors that will allow them to regain and maintain their health and to attain even higher levels of wellness.

3. The identification of learning needs and patient teaching based on these needs are integral parts of the nursing process and of excellent nursing care for every patient.

A component of patient education that is not often addressed is the requirement that the teacher—the nurse—must be knowledgeable about the content. The patient expects this, and the nurse who is not knowledgeable will experience anxiety, which will limit the educational process. Even though it is important for the nurse to be prepared, it is also important for the nurse to admit lack of knowledge and then to obtain the required information for the patient. Pretending to know may compromise the collaborative relationship and the health of the patient.

Education is a major component of psychiatric care and rehabilitation and, in many cases, it is the most important intervention. Three approaches to patient education as an intervention are[4]

1. *Relating serious consequences and high risk of recurrence of illness as incentive to learn.* Psychiatric patients often have a long history of relapses that frequently they and their families/SOs find very disturbing. Discussing with the patient the advantages to learning about symptom monitoring in order to prevent relapse may be helpful in encouraging the patient to participate actively in the learning process.
2. *Identifying major problem areas.* The patient should be asked to identify major problem areas. Then the nurse and the patient can determine if some of these problems have an educational component (few do not). Can learning more about the problem, its solution, or new skills help the patient with the problem? For example, does the patient understand why it is important to take medication as ordered? What happens in the patient's body when the medication is taken infrequently? What happens when the patient tries to make up a missed dose?
3. *Capitalizing on learner frustration and convincing the learner that positive benefits can result by initiating a specific behavior.* If the patient is having difficulty communicating a specific problem with his or her family/SOs and feels frustrated by this inability, it is probably affecting the patient's symptoms. The home care nurse should discuss this with the patient and point out that the patient can learn better communication skills to help the patient discuss immediate problems with the family/SOs.

Steps in the Learning Process

1. *Assessment.* Factors that need to be assessed for the patient and in some cases for the family/SOs include the following:

- What does the patient know, want to know, and need to know?
- What are the patient's fears about the illness and the treatment?
- What is the patient's ability to learn? Does the patient understand easily? Does the patient ask questions? Does his or her body language indicate confusion about the information? Can the patient follow directions? Can the patient concentrate? Can the patient recall information? Can the patient hear, see, and communicate? Is the patient easily distracted? Does the patient understand abstract ideas?[5]
- What is the patient's past compliance history?
- What is the patient's educational history?
- Are there cultural issues that should be considered?
- Are there physical problems that may interfere with learning?

2. *Outcome identification.* Following the assessment, the home care nurse and the patient should identify expected outcomes. The outcomes describe the behavioral change that the patient will exhibit at the conclusion of the learning. As is true of treatment outcomes, educational outcomes must be stated from the patient's viewpoint (e.g., The patient will . . .). To be successful, there must be collaborative identification of outcomes. The nurse should encourage the patient to express his or her feelings about what needs to be accomplished. The nurse acts as the "reality checker" but cannot force an outcome on the patient.

3. *Implementation.* Implementation is the actual teaching that occurs. Factors that affect implementation include the following:[6]
   - *Anxiety.* Anxiety that is experienced by the patient, family/SOs, and the home care staff is always important. Mild anxiety is helpful; however, severe anxiety prevents any learning from taking place.
   - *Motivation.* Motivation can be internal, with the patient feeling that he or she wants to change. It can also be external, with the pressure for change originating outside the patient (e.g., the family/SOs, physician, home care nurse, fear of rehospitalization, legal authorities).
   - *Control.* Some patients may feel they have lost all control over themselves and their lives and feel helplessness. This can make it very difficult for the home care staff to teach the patient, and it is very important for the staff to work with the patient to communicate that the patient can gain control.
   - *Trust and honesty.* Continuity and consistency will be very important in developing trust and honesty between the patient and the home care staff. Trust and honesty are also influenced by the home care staff's knowledge and their ability to admit when they are wrong or lack information.

- *Current physical and emotional status.* Is the patient hungry or in pain? Is the patient tired or on drugs that alter his or her cognitive functioning? Is the patient's mobility limited? Is the patient lonely? How much are others pressuring the patient to perform? What is the stage of illness? Are there additional family stresses or crises occurring? Is the patient's behavior escalating, so that concentration is decreased? Is the subject matter disturbing the patient?
- *The home environment.* Is the home environment conducive to learning? Is it quiet? Are there distractions? Is there privacy? Are the important people present or absent?

Teaching takes place during every home visit. Much of it is informal, but there must also be a formal component that is planned and well thought out. Home care staff must always take advantage of the "teachable moment" that is a part of a patient education plan. Liberman, who has written extensively about psychiatric rehabilitation with a major focus on education, describes some critical aspects of the learning process and the treatment process:

> A good behavioral family therapist is a good teacher. In explaining principles and guidelines to patients and relatives, therapists frequently overestimate their capacity for processing information. Even highly educated patients and relatives, because of the stress they are experiencing and other intrinsic learning disabilities, need information that is transmitted simply and clearly in their own language. Frequent repetition is required, along with inquiries that ascertain how well the therapist's communications are being decoded by family members. In addition, the therapist must make sure that patients and relatives are learning principles rather than simply enacting new behaviors in response to the expectation of the therapy program.[7(p.234)]

The home care nurse will confront similar issues as care is provided in the home and the patient is taught.

Teaching Methods

Teaching methods that can be used in the home are varied and will depend upon the skills of the home care staff, the needs of the patient and family/SOs, the home environment, the time frame, and the content. Some of these methods are individual discussion, group/family/SOs discussion, demonstration, problem solving, role play, simulation, behavioral modification, contracting, audiovisual materials (e.g., audiotapes or videos), literature (e.g., pamphlets or books), diaries and logs, worksheets focused on a particular topic, and homework assignments. Methods that may be less familiar to the nurse are role play, simulation, and behavioral modification.

- *Role play.* This method allows the patient or family/SOs to play a role without rehearsal and then discuss it. The person should not play himself or herself. There is no script other than a general description of who the person is (such as mother, father) or other characteristics (e.g., mother who is angry about . . .). After the role play, there must be time to discuss it.
- *Simulation.* In a simulation, the patient acts out with the nurse a real situation to help the patient learn specific skills. Examples might be using the bus, calling for a medical appointment, or discussing a change of medications with the physician.
- *Behavior modification.* The patient is given positive reinforcement for a specific behavior, which will then cause the desired response to happen more frequently. The nurse identifies positive reinforcers for the individual patient. This method requires active family/SOs participation and explanation, because the family/SOs will be providing the reinforcement when home care staff are not present.

EDUCATION CONTENT

Education for the psychiatric patient and family/SOs at times tends to be narrowly focused on psychiatric content. However, according to Nigro and Maggio, "[a] health education approach that incorporates psychiatric issues, environmental safety, physical health information, and lifestyle modifications for wellness can best address the inter-related physical and mental health needs of this population."[8(p.15)] Exhibit 5–1 identifies some recommended focus areas for patients and for families/SOs. Exhibit 5–2 provides examples of educational materials and publications for patients and families/SOs. Appendix 5A describes content for major patient and family/SOs education topics.

SUMMARY

Psychoeducation is a major component of psychiatric home care for all patients and their families/SOs. It should be based on their needs and their readiness to learn. The home care nurse cannot assume that the patient learned information in the hospital or at an earlier time during the illness. It is also important to educate the patient about other medical problems he or she may have and general health habits.

Exhibit 5–1 Educational Focus Areas for Patients and Families/Significant Others

Patients, Families/Significant Others	Patients	Families/Significant Others
• nature of illness, etiology, treatment • relationship of illness and stress • identification of early symptoms of acute episodes of illness • medications—their purpose, importance • aftercare visits—using staff for consultation on problems • communication and problem-solving skills	• monitoring stress; balancing stimulation with caution about adding stressors • self-regulation of specific symptoms of illness • learning to understand others; empathy development • developing social and leisure skills; balancing with constructive activity • learning to live with stigma; self-help groups for the mentally ill	• maintaining simple, structured, consistent environment • management of specific behavioral problems • importance of low-key, noncritical attitude and communication • including the client in activities • importance of developing own life • support groups for families; advocacy for mentally ill

Source: From *Issues in Mental Health Nursing*, Volume 15, H. Holmes, Taylor & Francis, Inc., Washington, D.C. Reproduced with permission. All rights reserved.

Exhibit 5–2 Educational Materials for Patients and Families/Significant Others

---

Backlar, P. 1994. *The family face of schizophrenia.* New York: G.P. Putnam's Sons.

Baer, L. 1991. *Getting control: Overcoming your obsessions and compulsions.* Boston: Little, Brown & Company.

Burke, R. 1995. *When the music's over: My journey into schizophrenia.* New York: Basic Books.

Carter, R. 1994. *Helping yourself help others: A book for caregivers.* New York: Times Books.

Copeland, M. 1992. *The depression workbook.* Oakland, CA: New Harbinger Publications, Inc.

Cronkite, K. 1994. *On the edge of darkness: Conversations about conquering depression.* New York: Doubleday.

Dinner, S. 1989. *Nothing to be ashamed of: Growing up with mental illness in your family.* New York: Lothrop, Lee, & Shepard Books.

Falloon, I. et al. 1984. *Family care of schizophrenia.* New York: Guilford Press.

Gruetzner, H. 1992. *Alzheimer's: A caregiver's guide and source book.* New York: John Wiley & Sons.

Hatfield, A. 1990. *Family education in mental illness.* New York: Guilford Press.

Kass, F. et al. 1992. *Columbia University College of Physicians and Surgeons complete home guide to mental health.* New York: Henry Holt.

Laskin, P., and A. Moskowitz. 1991. *Wish upon a star: A story for children with a parent who is mentally ill.* New York: Magination Press.

McCue, K. 1994. *How to help children through a parent's serious illness.* New York: St. Martin's Press.

Mueser, K., and S. Gingrich. 1994. *Coping with schizophrenia: A guide for families.* Oakland, CA: New Harbinger Publications, Inc.

Peterkin, A. 1992. *What about me? When brothers and sisters get sick.* New York: Magination Press.

Roberts, D. 1991. *Taking care of caregivers: For families and others who care for people with Alzheimer's disease and other forms of dementia.* Palo Alto, CA: Bull Publishing.

Wurtzel, E. 1994. *Prozac nation: Young and depressed in America.* Boston: Houghton Mifflin.

Yudofsky, S. 1991. *What you need to know about psychiatric drugs.* Washington, DC: American Psychiatric Press, Inc.

In addition to the above materials, the U.S. Department of Health and Human Services has published pamphlets, including the following:

- *If you're over 65 and feeling depressed.* 1990.
- *The 14 worst myths about recovered mental patients.* 1990.

continues

Exhibit 5–2 continued

- *Bipolar disorder.* 1993.
- *Understanding panic disorder.* 1993.
- *Helping the depressed person get treatment.* 1990.
- *Diagnosis and treatment of depression in late life.* 1991.
- *Depressive illnesses: treatments bring hope.* 1993.

NOTES

1. J. McCloskey and G. Bulechek, *Nursing Interventions Classification (NIC).* (St. Louis, MO: Mosby–Year Book, 1992), 483.
2. American Nurses Association, *Psychiatric Mental Health Nursing Psychopharmacology Project* (Washington, DC: American Nurses Publishing, 1994), 33.
3. J. Rorden, *Nurses as Health Teachers: A Practical Guide* (Philadelphia: W.B. Saunders Company, 1987), xi.
4. K. Hellwig, "Health Teaching: The Crux of Home Care Nursing," *Home Healthcare* 8, no. 4 (1990): 35–37, at 35.
5. R. Ford, *Patient Teaching Manual, II* (Springhouse, PA: Springhouse Corporation, 1987), 5.
6. Ford, *Patient Teaching Manual, II*, 6–7.
7. R. Liberman, "Behavioral Family Management," in *Psychiatric Rehabilitation of Chronic Mental Patients*, ed. R. Liberman (Washington, DC: American Psychiatric Press, Inc. 1988), 199–244, at 234.
8. A. Nigro and J. Maggio, "A Neglected Need: Health Education for the Mentally Ill," *Journal of Psychosocial Nursing* 28, no. 7 (1990): 15–19, at 15.

SUGGESTED READING

Bisbee, C. 1991. *Educating patients and families about mental illness: A practical guide.* Gaithersburg, MD: Aspen Publishers, Inc.

Daudell-Streje, D., and C. Murphy. 1995. Emerging clinical issues in home health psychiatric nursing. *Home Healthcare Nurse* 13, no. 2: 17–21.

Dispenza, D., and A. Nigro. 1989. Life skills for the mentally ill: A program description. *Journal of Applied Rehabilitation Counseling* 20, no. 1: 47–49.

Hatfield, A. 1990. *Family education in mental illness.* Washington, DC: American Psychiatric Press, Inc.

Heyduk, L. 1991. Medication education: Increasing patient compliance. *Journal of Psychosocial Nursing* 29, no. 12: 32–35.

Keating, S., and G. Kelmer. 1988. *Home health care nursing: Concepts and practice.* Philadelphia: J.B. Lippincott Co.

Maynard, C. 1993. Psychoeducational approach to depression in women. *Journal of Psychosocial Nursing* 31, no. 12: 9–14.

Moller, M., and J. Wer. 1989. Simultaneous patient/family education regarding schizophrenia: The Nebraska model. *Archives of Psychiatric Nursing* 3, no. 6: 332–337.

Nigro, A., and J. Maggio. 1990. A neglected need: Health education for the mentally ill. *Journal of Psychosocial Nursing* 28, no. 7: 15–19.

Pollack, L. 1995. Information needs of patients hospitalized for bipolar disorder. *Psychiatric Services* 46, no. 11: 1191–1194.

Rorden, J. 1987. *Nurses as health teachers.* Philadelphia: W.B. Saunders Company.

Torrey, E. Fuller. 1988. *Surviving schizophrenia: A family manual.* New York: Harper & Row.

Zind, R. et al. 1992. Educating patients about missed medication doses. *Journal of Psychosocial Nursing* 30, no. 7: 10–14.

Appendix 5-A

Patient and Family/Significant Others Education Content

Specific content for some topics is provided; however, this content must be adapted to individual patient and family/SOs needs.

ANXIETY

Definition

Person feels uncomfortable and tense and unable to clearly identify the threat. There are four levels: mild, moderate, severe, and panic. When experiencing severe or panic levels of anxiety, the person needs immediate help from others.

Etiology

There is no known specific cause of anxiety. There is, however, some evidence that benzodiazepine binding sites in the brain may have something to do with anxiety, due to the responsiveness of these sites to benzodiazepine medications.

Signs and Symptoms

- sleeplessness
- restlessness
- pacing
- shaking
- increased pulse and respirations
- sweating
- irritability
- inability to problem solve or learn (this is not a problem with mild anxiety and sometimes not with moderate anxiety)
- uneasiness
- powerlessness
- helplessness

Treatment/Interventions/Important Issues

- medications
- relaxation
- deep breathing
- imagery
- exercise
- problem solving
- stress reduction
- monitoring symptoms
- problems with use of nonprescription medications and alcohol
- decreasing environmental stimuli
- role play and simulation of anxiety-provoking situations

Provide more detail for those issues that are relevant to the individual patient or family/SO. See Chapter 20 for an in-depth discussion of anxiety disorders.

DEPRESSION

Definition

Person feels low self-esteem and generally slowed down, physically and psychologically. Depression is a disturbance of affect.

Etiology

Biochemical factors with a focus on neurotransmitters that regulate mood, behavior, and bodily functions are very important in relation to the etiology of depression. Proposed hypotheses include a deficiency of norepinephrine, changes in serotonin, and abnormal cortical secretion. There is significant evidence supporting the importance of genetics. Physical illness and some medications can lead to depression. Loss also affects a person who may be vulnerable to depression.

Signs and Symptoms

- sadness
- hopelessness
- increased worry
- guilt
- loss of interest
- decreased self-esteem

- increased fatigue
- irritability
- decreased or increased sleep
- change in appetite
- poor hygiene
- unrealistic expectations
- suicidal feelings and behavior

Treatment/Interventions/Important Issues

- medications
- nutrition
- sleep/rest
- exercise
- personal hygiene
- stress reduction
- realistic and unrealistic expectations
- role of thoughts and feelings
- monitoring symptoms
- problem solving
- thought stopping
- socialization and activities: gradual increase
- assertiveness training
- increasing self-esteem
- problems with use of nonprescription drugs and alcohol
- increasing environmental stimuli
- electroconvulsive therapy (if appropriate for the patient)

Provide more detail for those issues that are relevant to the individual patient or family/SO. See Chapter 21 for an in-depth discussion of depression.

BIPOLAR DISORDER

Definition

Person experiences episodes of mood swings, mania and depression, with possible periods of normal mood; some experience more depression or more mania.

Etiology

Genetics is an important factor with this illness. Two neurotransmitters, serotonin and norepinephrine, are also thought to be related to the etiology.

Signs and Symptoms

- *Depression:* sadness, hopelessness, increased worry, guilt, loss of interest, decreased self-esteem, increased fatigue, irritability, decreased or increased sleep, change in appetite, poor hygiene, unrealistic expectations, suicidal feelings and behavior
- *Mania:* obnoxious or intrusive behavior, distractibility, irritability, decreased sleep, increased energy, poor judgment, racing thoughts, agitation, hallucinations, talkativeness, poor personal hygiene, unrealistic ideas or expectations, excessive behavior (eating, sexual, spending money, etc.)

Treatment/Interventions/Important Issues

- medications
- laboratory testing
- nutrition
- exercise
- monitoring symptoms
- personal hygiene
- stress reduction
- rest/sleep
- use of nonprescription drugs and alcohol
- decreasing environmental stimuli
- safety: accidents, assaultive behavior
- self-help groups

Provide more detail for those issues that are relevant to the individual patient or family/SO. See Chapter 22 for an in-depth discussion of bipolar disorder.

SCHIZOPHRENIA

Definition

Schizophrenia is an illness with alterations in thinking—both content and process—that affects a person's total functioning.

Etiology

Schizophrenia is considered to be a brain disease with a focus on the limbic system in the brain. There are problems with brain structure and function.

Signs and Symptoms

- hallucinations
- delusions
- lack of initiative
- inappropriate affect
- inability to think clearly
- apathy
- decreased activity
- poor personal hygiene
- paranoia
- social withdrawal and isolation

Treatment/Interventions/Important Issues

- medications
- nutrition
- personal hygiene
- reality orientation
- coping skills
- socialization, as tolerated
- monitoring symptoms and relapse prevention
- supporting compliance
- decreasing anxiety: stress in the home and learning coping skills
- coping with hallucinations
- decreasing or increasing environmental stimuli
- self-help groups

Provide more detail for those issues that are relevant to the individual patient or family/SO. See Chapter 23 for an in-depth discussion of schizophrenia.

ALZHEIMER'S DISEASE

Definition

Alzheimer's disease is a type of dementia leading to impairment of intellectual functioning that is a progressive disease of the central nervous system. It is irreversible.

Etiology

There is degeneration in nerve endings and brain cells.

Signs and Symptoms

- memory loss
- communication problems
- suspiciousness
- absentmindedness
- poor judgment
- irritability

See Chapter 28 for an extensive list of symptoms for the various stages of this illness.

Treatment/Interventions/Important Issues

- reality orientation
- need for routine and consistency
- compensation for memory loss; label items; label directions to bathroom, etc.; use reminder notes, calendars, clocks; state name when seeing patient
- safety: lighting, clear areas of obstacles, stove, stairways, throw rugs, hot water (tub and sink), matches, use of smoke detector, lock outside doors to prevent wandering from home, procedure for administration of medications
- medications
- personal hygiene
- nutrition
- rest/sleep
- exercise
- self-esteem: allow as much control as possible
- support group for family/SOs

Provide more detail for those issues that are relevant to the individual patient or family/SO. See Chapter 28 for an extensive discussion of psychiatric disorders and neurological diseases in the elderly patient.

MEDICATIONS

The following teaching guideline refers to all medications; however, specific information about each medication the patient is taking should be reviewed with the patient and family/SOs. Refer to Chapters 12 through 19 and other references regarding specific medications. For each medication, the home care nurse must include information about the following:

- the generic and brand names
- distinctive characteristics of the medication (e.g., color, shape, size)
- purpose and action
- dosage, route, and duration
- time schedule
- administration of the medication
- dietary restrictions
- action to be taken if dose missed (e.g., take another dose—appropriate time frame, skip a dose, call physician or home care nurse)
- adverse side effects and any interventions that may be used to prevent or relieve them
- responses for which the physician should be contacted
- required laboratory testing, importance, and how to obtain
- filling prescription (e.g., when, how to obtain prescription, where to obtain medication, financial issues)
- medication storage

In addition, the following should be discussed with each patient and as appropriate with the family/SOs:

- The patient should understand the importance of taking all medications as ordered, compliance, and relapse. The patient needs to be able to identify why the medication is being taken and what are the expected outcomes.
- The patient should understand the importance of discussing with the physician changes related to pregnancy, breastfeeding, use of nonprescription drugs or alcohol, and operation of machinery.
- Medications take time to work, sometimes several weeks.
- Safety is very important with young children (e.g., storage of medications, childproof caps).
- Do not share medications with anyone.
- The patient should have a reminder method to take medications (e.g., log or diary, calendar, medication dispenser box, routine time to take medication associated with some task).
- When a new prescription is obtained, the patient should read the label for accuracy and check the medication to see if it fits the label. Any questions should be referred initially to the pharmacist and then to the physician. Do not take medications that do not look "right."
- Symptom monitoring should be done by the patient because it provides information about responses to medications, possible relapse, and positive feedback to the patient.

- The patient should know how to contact the physician when there is a crisis and what information needs to be discussed with the physician. The patient may write down questions prior to calling the physician or before an appointment so that the information will not be forgotten. The patient needs to learn how to ask questions, and he or she can practice this with the home care nurse.
- The patient should carry with him or her a list of medications that are being taken. It is particularly important that the patient share this list with all of his or her health care providers.

For an in-depth discussion of medications, see Chapters 12 to 19.

SLEEP

Improving the patient's sleep pattern is important for the patient's overall health and for an opportunity for the family/SOs to obtain their own sleep. The following measures may be taught to improve sleep:

- Avoid sleeping during the day.
- Avoid caffeine (coffee, tea, chocolate, cola).
- Exercise regularly.
- Avoid eating before bedtime.
- Follow a bedtime routine.
- Use relaxation techniques before sleep.
- Sleep in a dark, quiet room.
- Avoid conversations about difficult subjects before sleep.
- Read before sleep.
- Use back rubs and warm baths to relax before sleep.
- Avoid use of hypnotics unless ordered by physician with appropriate periodic assessment.

REALITY ORIENTATION

Some patients need help with reality orientation, most of which will be provided by the family/SOs with guidance from home care staff. The following measures may be taught to the family/SOs:

- Use large calendars for making off the days.
- Use large clocks.

- Address the patient by name.
- Provide your name when speaking to the patient.
- Avoid treating the patient like a child.
- Listen to the patient when he/she speaks about past memories.
- Periodically mention the day and time while speaking with the patient.
- Use short, simple sentences, particularly when giving instructions.
- Discuss current events with the patient, even if the patient does not always seem to be aware of the facts.
- Use a photograph album with labeled pictures.

THOUGHT STOPPING

Chapter 20 describes thought-stopping techniques.

RELAXATION

Chapter 20 describes relaxation techniques.

IMAGERY

Chapter 20 describes imagery techniques.

PROBLEM SOLVING

Chapter 10 describes effective problem-solving techniques.

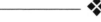

Administration of Psychiatric Home Care Services

6

Administration of Psychiatric Home Care Services

INTRODUCTION

According to Trimbath and Brestensky, "Home care services must not be over-looked as an effective part of the treatment of mental disorders. The home and community provide the most realistic environment for the patient as he or she reaches for recovery."[1(p.1)] Recognizing the importance of health care in the home for the psychiatric patient is often not difficult for staff who work in home care and have seen many patients who could benefit from psychiatric home care; how-ever, developing services for this patient may seem overwhelming as well as fright-ening. Staff may harbor many fears about the psychiatric patient and feel incom-petent to provide care for this patient in the home setting. When a home care agency decides to develop or expand psychiatric services the first step is to con-sider what that care will be. This should consist of a shared vision of what services will be offered to patients and how they will be operationalized. This process is not so critical for the care of medical patients (such as a patient with diabetes or a cardiac problem) in the home, because medical patients require very specific interventions that are usually well established. Psychiatric nursing does not always appear to be as clear-cut as medical nursing. Describing what the staff and the home care agency mean by psychiatric home care or describing the treat-ment model provides the following:

- an understanding of staff roles and the roles of the patient/family/significant others (SOs)
- interventions and their rationales
- a framework that describes how quality of care will be supported
- support for the identification of patient outcomes
- clarification of documentation requirements
- identification of relevant standards

Because the treatment model describes the services that staff will provide to psychiatric patients, it provides important information for physicians, patients/ family/SOs, referral sources, community resources, accrediting agencies, and third-party payers. In addition, it delineates philosophy, goals, policies, procedures, services, and job descriptions. The agency cannot, however, simply lift a treatment model from another psychiatric setting or home care agency. The model needs to be developed by the agency and be applicable to the home setting. Staff should participate in the development of the treatment model, understand it, periodically evaluate it, and—most of all—apply it. A description of a treatment model is more than words. How it is applied is the critical issue.

PHILOSOPHY OF TREATMENT

As the home care agency and staff develop a philosophy of treatment for the care of the psychiatric patient, consideration should be given to the following:

- Psychiatric home care is part of the psychiatric treatment continuum. The continuum includes the inpatient settings, partial hospitalization, outpatient treatment, and home care. Patients may go back and forth between these settings, because they require comprehensive care for very complex problems.
- Treatment needs to be stable, predictable, and consistent.
- Care focuses on facilitating healthy functioning rather than pathology. This does not mean that pathology is denied or ignored, but rather that staff are also very concerned with patient strengths and positive goals/outcomes.
- Patients are psychiatrically homebound.
- The patient's coping skills are assessed and developed as needed.
- Treatment and rehabilitation services are offered in place of hospitalization or as after-care.
- Most adults want to remain in their homes and communities and, whenever possible, should be permitted to do so.
- Patients with serious mental illness usually have complex problems, both psychological and physical.
- Services must be integrated and coordinated.
- Case management is integral to the psychiatric home care program and must emphasize collaboration and planning.
- Criteria for admission are clearly stated.
- Boundaries for patient, family/SOs, and nursing staff are clear and provide structure.
- Many patients will experience relapse, and this is not seen as failure. Staff must be prepared to help patients/families/SOs cope with compliance and relapse.

- Cure is not the focus, as it is currently not possible for most patients with serious mental illness.
- Each patient/family/SO is treated with respect.
- The staff are guests in the patient's home.
- Shared goals are developed with the patient, and when appropriate with family/SOs.
- Patient rights are considered at all times.

In addition, many forces affect the content of the agency's philosophy such as standards, regulations, staff philosophies, and community needs. According to Reif and Martin, "Medicare regulations substantially affect the philosophy of care and the manner in which services are provided. While consumers are informed of their rights and consulted during treatment planning and implementation, care recipients and their families are typically given less choice about the type and amount of services provided, and less control over the persons who deliver care in the home. In such situations, it is the agency, not the patient, that directs the care."[2(p 6)]

GOALS OF PSYCHIATRIC HOME CARE

As part of the treatment model, goals are identified that support the philosophy. These goals assist in providing direction and assessment for the services delivered by the home care agency and its staff. Several authors have identified goals. Pelletier identified these goals as follows:[3(p.24)]

- Develop collaborative relationships with all health care providers.
- Provide care by highly qualified staff members who are current with psychiatric nursing trends.
- Respect the integrity of the patient/family/SO relationships as well as the patient/health care professional relationships.
- Provide comprehensive care as an alternative to hospitalization by assisting the patient to remain in the community and use community resources.
- Ease the transition from the hospital to the home.
- Act as an educational resource for the patient/family/SOs on such issues as medication and diet regimens, self-care, interpersonal relationships, social skills, individual coping strategies, problem solving.
- Help decrease symptoms and increase feelings of self-esteem, self-confidence, and control.

McFarland and Thomas identified the following additional important goals:[4(p.897–898)]

- Promote the highest level of functioning and decrease recidivism.
- Promote early detection of exacerbation of symptoms.

- Provide care specific to the needs of the patient or family.
- Ensure the transfer of learned behaviors from the hospital to the home and community setting.
- Evaluate patient and family progress relative to the overall interdisciplinary plan.

Klebanoff has developed other goals:[5(p.759)]

- to gain, regain, maintain, or restore the patient's state of health and independence
- to minimize and rehabilitate the effects of illness and disability either before or after institutionalization
- to provide least-restrictive alternative to treatment

ORGANIZATION OF STAFF

In general, home health care services are provided by[6(p.758)]

- official or public agencies operated by state or local governments
- private and voluntary nonprofit agencies operated by boards of directors
- combinations of official and voluntary nonprofit agencies operated by both sources or a separate board
- hospital-based agencies administered by the hospital's board of directors.

These factors affect the organization of staff and services offered to the home care patients. The organization of staff includes staff qualifications, staff assignment, and models of practice.

Qualifications of Staff

Qualifications for the psychiatric home care nurse should include psychiatric experience or a psychiatric degree and knowledge about medical problems. The following skills are important:

- psychiatric and physical assessment, diagnosis, and treatment planning
- outcome identification and monitoring of progress
- patient education
- family dynamics and communication
- communication skills
- specific interventions for psychiatric problems
- knowledge about required diagnostic testing, obtaining laboratory specimens, and assessing laboratory results

- medications including types and their use, side effects and interventions, administration, dietary interactions, interactions with other medications, and compliance
- psychiatric rehabilitation and self-management
- safety in the home
- legal and patient rights issues
- documentation of psychiatric issues
- interviewing process
- activities of daily living
- utilization of intermittent care rather than continuous care provided in the hospital

In addition, many agencies require a bachelor's degree in nursing and certification from the American Nurses Association (ANA) in psychiatric-mental health nursing. The following characteristics are helpful for the nurse who cares for the psychiatric home care patient:[7(p.92)]

- self-starter
- good physical assessment skills
- superb clinical judgment
- the ability to communicate effectively with patients, family/SOs, other health team members, and others in the community
- efficient organizational skills
- well-honed time-management techniques
- the ability to prioritize one's work
- the ability to function independently, with minimal supervision
- a good and growing working knowledge of community, state, and national resources and referral sources

The various reimbursement sources, particularly the Health Care Financing Administration (HCFA), have identified the qualifications for the psychiatric nurse in the home setting. According to the *Medicare Home Health Manual*, "the evaluation and psychotherapy needed by a patient suffering from a diagnosed psychiatric disorder that necessitated active treatment in an institution requires the skills of a psychiatrically trained nurse and the costs of the psychiatric nurse's services may be covered as a skilled nursing care. Psychiatrically trained nurses are nurses who have special training and/or experience beyond the standard curriculum required for an R.N."[8(p.15)]

In addition, HCFA agrees to a psychiatrist prescribing services of a nonpsychiatric nurse to administer intramuscular injections or behavior-modifying medications.

For all home care nurses, clinical supervision is very important, particularly if the nurse has limited psychiatric experience. Medicare defines supervision as "authoritative procedural guidance by a qualified person for the accomplishment of a function or activity."[9(p.451)] This supervision, according to Medicare, must be on-site if the staff member does not meet Medicare qualifications and supervision is available during working hours.[10] Nursing supervision can be provided by a psychiatric nurse consultant. The nurse may contact this consultant on an as-needed basis; however, it is also important to have scheduled times for contact, preferably with individual supervision. This time is used to review each patient's status and care and, if required, develop new plans. This can also be time for staff development focused on the needs of an individual staff member. If there are a number of nurses seeing psychiatric patients, group supervision can also be conducted. This allows time for sharing and learning from one another. Due to the lack of time, each agency must determine the frequency of formal supervision times; however, informal or as-needed supervision must be provided and can be done by telephone. Team meetings about a patient also provide clinical supervision, as team members share their experiences and develop the treatment plan.

The patient needs to have a physician, and some patients require a psychiatrist. If the patient does not have a psychiatrist and requires one, the home care agency can supply a list of potential psychiatrists from which the patient may choose. The patient's medical physician may recommend a psychiatrist. The home care nurse should communicate frequently with all physicians who are working with the patient.

The home health aide needs to be oriented to the patient's needs and problems before visiting the patient. Consistent assignment is very important for the psychiatric home care patient. Changing staff will interfere with the development of a patient-staff relationship that can be an effective tool in caring for the patient. The home health aide should be a good role model for the patient. Supervision from a nurse who meets the qualifications for psychiatric home care is critical. At all times, the home health aide must feel comfortable asking for help. The home health aide must have successfully completed a state-established or other training program that meets the requirements and a competency evaluation program or state licensure program to receive Medicare reimbursement.[11]

The medical social worker is a person who has a master's degree from a school of social work accredited by the Council on Social Work Education and has one year of social work experience in a health care setting. The social worker's role may vary from one agency to another. Usually the services provided include assistance with housing, financial issues, employment, accessing community resources, and—if the patient requires other treatment—disposition.

Occupational, speech, and physical therapists are used when the patient can benefit from their services. These staff members should meet the professional requirements for their individual professions, including appropriate education, clinical training, licensure, and certification. Patients are referred for these services after an assessment by the nurse.

Assignment of Staff

To promote stability and predictability, consistency of assignment is important for the psychiatric patient. There are many methods that can be used to assign staff to a patient. A nurse may have overall responsibility, completing the assessment, establishing the treatment plan with the physician or psychiatrist, and teaching and supervising a home health aide who may have direct and frequent contact with the patient. Other staff, such as the medical social worker or occupational therapist, may join the team as required for the patient's needs. The nurse and home health aide will be the consistent staff.

MODELS OF PSYCHIATRIC HOME CARE

There are many models that the home health agency may use as psychiatric services are developed. Models can differ in treatment focus, base of operations, and time allotment.

A model with a crisis or outreach orientation focuses on the treatment.[12] This type of model has a very narrow and specific range of services. A multidisciplinary team that might include a nurse, psychiatrist, and social worker provides a one- to two-visit comprehensive evaluation of a homebound patient. This type of model often focuses on elderly patients. The goal is to link the patient with appropriate medical, mental health, and social services. Other uses of teams for home evaluations are for crisis calls about potential or real threats of physical harm to self or others. The goal is to defuse the situation and, when required, facilitate more intensive treatment such as hospitalization. This model does not encourage further contact with the patient after the prescribed evaluation and determination of specific interventions.

Another model uses the hospital as the base of operations, with home visits built into the hospital's after-care program.[13]

The time-allotment model focuses on time spent in the home.[14] The most common schedule is intermittent visits based on the patient's needs and, in some cases, reimbursement guidelines. More than intermittent care may be approved by the reimbursement source, such as Medicare, but usually this level of care triggers the source to question the appropriateness of home care for the patient.

A question that might come up as psychiatric services are developed is whether psychiatric nursing services should be provided in conjunction with medical nursing services or separately. The reality is that often the same nurse delivers both types of services. This may be confusing for a psychiatric patient who may be accustomed to psychiatric nurses who do not provide physical care; however, this is the most efficient method for providing nursing care. It also recognizes a holistic view of the patient—the psychological, sociological, and biological. This type of assignment also decreases the need for communication between two nurses and reduces the chance of errors and complications that might occur when psychiatric and medical care are separated.

ADMISSION CRITERIA

Criteria for admission to psychiatric home care are developed by the agency based on the services that can be offered, the community needs, payer requirements, and—in some cases—geographic areas. The purpose of admission criteria is to identify patients who are appropriate for the services offered and their reimbursement requirements. The patient needs to consent to treatment and agree to payment of treatment. Typical payer reimbursement requirements indicate that the patient meet the following criteria:

- Patient has a psychiatric diagnosis based on *Diagnostic and Statistical Manual of Mental Disorders (DSM-IV)*.[15]
- Patient is receiving active psychiatric treatment.
- Patient is under the care of a psychiatrist who establishes and reviews the treatment plan.
- Patient requires skilled nursing, physical therapy, speech therapy, or continuing occupational therapy.
- Patient requires part-time or intermittent care.
- Patient is psychiatrically homebound.

Homebound status reflects on the patient's ability to safely, independently, and consistently access mental health follow-up care. The patient does not have to be bedridden. The patient may even be able to visit the physician's office, but this must require great effort. The patient cannot go to work or school, drive, take long walks, attend day care for nonmedical reasons, or frequently leave home for nonmedical reasons. Documentation must explain why the patient is homebound and how the patient's symptoms keep him or her homebound. Examples might be patient refuses to leave home; patient is unsafe in a specific way when he or she leaves home without assistance; symptoms escalate when patient leaves the home; delusions keep the patient from functioning (e.g., patient cannot cross street or take bus because he states he is being watched); vegetative symptoms of depression prevent patient from dressing appropriately and having energy to leave the home; patient's judgment is impaired; patient is disoriented; or patient is a risk to self or others. It is particularly difficult to establishing homebound status when the patient is young with no medical problems that might keep the patient in the home. With such a patient, it is even more important to be specific about the homebound status. The patient's plan of care should specify criteria that will be used to determine when the patient demonstrates a consistent pattern of receiving mental health care outside the home.

TYPICAL PATIENTS

Generally, psychiatric patients fall into three groups. The first group includes patients who have a medical or surgical diagnosis and a secondary psychiatric diagnosis. The second group includes patients who have a primary psychiatric diagnosis that requires ongoing treatment and monitoring. Examples might be schizophrenia, major depression, bipolar disorder, severe anxiety disorder, Alzheimer's disease, agoraphobia, and paranoia. Many, but not all, of these patients have been hospitalized or at least have had some type of outpatient psychiatric treatment. Today, hospitalizations tend to be short and many patients have histories of several hospitalizations. There is a third group that is made up of patients with medical or surgical diagnoses who have emotional problems or reactions to their illnesses or stress but do not have an official psychiatric diagnosis.

Other characteristics that might identify patients who need psychiatric home care assistance include the following:

- lives alone
- family/SOs require support and respite to facilitate patient's treatment
- is noncompliant with treatment, particularly medication, and has poor follow-through with treatment appointments or partial hospitalization
- refuses to leave home to receive injectable neuroleptics
- requires facilitation of transfer to a temporary or permanent facility
- needs preadmission screening and triage to assess functioning in the home environment
- requires more structure but does not need partial hospitalization or hospitalization
- has frequent relapses of unknown cause after hospitalization
- has high rate of readmissions
- needs assistance with activities of daily living
- needs long-term planning for transition back into community
- needs ongoing monitoring for chronic suicidality

- experiences multiple situational stresses in addition to psychiatric illness (e.g., divorce, children leaving home, death of spouse, loss of a job)
- needs assistance coping with a disabling medical condition
- has substance abuse problem in addition to psychiatric problem

The home care agency may decide to exclude the patient with a history of violence. This must be thought through very carefully. Developing a policy and specific assessment parameters will assist staff in determining which patients to exclude. Some decisions will be wrong, as it is impossible to be correct on all assessment decisions. Prediction of violence is not easy to do under any circumstances. When incidents do occur, the assessment process should be reviewed so that staff may learn more about the decision-making process.

SERVICES AND ACTIVITIES

Each psychiatric home care agency develops its own list of specific services and nursing activities that it will provide to its patients. This list is important to the patients, families/SOs, referral sources, reimbursement sources, accrediting agencies, and the staff who provide the care. The list determines the types and qualifications of staff who will be required on a full-time or part-time basis. The term *skilled nursing* is found in some reimbursement requirements. Jackson and Neighbors explain that a service is considered *unskilled* "when the nature of a service is such that it can safely and adequately be self-administered or performed by the average non-medical person without the direct supervision of a licensed nurse or therapist."[16(p.40)]

The following are examples of services and nursing activities that may be provided by a home care agency:

- *Assessment and diagnosis.* Assessment and diagnosis must be done during admission and throughout the patient's treatment. It provides information to determine the appropriateness of the patient for home care services and the focus for the treatment plan.
- *Suicidal assessment/escalating behavior assessment.* This assessment must be done for all patients, and it is particularly important for those patients with a history of this behavior.
- *Mental status exam.* This exam is part of the admission assessment and ongoing assessment as needed.
- *Medication assessment.* For each psychiatric home care patient, it is critical to identify medications taken (including nonpsychiatric medications), their interactions, past history with medications, patient's and family/SO's knowledge of medications, and educational needs.

- *Home environment assessment.* Assessing the patient in the home allows for the evaluation of additional information that can only be obtained in the home and the patient's interactions with others in the home.
- *Treatment planning.* Treatment planning includes identification of medical and nursing diagnoses and problems, development of interventions, and outcome identification and monitoring.
- *Skilled nursing care.* Skilled nursing care includes nursing care for medical and psychiatric problems.
- *Medication administration and management.* Medication administration and management has many components including obtaining prescriptions, identifying schedules and any specific requirements for taking medications, developing reminder systems for the patient, assessing side effects and suggesting interventions to alleviate or decrease them, modifying patient teaching based on medication use and response, and assessing response to medications and documentation. In the case of injectable neuroleptics, the nurse administers the medication.
- *Management of specific behavior.* Management of specific behavior requires skilled nursing care that is either provided directly by a nurse or provided by another staff member under a nurse's supervision. The goal typically is to assist the patient in coping with a specific behavior.
- *Activities of daily living.* Activities of daily living (including personal hygiene, nutrition, sleep, exercise, and relaxation and leisure activities) must be maintained. If the patient is unable to meet activities of daily living needs, the patient must be assisted to meet these needs.
- *Follow-up care for outpatient electroconvulsive therapy (ECT).* Patients who received ECT in the hospital require assessment and support if they continue to have side effects at home such as memory loss. Education about the treatments and their effects may need to be repeated. Patients who are receiving outpatient ECT will require follow-up care, assessment of response, and further education.
- *Case management.* Because the psychiatric patient frequently has complex problems that require coordination with community mental health and other health care services, case management is a critical component of psychiatric home care.
- *Patient/family/SO education.* Patient education is part of skilled nursing care. Chapter 5 discusses patient and family/SO education. It is very important to provide education that is appropriate to the patient's needs to assist the patient to become more independent. With early discharges from the hospital, patient education in the hospital can only be done superficially. The outpatient psychiatrist usually provides little patient/family/SO education.

- *Psychiatric rehabilitation.* Psychiatric rehabilitation assists the patient in strengthening or developing skills needed for living, working, and socializing that will increase the patient's ability to cope with daily stresses.
- *Assisting with transition from hospital to home.* Patients who have short hospital stays will have little time to prepare for discharge; they may have just become comfortable in the hospital and may not feel much better. Support will be required when they return home. Patients who have had a longer stay in the hospital will require assistance adjusting to living in the community again. Families/SOs will need support and education about the transition process and postdischarge problems.
- *Assisting with transition to and/or compliance with outpatient treatment.* Many psychiatric patients have difficulty getting to outpatient treatment, and some refuse it. Helping the patient to develop coping skills and to take medication may assist the patient to participate in treatment.
- *Documentation.* Documentation of treatment is important to provide information about the patient's problems and treatment as well as for the purpose of receiving reimbursement for care provided.
- *Nursing home and residential living facilities consultation.* A home care agency may receive referrals from a nursing home or residential living facility for a psychiatric assessment of a patient and recommendations for interventions.
- *Individual and family therapy.* Intensive psychotherapy is not usually done in the home; however, supportive brief psychotherapy may be part of the patient's treatment. Usually the focus is on the here-and-now and psychoeducation.
- *Education and support for the caregiver.* Education and support for the caregiver is particularly important when the patient requires a considerable amount of care and supervision and the family/SO carries most of the burden of the care (such as with the patient who has Alzheimer's disease).
- *Occupational therapy.* This therapy can be helpful because it can focus on activities with which many patients with serious mental illness need help (such as self-care, home management, and vocational skills).
- *Vocational services.* Vocational services focus on the needs of the patient who may be returning to or beginning work; this work may be employment with pay or a volunteer, sheltered type of employment.
- *Social services.* Social services may be used to assist with community referrals and assistance (such as financial, food, housing, and transportation) directed at long-term care planning and discharge from home care.
- *Speech and physical therapies.* These interventions may be required for patients with psychiatric and medical problems.

- *Diagnostic testing.* Testing may be required for medical and psychiatric problems. The nurse provides patient education about the testing and results; prepares the patient; obtains the specimen; ensures that the specimen reaches the appropriate laboratory; receives the report; discusses results with the physician and, as appropriate, with the patient.
- *Pharmacy.* The home care agency will need resources to obtain medications that the nurse administers and may need to help patients find resources for their prescriptions.
- *Equipment and supplies.* These may be required for the psychiatric patient. The agency should have resources to obtain these supplies and charge them to the patient.
- *Intravenous and parenteral therapy.* These may be required for the psychiatric patient. The agency should have resources to obtain these supplies and charge them to the patient.
- *Homemaker/home health assistant/companion services.* These staff provide personal assistance services (e.g., bathing, ambulation, dressing, eating) or assistance with instrumental services (e.g., cooking, cleaning, laundry, shopping, and transportation). About 80 percent of the formal home care provided in the United States is provided by paraprofessionals. This is the area of health care that has the greatest need for improvement.[17]
- *Transportation services.* The home care agency should develop a list of transportation resources for the patient who needs assistance with getting to medical appointments.
- *Respite care.* Families/SOs may need time away from the patient. Twenty-four-hour responsibility may lead to excessive stress that can cause burnout, patient abuse, and even medical and emotional problems for the family/SOs. The patient will also benefit from time away from the caregivers to develop more independent skills.
- *Preadmission screening and triage.* Preadmission screening and triage are additional services that may be offered. They are helpful in determining the best intervention for a patient, because they allow clinicians to evaluate the patient in the home environment.
- *Crisis intervention.* Home health agency staff may be called to the patient's home during times of crisis to determine the best intervention for the patient and the family/SO. Some agencies provide 24-hour coverage, while others tell patients to use appropriate emergency health care facilities in the community during the agency's nonoperating hours. Patients should be given written information about these resources.
- *Patient advocacy.* Consumers, the patients, and providers have had considerable differences in perspectives and priorities of treatment. The nurse plays a

critical role in making home care more consumer-responsive by acting as the patient's advocate.

- *Family/SO support.* This is a critical service that is ongoing during the patient's care. The range of interventions vary greatly, from specific interventions to less intensive support.

Care in the home is part-time or intermittent. The focus is short-term. The frequency of visits varies from agency to agency and also depends on the patient's needs and reimbursement guidelines. Typically, nursing visits are made two to three times per week, and a visit lasts from 45 to 60 minutes. Assessment usually requires the most time, and other visits may extend to 90 minutes if there is a crisis that requires more complex interventions. Home health aide visits may also occur two to three times a week, with a visit lasting one to two hours.

STANDARDS[18]

Many questions arise about standards and, as a consequence, there is confusion. What do the standards mean? Where do they come from? Why should they be followed? Professional ethics, values, and legal issues are important in the understanding of standards, their development, and their implementation.

Critical Definitions

The confusion about standards often centers around definitions that are found in nursing and other health care literature. The definitions adopted by the American Nurses Association (ANA) are as follows:[19(pp.1–3)]

- *Standard*—A standard is an authoritative statement by which the nursing profession describes the responsibilities for which its practitioners are held accountable. A standard reflects the values and priorities of the profession.
- *Standards of clinical nursing practice*—These are statements that delineate the professional responsibilities of all registered nurses engaged in clinical practice regardless of setting. They include both the standards of care and standards of professional performance. Nurses who are practicing in a specialty area are still accountable for meeting the standards of clinical nursing practice as well as the appropriate specialty standards.
- *Standards of care*—These standards describe a competent level of care as demonstrated by a process of accurate assessment, diagnosis, outcome identification, planning, implementation, and evaluation. These standards delineate care that is provided to all patients.

- *Standards of professional performance*—These standards describe a competent level of behavior in the professional role including activities related to quality of care, performance appraisal, education, collegiality, ethics, collaboration, research, and resource utilization appropriate to education, position, and practice setting.

Three types of standards are generally used: structure, process, and outcome standards. *Structure standards* focus on determining what needs to be done in order to provide care. They include standards related to number and qualifications of staff, resources, equipment and supplies, and productivity. An example of a structure standard is one that states that there is an appropriate number of qualified staff to meet the needs of the census and the patient's acuity level. *Process standards* describe how the care is provided or the nursing actions used in providing the care. They include standards related to all aspects of the nursing process. An example of a process standard is one that states when a suicidal patient should be discharged from home care to more intensive treatment. *Outcome standards* identify the desired outcome of the nursing care. This has always been the most difficult type of standard to describe and to evaluate for psychiatric nursing care. An example of an outcome standard is one that states the patient will assess his or her anxiety level and institute specific anxiety-relief interventions.

Purpose of Standards

With so many standards to consider on a daily basis, home care staff might realistically ask why standards exist. The major purpose of professional standards is self-regulation of the profession. Standards are developed to identify the baseline of nursing practice. They help nurses to clarify their values, and the standards become agreed-upon levels of excellence or norms. When this level of excellence is not met, the standards identify areas for improvement of care and practice. Standards benefit nurses, patients, and families/SOs by[20(p.vii)]

- assisting nurses in evaluating and improving their own practice
- providing satisfaction to nurses when they provide excellent nursing care
- providing objective criteria for the assessment of nurses' performance
- determining the staffing needs to meet the needs of home care patients
- identifying the need for and content of orientation and staff development programs
- delineating the content of curricula and the criteria for evaluation of students
- improving health care delivery
- identifying the focus of research

Sources of Standards

Standards originate from many sources, and this is probably why there is some confusion about what they are and which ones are relevant. Some standards are internal and specific to the home care agency and its nursing practice, and some are external or generic standards that affect the home care agency and the care provided but are developed by sources outside the agency.

Internal Standards

Internal standards are developed by the home care agency and are related to issues that are important to the services provided to the agency's patients and families/SOs. These standards are found in position descriptions, standards of care, policies, procedures, and various guidelines. The performance-appraisal process also is dependent on standards. Position descriptions describe the standards for each job category or position. Goals identified by individual staff members during performance appraisal as important to their own individual performance are also standards.

Nursing staff are involved in the development of all of these standards, but these standards should not conflict with any external standards. Resources for content may come from other standards, or their content may come from nursing research results, clinical experience, nursing and health care literature, and accrediting and regulatory agency requirements and reviews. As the home care agency begins to develop its own nursing practice standards, it must follow certain guidelines.

- Standards should be consistent with national norms established for nursing practice (e.g., *A Statement on Psychiatric-Mental Health Clinical Nursing Practice and Standards of Psychiatric-Mental Health Clinical Nursing Practice*[21] and *Standards of Home Health Nursing Practice*[22]).
- Standards should complement expectations of regulatory and accrediting agencies, such as the Joint Commission on Accreditation of Healthcare Organizations.
- Standards must be consistent with legal guidelines for practice (e.g., nurse practice acts).
- Standards must reflect the philosophy of the home care agency.
- Standards must be achievable.
- Standards must be measurable through well-defined criteria.
- Standards must be understood and valued for effective integration into daily nursing care.

As internal standards are developed and periodically evaluated, these seven guidelines are used to measure the quality of the standards.

External Standards

All nursing staff must be aware of and apply appropriate external standards from the ANA (the nursing professional organization), psychiatric nursing specialty groups, and home care nursing groups. Professional nursing standards that are relevant to psychiatric home care are found in *A Statement on Psychiatric-Mental Health Clinical Nursing Practice and Standards of Psychiatric-Mental Health Clinical Nursing Practice*, found in Appendix B and *Standards of Home Health Nursing Practice*, found in Appendix C. These professional standards provide a place for the home health agency to begin as staff develop specific standards.

Standards are also promulgated by local, state, and federal laws. It is important to be aware of changes in these laws that might affect psychiatric home care. Regulatory agencies, both state and federal, identify standards that must be followed by home care agencies. These are often used to control health care costs. With so many different standards that are never static, staff must continually update information about these requirements.

The consumer is also a source of standards. Patients and their families/SOs have become more involved in identifying their own expectations of care. Seeking this information from consumers is critical; however, it is a relatively new idea for health care and particularly for psychiatric care. Health care providers have much to learn about how to identify these expectations, how to assess their relevance, and how to use them in the practice setting. Another new source of standards is third-party payers; they are especially important in managed care, which has created its own expectations of patient care. This particular source of standards has caused many conflicts in health care.

Legal Implications of Standards

Standards of care or guidelines that identify recommendations for patient management have mushroomed. These standards may play an important role in malpractice cases. In nursing malpractice cases, the actions of the nurse defendant are measured against the appropriate nursing standard of care. Clearly, not having standards or policies is dangerous, but having them and not following them can lead to major problems and increase liability. As the legal implications of standards in medicine increase, there will be increased focus on the legal implications of nursing standards. In a court case, "the weight given to the guideline in establishing the standard of care will be influenced by a number of factors, including whether or not the guideline reflects officially sanctioned practice by the profession; the specificity of the guideline to the case in question; the validity of the scientific evidence for the recommendations outlined in the guideline; the methods used in developing, disseminating, and evaluating the guideline, and most important, the purpose of the guideline."[23(p.309)]

These factors may also be used to help the home care nurse administrator evaluate the available standards to determine which standards to adapt and to guide the agency in the development of standards, policies, and procedures. Nursing staff often do not recognize the importance of standards and view them as more written information to be filed away in a manual. It is the responsibility of the home care nurse administrator and supervisors to emphasize the legal implications of standards in daily practice. It is not helpful to have nurses practice in fear of malpractice, but it is important for them to understand that standards represent minimum expectations that should be met and should not be taken lightly. Developing and reviewing agency standards, policies, and procedures cannot be done in isolation. External relevant standards should be reviewed and incorporated, as appropriate to the home care agency, patient, the treatment model, and services. Home care nurses practice in highly independent roles with minimal direct supervision, and they also provide supervision to many paraprofessionals. Most of the supervision is not provided as care is given. As the use of home care increases, malpractice issues will become more important.

Implementation of Standards

Active nursing staff participation helps the staff feel that the standards are theirs, and this will increase standard compliance. Standards describe what the patient can expect from nursing care provided by the home care nurse and other agency staff and, thus, it is important for home care staff to implement these expectations in their daily practice. Bleich and Bratton identify three strategies that can be used to make standard implementation real to nursing staff.[24] The first strategy is to help staff recognize that they have personal standards that they use in their practice and to compare these with the agency's standards. The following are some examples of psychiatric home care nursing standards:

- A suicidal patient develops a no-harm contract with the nurse that is reviewed at each visit.
- The patient identifies his medications including name of medication, purpose, dosage and frequency, side effects and appropriate interventions, and critical responses that require medical consultation.
- The patient participates in planning his or her care.
- The patient is informed of the visit schedule and the procedure for canceling appointments.
- The patient on medications has vital signs assessed at each visit.

A second strategy to encourage implementation of standards emphasizes the importance of using specific clinical standards in the competency-based evaluation for each staff member. This strategy is used to assess competency in assessment, priority setting, intervention, and evaluation. Using standards in evaluation communicates to staff the importance of implementing standards.

A third strategy recognizes the importance of monitoring and evaluating standards routinely as part of the quality assessment and improvement process. To encourage implementation, agency supervisory staff should take every opportunity to demonstrate that standards are not just written for accreditation or other requirements but are written to be applied. When staff development is planned, consideration is given to discussing any relevant standards. When care is discussed in staff meetings, standards are identified. Medical record reviews also include an assessment of the use of standards. Staff discussions about potential changes in the agency include relevant standards. The supervisory staff should establish the environment that supports and emphasizes the importance of implementing standards in daily practice.

LEGAL AND ETHICAL ISSUES[25]

Discussing legal issues and nursing care often increases staff anxiety; however, it is important that all nurses discuss and understand basic legal and ethical principles and their impact upon administrative and clinical decisions. This will reduce liability exposure for the home care agency and the staff. Legal issues frequently change, because they are dependent upon court decisions and changes in local, state, and federal laws. The home care nurse must be well informed about these changes and their implications for clinical practice.

Basic Legal Issues and Psychiatric Nursing

Legal terminology may be confusing to those in health care. There is much to understand; however, some terminology and concepts are particularly relevant to nursing management and psychiatric nursing practice. These are *confidentiality and privilege, release of information, access to records, duty to warn third parties, right to refuse treatment, informed consent, confidentiality and disclosure of human immunodeficiency virus (HIV) status*, and *disability*.

Confidentiality and Privilege

Confidentiality and privilege are not the same. Nurses often have heard more about confidentiality; however, understanding both of these terms and their implications will assist in protecting patients' rights. According to Laben and McLean, "Confidentiality is the legal and ethical responsibility to keep all information concerning patients private.[26(p.7)] Staff may not reveal that an adult patient is receiving care to anyone without the patient's permission. In the case of a minor, the minor's parent or guardian must give this permission. The exception is the duty to warn third parties. Confidentiality affects all aspects of sharing information such as telephone conversations, casual or personal discussions, or information provided to the family/SO. The latter is particularly problematic, and it has been recently discussed in two editorials in *Archives of Psychiatric Nursing*.[27,28] Most psychiatric nurses have confronted this dilemma, and many have crossed the line and shared confidential information without the patient's consent. How often does a nurse obtain an adult patient's permission prior to talking with the patient's family/SO? How does a nurse encourage family/SO participation in the home without sharing information? How does a nurse plan for discharge from home care without the family/SO? In many cases, the patient provides consent; however, with some patients (such as the seriously ill, long-term patient), the nurse may not have this consent. There are times when confidentiality works against the patient and the care required. As Krauss has stated: "Don't misunderstand me. I am not opposed to confidentiality. And, I don't think that everyone who claims to have the patient's best interest in mind should necessarily be given immediate access. But, it seems to me that we need to take another look at confidentiality and ask whether it is still working toward the purposes for which it was originally intended."[29(p.256)] The definition of this term or its legal definition cannot be changed by staff; however, these issues will come up in practice and should be discussed. All efforts to obtain the patient's consent to share information with the family/SO should be made during the initial visit with an explanation of its importance given to the patient. Home care will not be successful if there is not open communication. If staff consider that it is important for the patient to participate in treatment planning and its implementation, then the staff must work to increase the patient's awareness of the importance of family/SO participation when appropriate. Staff should take care to share only the information that is absolutely required. Staff will need frequent guidance about confidentiality from the home care nurse administrator.

Privileged Communication

Privileged communication refers to communication between the physician and the patient, and it "is a legal statute that protects patients from having their confidential communications disclosed in court without their permission."[30(p.22)] This does not apply to medical records as they can be disclosed in court. There are times when professionals for whom privileged communication applies may be subpoenaed for court proceedings. Most states have not granted privileged communication by law to nurses, and thus it is important to recognize that psychiatric home care nurses can be asked to reveal information about patients in a court of law. Each nurse should know the state laws related to this issue. This is particularly important for nurses who may establish clear psychotherapeutic relationships with patients. These nurses should clearly discuss the lack of privileged communication with their patients, because patients may assume that since privileged communication applies to the psychiatrist it applies to the nurse psychotherapist or psychiatric home care nurse. Exceptions to privileged communication are information related to child abuse, which must be reported; information related to the patient's competency to stand trial as the nurse acts as a "friend of the court"; and the duty to warn.[31] Even in states that include nurses in privileged communication, the law applies only to situations in which the nurse is performing nursing functions and not some other function such as clerical duties.

Release of Information

Release of information is directly related to confidentiality and privileged communication. Patients receiving psychiatric home care reveal highly personal information and feelings. Even though continuity of care is important, this information cannot legally be shared without the patient's consent and proper authorization. Information is never released by telephone. The home care agency's release form with the patient's signature is used for release of information to other health care providers, hospitals, agencies, etc. This form specifies to whom the information is to be released, the specific information to be released, and for what time period. Release of information that has not been authorized by the patient or by statutory, regulatory, or other legal authority may lead to civil or criminal liability. Cazalas defines liability as "an obligation one has incurred or might incur through any act or failure to act."[32(p.258)] Most states via their confidentiality statutes authorize the release of information by court order, even if the patient objects.[33]

Regardless of confidentiality and privileged communication, states have statutes that identify reporting requirements. These obligate the home care agency and its staff to report specific types of information to a designated state agency. Common examples include the following:

- child abuse
- adult abuse
- substance abuse
- specific communicable diseases
- injuries that appear to have been caused by a dangerous weapon
- deaths of uncertain nature
- animal bites

Home care nursing staff need to know the specific state requirements so that they do not release information that might lead to problems with confidentiality and privileged communication statutes but yet they report information that is required by law. Adult abuse may be confusing to staff. Calfee has identified three categories of adult abuse: an adult who is not taking care of himself or herself, suspicions of adult physical abuse, and manipulation of an adult financially (e.g., forcing the patient to sign over property or Social Security checks to family/SOs).[34]

Access to Records

The first question that often comes up regarding release of information is who owns the medical record? Medical records are owned by the home care agency, but the patient has a right to the information. States usually include rules related to this ownership in their licensing regulations. There has been a tendency to grant patients greater accessibility to their medical records. Patients or their representatives may review the record. Third-party payers are the most frequent requesters for access, because this information is used to determine reimbursement. Medical records are also reviewed for QA purposes, but staff must take every possible measure to ensure individual patient confidentiality.

Duty To Warn Third Parties

The duty to warn third parties was established in *Tarasoff v. Regents of University of California* (1976) and has since been expanded.[35] It includes the duty to warn endangered third parties if a patient intends to harm them, duty to warn about possible property damage, failure to commit a patient who later harmed an unknown third party, and notification of law enforcement agencies when a patient with known violent propensities is released from treatment. Home care nurses should know the state statutes related to the duty to warn.

Right To Refuse Treatment

The right to refuse treatment is closely related to informed consent. Most states allow emergency use of forced medications, seclusion, and restraints only until the emergency situation is resolved. According to Trudeau, "Mental illness is not equivalent to incompetence, which renders one incapable of giving informed consent to treatment."[36(p.10)] All patients, regardless of their clinical status, should be given as much control over their treatment as possible. Informed consent policies vary, based on statute, litigation, administrative rule, and agency policies; however, it is important to consider if an individual patient has the capacity to make reasoned decisions regarding treatment.

Informed Consent

Informed consent is not a piece of paper, which is the common view of it. Rather it is the educational process and communication interchange between the patient and the physician that provides information to a competent adult enabling him or her to make decisions about his or her body.[37] Home care agency policy should describe what is required for informed consent; the usual components are a description of the procedure, benefits and risks, possible complications, and alternatives. For specific procedures, it is very helpful to have a form that is located in a specific place in the medical record. Even though it is the physician's responsibility to talk with the patient and obtain consent, the home care agency is responsible for monitoring this process. According to Fiesta, "A nurse who becomes involved in the process of documenting informed consent through obtaining the patient's signature on the form may become part of an informed consent litigation."[38(p.17)]

Psychiatric care has been and continues to be an area of health care in which there is conflict about the patient's competence to make decisions about his or her care or forced treatment. Patient participation and patient control over treatment does affect compliance and outcome. Nurses must understand applicable state statutes and act as the patient's advocate within state statutes. As a patient's competence to provide informed consent is considered, staff can ask if the patient possesses the capacity to make such a decision. Lack of capacity is the inability, due to mental impairment, to make reasoned decisions regarding the procedure or medication by evaluating the information about the likelihood of therapeutic benefit, the risk of side effects, and the availability of alternative treatments.[39] Information about the procedure or medication is given to the patient in language that can be understood by the patient and, if required, repeated. Initially, the physician discusses the information with the patient; nursing staff may be involved in the initial discussion, or later the patient may ask them questions or for more information. To assess the level of the patient's competence, the patient may be asked to paraphrase the information or questioned specifically about the information.

Because the patient's condition is constantly changing, competency assessment is ongoing. Whenever a nursing staff member hears something from the patient that indicates the patient might not adequately understand, this information must be shared with the physician. Patient participation is directly tied to informed consent. In addition, documentation is critical for legal reasons and to prevent staff communication problems.

Confidentiality and Disclosure of Human Immunodeficiency Virus Status

Human immunodeficiency virus (HIV) status is a growing concern for psychiatric patients. It is a complex medical, ethical, and legal issue. The American

Psychiatric Association (APA) published *Guidelines for Care of HIV-Infected Inpatients* in 1993.[40] The guidelines indicate that HIV-infected patients are entitled to the same standard of care as all other patients. Hospitals need to develop strategies to safeguard patients while they are in the hospital and to help patients protect themselves after discharge. Questions about confidentiality about HIV testing and acquired immune deficiency syndrome (AIDS), of course, have come up on many inpatient units. Disclosure must be limited to staff directly involved in the patient's care. The only way the patient community should know about an HIV-infected patient is if that patient shares the information. If the patient's behavior puts others at risk, the treatment team must develop interventions to help the patient control that behavior; however, disclosure is not the only intervention. According to the APA guidelines: "Psychiatrists have an ethical obligation to preserve the confidences of their patients, but that confidentiality may be breached in cases in which there is danger to self or others."[41(p.296)] Nurses should not reveal the HIV status of any patient, except to those who are caring for the patient. All states require that AIDS cases are reported but not all require the patient's name. The nurse in home care must follow the agency's policy as well as the state statutes related to confidentiality and HIV. The home care nurse may care for a patient who has had a negative experience in the hospital related to confidentiality. It is important to understand how the hospital should handle this problem in order to help the patient in the home.

Disability

The Americans with Disabilities Act of 1990 (ADA), effective July 26, 1992, has direct implications for the rights of persons with mental illness.[42] According to Ravid and Menon, "Disability is defined as a physical or mental impairment that substantially limits one or more major life activities, a record of such impairment, or being regarded as having such impairment."[43(p.280)] Exclusions in this definition are sexual behavior disorders, compulsive gambling, kleptomania, or psychoactive substance abuse disorders resulting from current illicit drug use. There are several important points in ADA that nursing staff should be aware of that affect patients and their employment. The ADA offers protection once employed. It is not affirmative action. Suggested specific guidelines related to ADA follow:[44]

- Employers may not ask questions about medical conditions or disabilities on job applications and tests. They may ask, "Can you perform the essential job function(s)?" not "How will you perform the essential job functions?"
- Medical exams may be required for employment; however, all potential applicants must meet the same requirements.

- A person should not reveal a disability during the preemployment period; however, after employment it is to the person's advantage to admit that he or she has a disability. No more details are required. This will help to ensure that the person will not lose the job at a later date due to the disability.
- The employer is required to make reasonable accommodations to the disability if necessary.
- Drug testing requirements must not conflict with ADA. This testing must only test for illegal drugs, not drugs taken under medical supervision.
- Patients must be informed about possible side effects from psychotropic drugs that might impair cognitive and motor functioning, and this should be documented. These drugs can also be detected in drug screens and may cause a false-positive result.
- The disabled person has the right to attend any local and state program or service, and this should be encouraged. For example, the person may receive rehabilitation in all public rehabilitation programs, not just those that focus on patients with mental illness.
- Another part of ADA focuses on public accommodations or access to services in a format usable by the person. This applies to such public places as transportation, health care institutions, theaters, and restaurants.

Staff Assignments

When assigning staff to patients, the home care nurse administrator and supervisors must consider not only clinical and administrative issues but also the legal implications. Some examples of staff assignment liability exposure are

- incompetent staff assigned to perform a task or job
- agency lack of knowledge about staff competency and qualifications
- inadequate supervision
- failure to meet state or federal requirements
- unjustified refusal of an assignment or inadequate referral of the patient, which is seen as patient abandonment

When there are assignment problems, they often affect staff morale. Anything that affects staff morale affects patient care and consequently increases liability exposure for the staff and the home care agency. The agency's policies and procedures should include information related to staffing levels, staffing assignments, refusal of assignments, staff training and competency, coverage during emergencies such as inclement weather, supervision of staff, and specific position descriptions. During orientation, and as needed, these policies and procedures should be reviewed and discussed. Staff need time to discuss their concerns regarding assignments, relevant information about the legal implications, and time to honestly discuss their ethical concerns.

Least-Restrictive Alternative

The patient should receive the least-restrictive treatment or care in the least-restrictive setting. This has great implications for psychiatric care in all settings. If a patient could benefit more from partial hospitalization, outpatient treatment, or home care and there is no reason for hospitalization, the patient should not be admitted to the hospital to receive treatment. Selection of the least-restrictive alternative should be considered every time a decision is made in the hospital to use seclusion or restraints. The home care nurse needs to understand least-restrictive alternative, as there may be times when patients need more intensive care. The home care nurse is the first health care provider to assess the patient in crisis to determine needs for treatment. The nurse may encounter many patients who want to discuss their feelings and experiences from their hospitalizations. Often these relate to restrictions placed upon them in the hospital. If the home care nurse has never worked in an inpatient psychiatric setting, it may be difficult for the nurse to understand the experience.

Types of Admissions

An admission for psychiatric treatment is far more complex than one for medical reasons, and the admission affects the patient's freedom of choice and rights. Home care nurses must understand the basic information about hospital admission in order to help the patient and family/SOs. Admission to a hospital for psychiatric treatment is more traumatic for patients than admission for medical problems. Patients and their families/SOs may require information about the meaning of the different types of admissions. Of course, at any time, the patient is free to consult an attorney. There are three types of admission: informal admission, voluntary admission, and involuntary admission. The elements of how the admission is initiated, the status of the patient's civil rights, justification, and the related type of discharge are described.[45]

1. *Informal admission* requires no formal application and occurs when a patient is admitted to an acute care hospital. The patient retains all civil rights and voluntarily seeks help. Discharge may be initiated by the patient, who may be asked to sign an "against medical advice" form but is not required to do so.

2. *Voluntary admission* requires a formal application from the patient and occurs when the patient is admitted to a public or private psychiatric hospital. The patient retains all civil rights and voluntarily seeks help. Discharge may be initiated by the patient; however, most states require that this is done in writing. In some states the patient may be released immediately, and in others the patient is required to wait anywhere from 48 hours to 15 days, depending upon state statute.

3. *Involuntary admission* is not applied for by the patient. The justification for the admission is made by others and varies according to state statute. Common justifications are that the patient is dangerous to self or others, or the patient needs treatment. The patient retains from none to all of his or her civil rights. This varies from state to state, depending on specific state statutes. Clearly, this type of admission causes the most problems for staff, ethically and legally. It also adds another burden for the staff, because the commitment process requires staff time and energy and creates increased stress for the patient and family/SOs. There are three types of involuntary admissions: emergency, short term, and long term.[46] The emergency involuntary admission is used to continue treatment for a patient who is a threat to self or others, and it usually lasts from 3 to 30 days. Short term involuntary admission is primarily used for diagnosis and short-term care; it lasts from two to six months. Long term involuntary admission is used for treatment that will continue until the patient is ready for discharge. State statutes determine who can make the decision, the process, and how long the patient may be hospitalized. Holding patients without following the state statutes opens the hospital to liability.

The commitment process varies from state to state, and home care nurses should know about their state's requirements and the commitment process if they care for psychiatric patients in the home. There are some key terms that are similar in all states.[47]

- *Medical certification*—A specified number of appointed physicians, not just psychiatrists, may make the commitment decision.
- *Court or judicial commitment*—The commitment decision is made by a judge or jury in a formal hearing. In most states, the patient may have legal counsel present for the commitment hearing. The state may or may not appoint one.
- *Administrative commitment*—The commitment decision is made by a special group of hearing officers. Administrative commitment is subject to judicial review in order to give patients due process, or their rights under the Fourteenth Amendment.

Discharge from the Hospital

There may not be a law that states that after-care must be provided, but there are many standards stating that this must be done. Some of them are the Joint Commission on Accreditation of Healthcare Organizations standards and the ANA standards. As patients are discharged earlier and earlier from the hospital, after-care is increasingly more important. Many patient outcomes are not fully realized in the hospital, and the patient requires additional support and treatment after discharge. Nursing staff must play an active role in developing and implementing plans for after-care; as a consequence, home care nurses should have contact with hospital nurses. In addition, they need to understand the type of discharge from the hospital that the home care patient has had when admitted to home care.

When a patient has voluntarily admitted himself or herself, discharge may occur when staff and the patient believe that maximum benefit from treatment has been reached. This is a regular discharge. However, if a patient requests a discharge and staff believe the patient is not ready for discharge and might be a danger to self or others, the against medical advice process may begin. This process is described in state statutes. Most states require that the patient make the request in writing, and most hospitals have a specific form for this purpose. The written request becomes part of the medical record. The patient may be discharged against medical advice from 24 to 72 hours after the request, depending on the specific state requirements. A committed patient may not leave the hospital when he or she wishes.

A voluntary patient who elopes (absent without leave, or AWOL) from the hospital may be discharged without forcing the patient to return. The hospital should have a policy and procedure to follow for these situations. It is usual to try to talk with the patient about returning to the hospital prior to initiating the discharge. If it is appropriate, the hospital provides information about after-care. Documentation of these recommendations is critical. If the physician believes the patient should be in the hospital, then commitment proceedings would be initiated. A patient who goes AWOL and then agrees to home care needs to discuss the decision to go AWOL from the hospital and his or her commitment to treatment in home care. It is important to assess whether the patient will comply with home care treatment.

Risk Management

The goal of risk management is to identify, reduce, or avoid those situations in which the home care agency may incur financial loss. Whenever there is potential malpractice or an actual malpractice suit, the agency loses money. Such a suit can be extremely costly and highly stressful for all involved. The home care agency should have a plan for coping with these situations. Incident reports, their track-ing, and analysis are the major forms of data collection. The goal is to prevent high-risk situations from developing. Nurses play an important role in this pro-cess by

- following agency standards, policies, and procedures
- using sound clinical judgment
- communicating
- documenting
- following the policies and procedures related to incident reports
- reporting any statements by patients and families/SOs about "suing" or mal-practice

What can the home care nurse do about "potentially contributing" patient acts? These are patient acts that might contribute to a failure to respond to treatment or an injury. In a sense, this is practicing defensive documentation or being alert to those situations that might lead to problems. Iyer and Camp identify several of these "red flags."[48] Staff can be taught about them, and the following suggested documentation guidelines can be used:

- Describe a patient's refusal or inability to provide accurate or complete in-formation regarding health status, history, and current medications and treat-ments. Whenever possible, it is important to distinguish between refusal and inability to provide information. Patients are told about the importance of sharing information and the effect it has on their treatment. It is not uncom-mon during a psychiatric nursing assessment for a patient to refuse to re-spond to questions, such as those related to substance abuse, suicidality, or violent behavior. This should be noted in the assessment, as it may prove significant if the patient is harmed later, and the information might have prevented the problem.
- Report noncompliance with medical and nursing interventions. State stat-utes provide patients with the right to refuse treatment under most circum-stances. Refusal of treatment should be documented. Any patient behavior that indicates the patient is not compliant with treatment should also be docu-mented, not judgmentally but factually. Actions taken by staff to assist the patient with noncompliance are also clearly described, as well as patient re-sponse to these actions.
- Document tampering with medical equipment. This is not a significant prob-lem in psychiatric home care, because little equipment is used; however, patients with additional medical problems may require equipment. Patient tampering should be documented, as well as instructions given to the patient about tampering and use of the equipment.

- When investigational drugs are used, ethical issues should be considered and investigational trials should be clearly described to the patient.
- Patient advocacy is important.
- Patient/family/SO education about illness, treatment, and health are continually assessed and plans developed and implemented for these needs.
- Serious mental illness has a biological component, and this information should be incorporated into the treatment plan and patient education.
- The program should identify useful and accessible community resources for the patient/family/SOs.
- Maintenance of normal role functioning should be promoted from the time of admission, with an emphasis on the patient's power and responsibilities.
- Crisis resolution is preferred over crisis intervention.
- The nurse should take the approach of "being with" and "doing with" the patient while expecting the patient to learn how to help himself or herself.[49]
- Recognize that symptoms are expressions of unmet needs.
- The focus is on what the patient wants rather than what the staff want for the patient.
- Remoralization and psychiatric rehabilitation are important parts of each patient's care.
- Outcome-based treatment should be supported.

These guidelines should be applied to all patients and should be periodically monitored through the home care agency QA process.

POLICIES AND PROCEDURES[50]

Pressures for improved quality of care, governmental regulations, and malpractice litigation increase the need to develop and implement policies and procedures. Because policies and procedures reduce decision-making time and increase staff productivity, they can help to increase efficiency. Furthermore, when procedures are written in a specific, logical, and sequential manner, the activity can be completed more quickly and effectively. This is particularly helpful in psychiatric settings such as home care, in which nonprofessional staff may be providing much of the direct care. In these cases, it is necessary to provide staff with guidance that will ensure that quality patient care is delivered in a safe manner. Content will be determined by professional standards, accrediting agencies, medical and nursing research and literature, reimbursement sources, state and federal regulations, legal issues, the community, the patient population, and the agency's treatment model and philosophy.

Policy and procedure development is a complex process that ultimately affects management and all nursing care provided. The entire process takes place in the context of the critical concerns and influences that have been described. All nursing staff should be involved in the process, and the process should flow from the home care nurse administrator through all nursing management staff and to all levels of nursing staff. Most policy and procedure development is done by a committee or several committees with additional staff input as necessary.

Objectives for policy and procedure development are identified prior to the development of policies and procedures. A committee needs to know its tasks. The following are examples of objectives:

- to promote quality care
- to implement the home care agency's mission, goals, objectives, and treatment model
- to incorporate health care changes into the home care agency
- to develop consistent decision making and action
- to maintain cost containment through efficient use of staff, time, and supplies
- to meet accrediting agencies' requirements
- to maintain professional nursing standards
- to increase the quality of organizational communication
- to promote a risk management program by preventing negligence and maintaining safety of patients, staff, and family/SOs
- to delineate lines of authority
- to increase interdisciplinary collaboration
- to assist in developing sound clinical and managerial judgment
- to identify expectations for the staff and promote job security
- to promote the resolution of problems closer to the job situation
- to act as a focus for discussion when differences occur and thus decrease the opportunity to personalize conflicts
- to decrease staff turnover due to poor communication and inadequate identification of expectations
- to assist with orientation of new, transferred, promoted, or temporary staff as well as nursing faculty and students
- to assist with staff development of all staff

Many definitions for the terms *policy* and *procedure* are found in the literature. These terms are different, but they are interrelated. A *policy* is a statement that communicates the expectations and philosophy of the home care agency. It provides a guideline for decision making. When staff require no further specific guidance, a policy may exist without a related procedure. Policies should not conflict with the home care agency's goals and objectives. Policies are usually not revised as frequently as procedures, but they require a minimum of an annual review. The agency's policy manual should provide a total picture of the agency's nursing and treatment beliefs. Identifying and describing a policy does not relieve the professional nurse from accountability for decision making, but it does provide some guidance in critical decision-making areas.

A *procedure* is a definite statement of the step-by-step actions required to obtain a specific outcome. It provides a recipe for reaching a specific goal, and that goal is usually a completed treatment or intervention that is safe; is efficient in the use of staff, time, supplies, and equipment; and meets the expected outcome. A procedure is more detailed than a policy. A minimum of an annual review of all procedures is required. Written procedures support quality care and assist in preventing errors.

Both policies and procedures help to maintain consistency and continuity; however, to do so, they need to be written in concise, easily understood language, and contain appropriate and up-to-date information. If policies and procedures are merely words on paper that are developed to meet external requirements, they will not be used by the staff. The effort, staff time, and financial resources used to develop them will be wasted. Asking nursing staff periodically to evaluate the policies and procedures will help to determine how realistic the policies and procedures are for the staff who use them daily.

The format for policies and procedures will vary from agency to agency; however, the format should be consistent within an agency. Certain elements are always included: the title of the policy or procedure, its purpose, effective date, review date, and administrator approval with signature. A consistent format helps staff use the policies and procedures effectively, with minimum time required for reviewing the organization of the content.

Before developing the content for a specific policy or procedure, the purpose of the policy or procedure is identified. What is the decision that needs to be made? Why make the decision? Who will make the decision or perform the procedure? As these questions are answered, the framework for the policy or procedure will be described. All information collected for each policy or procedure topic is kept in a designated file. The information in this file is then used to develop the content for the policy or procedure. If changes are required after a policy or procedure is implemented, the information is available for review. A staff member may be assigned the task of collecting reference information on a specific content area and may also write the first draft of the policy or procedure. This draft is then reviewed by all policy and procedure committee members, preferably prior to the meeting in which it will be discussed. To prevent confusion, each draft must be dated. If an agency is small and one or two staff members develop the policies and procedures, it is still important to ask for additional staff input.

As policies and procedures are written, several factors are important. First, terminology must be clear and concise. Because lengthy, cumbersome statements do not communicate information efficiently, short sentences are preferable. Abbreviations and acronyms may be used; however, they must agree with the agency's designated list of abbreviations and acronyms. This list should be included in the policy and procedure manual. Second, the information is organized in logical steps. Do the steps in the policy or procedure make sense? Can they be followed? Are they complete? Could the policy or procedure be stated more simply? The development of policies and procedures requires staff to be objective and willing to say that something does not work.

After the content is developed, the approval phase begins. Approval involves review of the entire content by the nurse administrator and/or agency administration and requires an approval signature and date. No policy or procedure is implemented without appropriate written approval. There may be several drafts, but staff need to know that the only draft that can be implemented must include an approval signature.

Implementation of a policy or a procedure requires planning and participation from the policy and procedure committee and all levels of the agency's management. The goal of implementation is to make all staff aware of the new or changed policy or procedure and to encourage staff to apply the policy or procedure at the appropriate time. With staff working alone in patient homes, communication is a very important part of the implementation process. Staff should know the purpose of the policy and/or procedure; its content; who may make the decision or perform the procedure; and the feedback mechanism for criticisms. Prior to implementation, it is important to identify what might interfere with staff use of the policy or procedure. There are many possible answers to this question, and assessment of these answers will help to combat underutilization or lack of awareness of a policy or procedure. Some of the most frequent reasons for not using policies or procedures are

- Staff do not have access to the policy and procedure manual.
- Staff do not know which policy or procedure to apply.
- Staff do not know what is in the manual.
- Staff do not know how to use the manual.
- Staff do not understand how policies and procedures reflect the philosophy of the home care agency.
- Staff do not feel that the policies and procedures are practical or helpful.
- Staff do not like someone telling them what to do and how to do it.
- Staff do not understand how the policies and procedures protect the patient and staff.
- Staff do not understand the relationship of policies and procedures to quality care.
- Staff feel that policies and procedures represent more paperwork.

Staff may have very realistic reasons for ignoring the policies and procedures. Each complaint is discussed and, if necessary, legitimate problems are resolved. It is, therefore, important to plan all steps in the development and implementation process. Anticipation of some of the possible problems before they occur may provide a better chance of successful implementation of a policy or procedure.

Evaluation and revision of policies and procedures is probably the weakest part of the development process. It is, however, critical to the success of implementation. An outdated policy or procedure can be just as detrimental to care and to the organization as no policy or procedure. Changes never come easily and usually involve some risk, but a system designed to ensure that every policy and procedure is evaluated regularly can ease change and prevent problems. Feedback from staff is critical. Policy and procedure development is never a task that is complete, because change is inevitable.

The following are examples of policy and procedure topics that a home care agency that provides care to psychiatric patients may need to develop:

- admission
- advance directives
- appointments
- assessment: nursing, initial and ongoing
- assessment: physician, initial and ongoing
- behavioral family management
- behavioral progress record
- canceling visits
- case management
- communication with referral sources (e.g., medical physician, psychiatrist, prehospitalization and postdischarge, other)
- community resources
- confidentiality
- consumer satisfaction
- continuity of care
- critical incidents
- diagnostic testing
- discharge
- documentation
- emergencies (crisis resolution)
- escalating behavior
- family/SO assessment
- family/SO problem solving
- family/SO support

- functional and behavioral approach to assessment and treatment
- home health aides
- homemakers
- homework assignments
- homework log
- incident reports
- informed consent
- interdisciplinary team collaboration
- interpreting services for hearing impaired
- medical problems
- medication compliance
- number and frequency of visits
- occupational therapy
- outpatient electroconvulsive therapy
- patient advocacy
- patient/family/SO conferences
- patient/family/SO education
- patient grievances
- patient outcomes
- patient property
- patient rights
- pharmacy
- physical therapy
- progress notes
- quality assessment and improvement
- rating scales
- referral to other health care services
- relaxation techniques
- skilled nursing care
- social services
- social skills training
- speech therapy
- staff safety
- suicidal patient
- target complaint scale
- teaching guides
- transition to other treatment modalities
- treatment contract
- treatment plan
- twenty-four-hour coverage
- vocational therapy

QUALITY ASSESSMENT AND IMPROVEMENT

The major focus of the quality assessment (QA) and improvement program should be outcomes. To accomplish this, each patient will need clear and measurable goals or outcomes. Critical questions to ask are: What do you do with the patient? Does it make a difference? QA focus areas that might be included in the home care agency's QA program include the following:

- treatment process: referral, assignment of staff, initial appointment schedule, frequency and length of visits, admission, discharge (Exhibit 6–1 provides an example of a tool that could be used to evaluate the referral process.)
- documentation reviews
- all types of communications
- patient/family/SO feedback
- patients who terminate home care prior to recommended time
- compliance with the patient's rights
- documentation that reflects treatment model and reflects what is considered to be important in the care of patients in the home
- licensure issues
- medication: administration, monitoring, education, documentation
- program planning
- relapses or rehospitalizations
- relationship and communication with referral sources
- review of open and closed cases: records, completion, appropriateness
- review of treatment model, philosophy, policies, procedures, job descriptions, staffing
- staff performance appraisals
- standards met
- use of case conferences and individual supervision
- critical incidents (e.g., suicidal behavior, escalating or assaultive behavior, accidents)

Other data that are collected and reviewed for trends include length of treatment, patient characteristics such as age, diagnosis, location of home, rate of readmission, services utilized, costs of services, reimbursement sources, referral sources. Examples of QA indicators that might be used in psychiatric home care are found in Exhibit 6–2.

McFarland suggests that the following general QA questions might be asked:[51(pp.898–899)]

- Does psychiatric nursing home care reduce the length of stay, prevent recidivism, and improve compliance with treatment protocols?

Exhibit 6–1 Psychiatric Home Care Referral: Quality Assessment

Patient Name _____

Physician(s) _____

Diagnosis _____

Referring Agency _____

Date of Referral _____

Date Home Care Began _____

Patients referred for psychiatric home care must meet one or more of the following criteria:

	Yes	No
1. Is the patient homebound with the exception of medical appointments?	____	____
2. Does the patient require monitoring of mental status?	____	____
3. Is noncompliance with treatment a potential problem?	____	____
4. Does the referral source feel that the patient will follow the recommended discharge plan?	____	____
5. Has the patient had repeated admissions to the hospital?	____	____
6. Does the patient have adequate family/significant other support in the home?	____	____
7. Are there potential problems with the patient's family/significant others/caregivers?	____	____
8. Does the patient require specific, skilled nursing care for a medical problem in addition to a psychiatric problem?	____	____

- Which patients benefit most from the home care program in terms of their diagnosis, age, sex, employment status, and family role?
- Does psychiatric home care reduce total health care costs for this population?

Other questions are more specific to an individual agency:

- Are patient referrals appropriate for the agency's services?
- Are discharge plans based on patient needs and realistic?
- Do patients comply with discharge plans?

Exhibit 6–2 Examples of Psychiatric Home Care Indicators

• number of patients with symptoms of suicidal ideation in a specific time period
——
all patients assessed in a specific time period

• number of patients with suicidal behavior identified in a specific time period
——
all patients seen in a specific time period

• number of patients with escalating behavior in a specific time period
——
all patients assessed in a specific time period

• number of injuries to patient/family/SOs/staff due to patients with escalating behavior for a specific time period
——
all patients with escalating behavior for a specific time period

• number of patients who comply with medications in a specific time period
——
all patients taking medications in a specific time period

• number of patients able to identify medications, side effects, dosage, frequency
——
all patients taking medications

• number of patients with complete suicide assessments in a specific time period
——
all patients admitted in a specific time period

• number of patients able to use a specific intervention to cope with a problem (e.g., relaxation technique)
——
all patients taught a specific intervention to cope with a problem (e.g., relaxation technique)

According to Reif and Martin:

> Coordination within the agency team, between the agency and the physician, and between the agency and other community providers is essential to assure high quality, patient-focused care yet an agency's professionals often feel they do not have enough time to communicate with each other, much less with providers outside the agency. As a result, the

goal of achieving a seamless system of health care delivery is rarely, if ever, achieved. Moreover, a steady decrease in the amount of time allowed per visit makes it difficult to include care recipients and their families in every phase of the planning, delivery, and evaluation of services.[52(p.10)]

Quality Assessment Methods

The evaluation process for Medicare patients should be continuous, with their records reviewed concurrently and retrospectively. According to Pelletier, "Concurrent review focuses on monitoring patient care, treatment plan review, medication administration review, patient care incidents, and monitoring adherence to documentation standards."[53(p.23)] Retrospective review occurs after the patient is discharged, and focuses on the quality of the documentation. Methods that might be used by a home care agency include the following:

- *Case review by a QA committee.* The committee should have representatives from the disciplines of medicine, nursing, social work, and the rehabilitation therapies such as occupational and vocational therapies. The sample should include open cases and closed cases monitored on a specific schedule. Results are shared with staff.
- *Critical pathways/disease management/protocols.* A critical pathway is a method used to manage patient care and can also be used for QA. A pathway identifies key activities for all disciplines providing patient care. These activities are described sequentially to achieve an appropriate number of visits.[54] This method identifies measurable and achievable outcomes, time frames, and resource utilization. Variances from the pathway can provide information about areas of care that need improvement.
- *Individual supervision.* Individual supervision can be used to assess QA issues and other areas that need improvement, both for an individual staff member and for the agency as a whole.
- *Patient and family/SO satisfaction.* Feedback from the patient and the family/SOs is very important. This should be obtained throughout the care process; however, a formal request for feedback should occur after discharge. This can be done in writing or by means of a follow-up telephone call. The written format is less threatening; however, obtaining a high rate of return may be difficult. Questions that might be asked include the following:
  1. What did you like about your care?
  2. What did you dislike about your care?
  3. Did you participate in your treatment planning?
  4. Did the staff listen to you?

5. How were your complaints handled?
6. Did the staff keep their appointments?
7. Did the staff give sufficient time when an appointment was changed or canceled?
8. Could you reach your home care nurse when you needed assistance?
9. Did your home care nurse teach you information that was useful to you?
10. Did you receive information you needed at the time of admission?
11. Were you told about the payment procedure?
12. Was our staff courteous on the telephone?

- *Outcome assessment.* If patient outcomes are to be used to assess the patient's progress, expected outcomes must be realistic and measurable. Focusing on the level of functioning is easier than on subjective data. Identifying expected outcomes and evaluating results should include the patient, the family/SOs, and the staff. In the ANA's recent review of home care, it is noted that "it is usually the agency, rather than the consumer, that takes the lead in establishing the goals for care, selecting the services and workers, and evaluating whether a satisfactory outcome has been achieved."[55(p.6)] Each home care agency should make changing this attitude a top priority.
- *Calendar worksheet.* The calendar worksheet can be used as a QA method as part of the record review. Harris notes that this can achieve several goals:[56(p.66)]
  - to determine whether the patients are receiving care as prescribed by the plan of care
  - to determine whether there was physician notification or an order for any deviation from the plan of care
  - to determine that the use of services was adequate to meet the patient's needs. For example, if a range was indicated, were services provided at the highest, mid, or lowest level of the range?

Discrepancies in the visit pattern must be documented with the reason for the discrepancy noted. Staff reviewing records should check to see if there has been a physician's order to change the visit schedule.

REIMBURSEMENT

Psychiatric home care is reimbursable by Medicare, Medicaid, and some private insurance providers. Private pay is also possible but, of course, not as common. Some coverage may be provided under home care benefits and some under psychiatric benefits. The agency must investigate and understand the common coverage sources in the community. According to the ANA review of home care, one of the most important changes made in the HCFA eligibility and coverage requirements involves "the expansion of the definition of skilled nursing to include observation and assessment of a patient's condition, teaching, and training activities, and management and evaluation of the care plan. . . . Because health monitoring and patient education now constitute a skilled nursing visit, patients requiring long-term management can continue to receive care, including more paraprofessional services."[57(pp.34-35)] As staff document, it is very important to understand the reimbursement requirements. This is not to say that the only reason to document is for reimbursement or that the documentation is false or limited due to these requirements, but rather that reimbursement requirements and clinical issues must be considered together. Identifying expected outcomes helps to identify services that will be provided. Third-party payers then have a better understanding of patient goals and patient care results. There is no doubt that the care for most psychiatric patients is low-tech, but it requires highly skilled staff. Third-party payers may need help in understanding this difference. Medicare considers the following services to be reimbursable:

- assessment
- patient education
- management of plan of care
- skilled nursing care
- psychotherapeutic interventions

Third-party payers may have staff credential requirements that must be considered when assignments are made.

Sources of reimbursement include the following:[58]

- Medicare, the program of the federal government, will pay for psychiatric home care services if the patient has a primary psychiatric diagnosis, has been evaluated by a psychiatrist and reevaluated every 60 days by one, and is homebound. Homebound status, in general, means that a patient is unable to leave the home due to illness or injury (e.g., physical reasons such as unsteady gait, shortness of breath after walking 10 feet, or a fracture, or because psychiatric illness makes it unsafe to leave home unsupervised or the patient refuses to leave the home).
- Medicaid, a federally and state-funded program, is a state-administered program of reimbursement that does not provide reimbursement for home care services. Each state has its own criteria for eligibility and reimbursement for psychiatric home care services.
- Many third-party payers, private health insurance companies, follow the guidelines established by Medicare. Others adhere to their own rules and regulations, which may or may not cover psychiatric home care nursing services. With the presence, increase, and benefit of home care services, some health insurance companies are paying for home care services on a

case-by-case basis, while others have included home care services as a general rule.

- Some patients pay directly for psychiatric home care services, mainly because they do not meet the criteria for Medicare, Medicaid, or private health insurance coverage or they do not have private health insurance. Some agencies or providers charge a flat rate, while others have a sliding-fee scale, based on the patient's ability to pay. A patient may also choose to pay directly for psychosocial home care services to continue desired services in the home beyond the period authorized by an insurance company or the government programs.

- Some agencies and persons have in their budgets funds to pay for home care on a charity basis for those in need of psychiatric home care services but for whom no funding sources exist.

MARKETING HOME CARE SERVICES

Marketing is a term that usually arouses complicated responses from staff, particularly nurses. In the late 1970s, the use of marketing in health care became more common, and its use rapidly increased in the 1990s. Today health care providers need to develop competitive readiness to prepare for the future. To meet the competition, the home care agency must communicate its uniqueness. While marketing yields positive results, it also carries negative connotations. Marketing has been seen as a business technique that is strongly motivated by financial gain. Marketing, however, is much more than obtaining patients for financial reward. Through a better understanding of the marketing process, this one-sided view of marketing can be changed. The marketing process drives major decisions in health care organizations.

The Marketing Process[59]

Marketing includes three elements: a means of identifying what is wanted and needed, a mechanism for bringing an individual or group with wants or needs together with an individual or group that can satisfy those wants and needs, and a focus on understanding and serving patients as consumers.[60] These elements are similar to the elements of the nursing process (e.g., assessment, diagnosis, outcome identification, planning and implementation, and evaluation). Comparing the marketing process to the nursing process makes it more understandable and acceptable to nurses. As is true of the nursing process, marketing is a complex process that is dependent on data, interaction between people, problem solving, decision making, and evaluating results.

A market consists of all actual and potential consumers or customers of a product or service. Segmentation of large markets may be necessary to divide the market group into subgroups. Then specific segments can be targeted in the marketing plan. Factors that might be considered in segmenting and targeting are diagnostic problems, age, sex, education, geography, accessibility, insurance coverage, and economic status.

Selling is part of marketing; however, selling is not the major focus of the marketing process. Distinguishing the differences between marketing and selling is part of the marketing educational program for the home care staff. Espy states that "Marketing is a consumer-based activity designed to allow you to identify actual and potential customers; assess their needs, attitudes, and preferences; and plan to serve their wants and needs. Selling is an organization-based activity aimed at motivating others to consume what your organization has to offer. It is geared toward filling the needs of the organization by selling programs and services in order to ensure survival and profitability."[61] The key difference between marketing and selling is that marketing is a consumer-based activity with the organization looking to the consumer for direction about needs; selling focuses on the organization's product or service first (e.g., We have a psychiatric home care program, and we need to find patients for it).

Selling requires specific skills. If staff are required to do selling, training that includes the information necessary to take on this task is critical. It is, however, very important to assess staff responses to selling before training begins. Their responses will affect their success in selling. Because many nurses have negative reactions to the selling component of marketing, this factor should be considered before deciding to use nurses in this position. Forcing staff to do selling may lead to problems of lowered morale, turnover, recruitment difficulties, and decreased quality of care. Even if nursing staff are not actively involved in marketing, they should be provided with information about the marketing process and its implications for clinical care.

As marketing is developed and implemented, the home care agency should ask who the consumers or customers are. They can be patients, psychiatrists, other clinical staff, nursing staff, other health care agencies and facilities, referral sources, third-party payers, families/SOs, and the community. An external relationship exists between the hospital and many of these consumers, such as the patient, family/SOs, attending psychiatrist, referral source, and the community. An internal relationship exists between all home care staff within the agency who participate in the work process and who depend on one another. The external relationships and their effects on marketing are easily understood by staff; however, the internal customer-supplier relationships may be a new concept. Identifying the needs of the consumer or customer requires more than just assessing the needs of the patient. If home care staff can begin to see the other staff that they work with as consumers or customers, more efforts may be made to improve all types of service—whether that service is providing direct patient care, obtaining laboratory reports on time, or providing clerical support.

The marketing goals are important and need to be reviewed and revised routinely. Examples of these goals are as follows:

- to maximize the amount of products or services that are purchased or used by the consumer or customer
- to maximize consumer or customer satisfaction
- to develop a quality product and service
- to take responsibility for that product and service

Goals should be based on a thorough assessment of needs. Market research is the assessment of the internal and external environments in which the product or service is provided and the competitors. It provides data for the marketing plan. This assessment is not a one-time effort but rather an ongoing process. As the internal and external environments change, the marketing plan must be revised.

The focus of the internal assessment is to identify the agency's strengths and limitations, whereas the focus of the external assessment is to identify the agency's threats and opportunities in the marketplace. Examples of internal data are the number of visits per product line or diagnosis, referral patterns for specific referral sources, utilization review data, patient satisfaction data, referral source satisfaction data, staffing patterns, quality assessment data, response to promotion campaigns, and financial statements and budgets. External data might include the number of home care agencies in the community; types of services these agencies offer; size of these agencies; community demographic information such as age, sex, family constellation, economics, number of people moving into and out of the area, number of specific types of clinicians in the area, and insurance coverage typical for the area; medical and nursing research results; new medications; economic trends; social trends; legislative and legal trends; and political trends. Clearly, this process develops a considerable amount of data to analyze; however, successful planning necessitates detailed assessment and analysis. An important component of the external assessment includes an assessment of the competition. Who are the competitors? What are their strengths and limitations? How is the agency competing with them? Is the agency successful? How could the agency do better?

A home care agency might use the following activities to develop a customer service marketing approach.[62(p.22)]

- Conduct program activities with an eye to what the patients want or need.
- Pay attention to the user-friendliness of everything that is done.
- Consider customer or patient satisfaction as one of the most important values.

- Check frequently on operations to be certain that goals are achieved.
- Compile and use available information about the organization in program and service planning and evaluation.
- Keep track of changes in the community, state, nation, or world that might impact the way business is done.
- Provide information and ongoing education to staff on the value of marketing and the customer-centered approach.

This list of activities underscores that marketing is an integral part of direct care, quality assessment and improvement, risk management, utilization review, administrative decision making and planning, performance appraisal, staff development, and community relationships.

During monitoring and evaluation, issues may arise that help to identify the need for revisions. All staff must be willing to make changes and accept them as part of the process. Staying with a creative idea that does not work is not creative management. Revisions must be considered carefully; they should not be made without reliable data. Changes can generate new ideas that lead to improvement in organizational performance.

Referral sources need critical information in order to know who to refer for psychiatric home care, such as medical patients who might have psychiatric problems or develop them during the course of care. Questions to ask include the following:

- Who is appropriate?
- What services are provided?
- Who provides the services?
- What are the benefits of psychiatric home care?

According to Miller and Duffey: "Specifically psychiatrists and others often have concerns regarding potential duplication of services, focus of nursing interventions, and how this service will benefit the patient. It is important to be responsive to requests for service, starting with evaluation of new patients and ongoing feedback on progress."[63(p.38)] These authors also state that home care services should "stress the importance of compliance and slowing down of the 'revolving door syndrome' as key benefits of referring patients."[64(p.40)]

Referral sources will also be concerned about losing patients, and they must be reassured that this will not occur. Staff need to emphasize collaboration rather than competition. One-to-one contact with hospital staff in the community and third-party payers will do much to increase referrals. Referral sources will need to be educated about home care and its benefits. It is best to describe a service package rather than charges per visit. Referral sources may have difficulty recognizing the hidden costs of a visit, such as travel time or communication time. A service package might be described as providing home care services for a period of time with a menu of services for a set fee. This type of service might appeal to a managed care organization. Referral information that should be obtained for every referral for psychiatric home care includes the following:

- patient's name, address, telephone number
- family/SOs contact
- psychiatrist's name, address, telephone number
- medical physician's name, address, telephone number
- primary or secondary psychiatric diagnosis
- any medical diagnoses
- reason patient is homebound
- insurance coverage, name, address, telephone number
- start-of-care date
- requested services and visit frequency
- orders from psychiatrist

Additional information that is helpful if it can be obtained includes the following:

- previous hospitalizations
- previous home care
- problems with compliance
- patient's knowledge about home care referral and response

Letters sent to possible referral sources can be useful to introduce the home care agency and its services. The letter might highlight some of the following:

- introduction with specific reasons for referring patients for psychiatric home care that emphasize the need to assist patients to comply with outpatient treatment
- identification of the agency goals
- identification of what the agency can do for the referral source
- identification of specific services provided
- description of the range of the frequency and length of visits
- description of who provides the services
- identification of the admission criteria
- identification of reimbursement factors
- description of the referral procedure and an agency contact person
- identification of office hours and whether 24-hour coverage is provided

Letters should be followed up with a telephone call to determine if the psychiatrist or potential referral source has questions. In some cases, a visit to the psychiatrist or potential referral source may be beneficial. Staff who do this should be prepared to give specific examples of patient referrals, services the patient received, and outcomes of care provided by the agency. All written materials should provide the same information as included in the letter. This information may be in the form of a brochure or a fact sheet. It should be easily read and attractive. Methods for marketing might include attending hospital conferences and nursing conferences in the community, providing continuing education programs, and obtaining patient and family/SOs satisfaction data.

SUMMARY

According to Christopher et al., "Nurses need agency administrators with vision and a willingness to shift the agency's philosophical foundations from a view of care as primarily agency-directed to one of partnership with patients or even patient direction."[65(p.45)] Developing and implementing a psychiatric home care service requires many of the same administrative skills as would be used for any home care services; however, it is critical that the agency considers the type of treatment model that will be used and how it will be implemented in daily home care visits. What will actually be provided to the patient and the family/SOs? This is a question that must be repeated frequently in order to ensure that the psychiatric home care services are effective and meet the needs of the patient.

NOTES

1. M. Trimbath and J. Brestensky, "The Role of the Mental Health Nurse in Home Health Care," *Journal of Home Care Practice* 2, no. 3 (1990): 1–8, at 1.

2. L. Reif and K. Martin, *Nurses and Consumers: Partners in Assuring Quality Care in the Home* (Washington, DC: American Nurses Association, 1996), 6.

3. L. Pelletier, "Psychiatric Home Care," *Journal of Psychosocial Nursing* 26, no. 3 (1988): 22–27, at 24.

4. G. McFarland and M. Thomas, *Psychiatric Mental Health Nursing: Application of the Nursing Process* (Philadelphia: J.B. Lippincott Co., 1991), 897–898.

5. N. Klebanoff, "Psychosocial Home Care," in *Psychiatric-Mental Health Nursing: Adaptation and Growth*, ed. B. Johnson (Philadelphia: J.B. Lippincott Co., 1993), 758–773, at 759.

6. B. Johnson, *Psychiatric-Mental Health Nursing: Adaptation and Growth* (Philadelphia: J.B. Lippincott Co., 1993), 758.

7. W. Burgess and E. Ragland, *Community Health Nursing Philosophy, Process, Practice* (Norwalk, CT: Appleton-Century-Crofts, 1983), 92.

8. HCFA Medicare Home Health Manual, HCFA-Pub. 11 through T273, Rev 3/95, U.S. Department of Health and Human Services, 205.1.

9. 42 CFR 4, Part 484, Conditions of Participation in Home Health, Subpart A, General Provisions (October 1, 1993), 451.

10. 42 CFR 4, 450–455.

11. 42 CFR 4, 451.

12. K. Patusky, "Psychiatric Home Care," in *Psychiatric/Mental Health Nursing: The Therapeutic Use of Self*, ed. L. Birckhead (Philadelphia: J.B. Lippincott Co., 1989), 645–655, at 648–649.

13. Patusky, "Psychiatric Home Care," 649.

14. Patusky, "Psychiatric Home Care," 649–650.

15. American Psychiatric Association, *Diagnostic and Statistical Manual of Mental Disorders*, 4th ed. (Washington, DC: 1994).

16. J. Jackson and M. Neighbors, *Home Care Client Assessment Handbook* (Gaithersburg, MD: Aspen Publishers, Inc., 1990), 40.

17. Reif and Martin, *Nurses and Consumers*, 31.

18. A. Finkelman, *Psychiatric Nursing Administration Manual* (Gaithersburg, MD: Aspen Publishers, Inc., 1995), 4–1:1–4–1:14.

19. American Nurses Association, *Standards of Clinical Nursing Practice* (Washington, DC: 1991), 1–3.

20. B. Brown, "From the Editor," *Nursing Administration Quarterly* 12, no. 2 (1988): vii.

21. American Nurses Association, *A Statement on Psychiatric-Mental Health Clinical Nursing Practice and Standards of Psychiatric-Mental Health Clinical Nursing Practice* (Washington, DC: 1994).

22. American Nurses Association, *Standards of Home Health Nursing Practice* (Washington, DC: 1986).

23. S. Merz, "Clinical Practice Guidelines: Policy Issues and Legal Implications," *Journal of Quality Improvement* 19, no. 8 (1993): 308–313, at 309.

24. M. Bleich and M. Bratton, "Solving the Quagmire of Clinical Standards Development and Implementation," *Journal of Nursing Care Quality* 8, no. 1: 17, 20–22.

25. Finkelman, *Psychiatric Nursing Administration Manual*.

26. J. Laben and C. McLean, *Legal Issues and Guidelines for Nurses Who Care for the Mentally Ill* (Thorofare, NJ: SLACK, Inc., 1984), 7.

27. J. Krauss, "Sorry, That's Confidential," *Archives of Psychiatric Nursing* 4, no. 5 (1992): 55–56.

28. S. Jones, "More on Confidentiality," *Archives of Psychiatric Nursing* 7, no. 3 (1993): 123–124.

29. Krauss, "Sorry, That's Confidential," 256.

30. S. Stern, "Privileged Communication: An Ethical and Legal Right of Psychiatric Clients," *Perspectives in Psychiatric Care* 26, no. 4 (1990): 22–29, at 22.

31. Stern, "Privileged Communication," 27.

32. M. Cazalas, *Nursing and the Law* (Gaithersburg, MD: Aspen Publishers, Inc., 1978), 258.

33. Laben and McLean, *Legal Issues and Guidelines for Nurses Who Care for the Mentally Ill*, 32–33.

34. B. Calfee, "Confidentiality and Disclosure of Medical Information," *Nursing Management* 20, no. 12 (1989): 23.

35. *Tarasoff v. Regents of University of California*, 529 P.2d 553 (Cal. 1984) and 551 P.2d 334 (Cal. 1976), at 347; *Peck v. the Counseling Center of Addison County*, 449 A.2d 442 (Vt. 1985), at 422; *Peterson v. State*, 671 P.2d 230 (Wash. 1983); *Williams v. United States*, 450 Federal Supplement 1040 (D.S.D. 1978).

36. M. Trudeau, "Informed Consent: The Patient's Right to Decide," *Journal of Psychosocial Nursing* 31, no. 6 (1993): 9–12, at 10.

37. J. Fiesta, "Informed Consent Process—Whose Legal Duty?" *Nursing Management* 22, no. 1 (1991): 17–18.

38. Fiesta, "Informed Consent Process," 17.

39. Trudeau, "Informed Consent: The Patient's Right to Decide," 10–11.

40. "APA Updates Guidelines for Care of HIV-Infected Inpatients, Confidentiality and Disclosure of HIV," *Hospital and Community Psychiatry* 44, no. 3 (1993): 296–297.

41. "APA Updates Guidelines for Care of HIV-Infected Inpatients," 296.

42. Americans with Disabilities Act of 1990, Pub. L. No. 101-306.

43. R. Ravid and S. Menon, "Guidelines for Disclosure of Patient Information under the Americans with Disabilities Act," *Hospital and Community Psychiatry* 44, no. 3 (1993): 280–281, at 280.

44. Ravid and Menon, "Guidelines for Disclosure of Patient Information under the Americans with Disabilities Act," 281.

45. G. Stuart, "Legal Context of Psychiatric Nursing Care," in *Principles and Practice of Psychiatric Nursing*, ed. G. Stuart and S. Sundeen (St. Louis, MO: C.V. Mosby, 1995), 171–197, at 171–174.

46. Stuart, "Legal Context of Psychiatric Nursing Care," 174.

47. Stuart, "Legal Context of Psychiatric Nursing Care," 173.

48. P. Iyer and N. Camp, *Nursing Documentation: A Nursing Process Approach* (St. Louis, MO: Mosby–Year Book, 1991), 90.

49. L. Mosher and L. Burti, *Community Mental Health: Principles and Practice* (New York: W.W. Norton & Company, 1989), 377.

50. Finkelman, *Psychiatric Nursing Administration Manual*, 2:1–2:8.

51. G. McFarland and M. Thomas, *Psychiatric Mental Health Nursing: Application of the Nursing Process* (Philadelphia: J.B. Lippincott Co., 1991), 898–899.

52. Reif and Martin, *Nurses and Consumers: Partners in Assuring Quality Care in the Home*, 10.

53. Pelletier, "Psychiatric Home Care," 23.

54. S. Meister et al., "Home Care Steps™ Protocols: Home Care's Answer to Changes in Reimbursement," *Journal of Nursing Administration* 25, no. 6 (1995): 33–42, at 33.

55. Reif and Martin, *Nurses and Consumers: Partners in Assuring Quality Care in the Home*, 6.

56. M. Harris, "Using the Calendar Worksheet as One Quality Assessment Tool," *Home Healthcare Nurse* 13, no. 2: 66–68, at 66.

57. Reif and Martin, *Nurses and Consumers: Partners in Assuring Quality Care in the Home*, 34–35.

58. Johnson, *Psychiatric-Mental Health Nursing*, 759.

59. Finkelman, *Psychiatric Nursing Administration Manual*, 1–7:1–1–7:3.

60. S. Espy, *Marketing Strategies for Nonprofit Organizations* (Chicago: Lyceum Books, Inc., 1993), 2.

61. Espy, *Marketing Strategies for Nonprofit Organizations*, 10.

62. Espy, *Marketing Strategies for Nonprofit Organizations*, 22.

63. M. Miller and J. Duffey, "Planning and Program Development for Psychiatric Home Care," *Journal of Nursing Administration* 23, no. 11 (1993): 35–41, at 38.

64. Miller and Duffey, "Planning and Program Development for Psychiatric Home Care," 40.
65. M. Christopher et al., "The Community as Partner," *Caring* 12, no. 1 (1993): 44–49, at 45.

SUGGESTED READING

American Nurses Association. 1986. *Standards of home health nursing practice.* Washington, DC.

American Nurses Association. 1994. *A statement on psychiatric-mental health clinical nursing practice and standards of psychiatric-mental health clinical nursing practice.* Washington, DC.

Andresen, P. 1995. Expanding services through student placements: Strategies for the home health administrator. *Journal of Nursing Administration* 25, no. 6: 29–32.

Birckhead, L. 1989. *Psychiatric/mental health nursing: The therapeutic use of self.* Philadelphia: J.B. Lippincott Co.

Brawn, B. 1991. The effect of nursing home quality on patient outcome. *Journal of the American Geriatrics Society* 39, no. 4: 329–338.

Brince, J. 1986. The psychiatric patient: Hospital care-home care. *Caring* 5, no. 7: 13–16.

Bruce, C. 1992. Financial concepts in home healthcare. *Journal of Nursing Administration* 22, no. 5: 29–34.

Davis, E. 1994. *Total quality management for home care.* Gaithersburg, MD: Aspen Publishers, Inc.

Fiesta, J. 1995. Home care liability—Part I. *Nursing Management* 26, no. 11: 24, 26.

Finkelman, A. 1994. *Quality assurance for psychiatric nursing.* Gaithersburg, MD: Aspen Publishers, Inc.

Finkelman, A. 1995. *Psychiatric nursing administration manual.* Gaithersburg, MD: Aspen Publishers, Inc.

Harris, M. 1994. Updates to home health and hospice regulations. *Home Healthcare Nurse* 13, no. 3: 78, 80.

Hawes, C., and R. Kane. 1991. Issues related to assuring quality in home health care. In *Advances in long term care*, ed. P. Katz et al., 200–251. New York: Springer Publishing.

Hekelman, F. et al. 1992. Clinical research in home care: A report of affiliates of the Visiting Nurse Associations of America. *Journal of Nursing Administration* 22, no. 1: 29–32.

Helwig, K. 1993. Psychiatric home care nursing: Managing patients in the community setting. *Journal of Psychosocial Nursing* 31, no. 12: 21–24.

Joint Commission on Accreditation of Healthcare Organizations. 1994. *1995 accreditation manual for home care*, Vol. 1. Oakbrook Terrace, IL.

Keating, S., and G. Kelmer. 1988. *Home health care nursing: Concepts and practice.* Philadelphia: J.B. Lippincott Co.

Koren, M., and H. Schrague. 1986. Psychiatric home care. *Caring* 5, no. 7: 29–35.

Kramer, A. et al. 1990. Assessing and assuring the quality of home health care: A conceptual framework. *Milbank Memorial Quarterly* 68, no. 3: 413–443.

Kruse, E., and M. Wood. 1989. Delivering mental health services in the home. *Caring* 8, no. 6: 28–29, 32–34, 59.

Lesseig, D. 1987. Home care for psych problems. *American Journal of Nursing* 87, no. 10: 1317–1320.

McFarland, G., and M. Thomas. 1992. *Psychiatric mental health nursing: Application of the nursing process.* Philadelphia: J.B. Lippincott Co.

Menosky, J. 1990. Occupational therapy services for the homebound psychiatric patient. *Journal of Home Health Practice* 2, no. 3: 57–67.

Miller, M., and J. Duffey. 1993. Planning and program development for psychiatric home care. *Journal of Nursing Administration* 23, no. 11: 35–41.

Miller-Hohl, D. 1992. Patient satisfaction and quality care. *Caring* 11, no. 1: 34–37.

Moffic, H. et al. 1984. Paraprofessionals and psychiatric teams: An updated review. *Hospital and Community Psychiatry* 35, no. 1: 61–67.

National League for Health Care, Inc., and Community Health Accreditation Program, Inc. 1993. *Standards of excellence for home care organizations.* New York: National League for Nursing.

Newton, N., and W. Brauer. 1989. In-home mental health services. *Caring* 8, no. 6: 16–19.

Pelletier, L. Psychiatric home care. 1988. *Journal of Psychosocial Nursing* 26, no. 3: 22–27.

Reding, K. et al. 1994. Home visits: Psychiatrists' attitudes and practice patterns. *Community Mental Health Journal* 30, no. 3: 285–296.

Ruch, M. 1984. The multidisciplinary approach: When too many is too much. *Journal of Psychosocial Nursing* 22, no. 9: 18–23.

Shaughnessy, P. et al. 1992. Developing a quality assurance system for home care. *Caring* 11, no. 3: 44–48.

Soltys, S. 1995. Risk management strategies in the provision of mental health services. *Psychiatric Services* 46, no. 5: 473–476.

Spilotro, S. 1995. Taking the leap of faith: Applying continuous quality improvement techniques to home care. *Home Healthcare Nurse* 13, no. 3: 38–45.

Stuart, G., and S. Sundeen. 1995. *Principles and practice of psychiatric nursing.* St. Louis, MO: C.V. Mosby.

Terkelson, K. 1990. *Family education in mental illness.* New York: Guilford Press.

Thobaben, M. 1989. Developing a psychiatric nursing home health service. *Caring* 8, no. 6: 10–14.

Twardon, C. 1992. Home care aide evaluation: Assuring competency and quality. *Caring* 11, no. 4: 16–20.

Walsh, M. 1986. The challenge of mental health home care. *Caring* 5, no. 7: 17–19.

7

The Role of the Nurse in Psychiatric Home Care

INTRODUCTION

According to the American Nurses Association (ANA): "Home health nursing refers to the practice of nursing applied to a patient with a health deficit in the patient's place of residence. Patients and their designated caregivers are the focus of home health nursing practice. The goal of care is to initiate, manage, and evaluate the resources needed to promote the patient's optimal level of well-being."[1(p.5)] Most home care nurses have cared for patients who had mental and emotional problems but were not diagnosed or would not seek treatment. Nurses who prepare to care for patients who are categorized as psychiatric patients may need to be reminded of this fact. Walsh stated in 1986:

> I can't stress enough that patients are already with us; they just aren't clearly diagnosed. We treat them when they have a physical need or require a skilled task. Most of us don't quite know what to do with the mental problem and avoid it. We try to step around it and get the physical, concrete service given and exit from the case. Reimbursement issues certainly push our staff in this direction. I am not saying we should keep a case of someone with mental illness open indefinitely but when we begin to deal head on with mental illness, there will be a qualitatively different interaction between our field staff and patient and the patient and home care system."[2(p.18)]

The last five years have brought a change; psychiatric home care is more available to patients because home care agencies are developing more services to meet the needs of psychiatric patients, and reimbursement is more available for psychiatric services in the home.

THE DEFINITION OF PSYCHIATRIC NURSING

The definition of psychiatric nursing is an important issue in the discussion of the role of the psychiatric home care nurse. The goal is to maximize functional ability within a collaborative relationship between the nurse and the patient and as appropriate with the family/significant others (SOs).

THE PATIENT'S ROLE

The role of the psychiatric home care nurse is greatly affected by the patient's role. The patient is more involved in his or her own treatment in the home setting, with increased control, independence, and responsibility for self-care. If the patient has recently been discharged from a hospital, this new role may be particularly stressful for the patient. The patient is still very sick, confused about the nurse's role when visiting the home, and nervous about being with his or her family/SOs. If the patient has never participated in home care, he or she may be distrustful and confused about this new form of treatment. The patient may expect or fear that it will be like the hospital. The patient will need help understanding the nurse's role, as well as the roles of other home care staff. This information must be shared at the beginning of home care. The patient must open the door to let the nurse in, and this may be the most difficult step. When the patient is confused about the nurse's role, this directly affects the nurse's role. To do what must be done, the nurse must educate the patient about the patient's own responsibilities as well as those of the nurse. There must be some flexibility, because no two nurse-patient relationships are the same. Another factor that will directly affect roles is the attitude of the family/SOs, because they are part of the treatment setting. If the ill family member lives with them, all family members' lives are directly affected 24 hours a day, every day. How they see their responsibilities and those of the patient will affect what the nurse is able to do in the home.

The two most critical dynamics directly related to nursing care and the nurse's role are *control* and *dependency*. The home setting changes these dynamics. Control moves from the nurse to the patient. The patient can choose if the nurse will visit, when the nurse will visit, how long the nurse will visit, and whether to be compliant and involved in treatment. This is not to say that the nurse does not set limits or that boundaries must not be clear. The nurse should never set lower standards but must make a greater effort to develop trust and to understand the patient. When the nurse enters the home, there is a fine line between being received as a health care professional and being welcomed as a pseudo-family member. Nurses need to be tuned into their own feelings and reactions in order to be clear about this boundary. If physical care is required, this may be new to a psychiatric patient; he or she may not see the psychiatric nurse as one who also provides nonpsychiatric nursing care. The home setting demands (and should demand) that the patient be as independent as possible; for the patient, this is a very different message from that received in a hospital setting. Even though nurses like to say that the hospital does not make the patient dependent, it does. The patient is told when to eat, dress, sleep, go to therapy, exercise, and even when to socialize. This relationship of dependency will be difficult to re-create at home.

PSYCHIATRIC HOME CARE NURSE QUALIFICATIONS

As position descriptions are developed and then revised, qualifications for the psychiatric home care nurse that should be considered include the following:

- knowledgeable about psychopathology, psychopharmacology, and medical and physical problems that might be interrelated with psychiatric problems
- able to assess the psychiatric patient and identify problems and diagnoses
- able to develop a treatment plan
- sensitive to changes in patient behavior
- able to develop a relationship with psychiatric patients that promotes patient independency and self-esteem
- able to work independently
- able to teach patients and family/SOs about mental and physical problems
- able to provide nursing care for psychiatric and medical problems in the home environment
- able to identify safety concerns and intervene appropriately
- able to administer and monitor medications
- able to use community resources appropriately for the patient's needs
- able to understand family/SOs' needs and assist them as they live with their ill family member
- able to work collaboratively
- confident

The ideal candidate for this position has a minimum of one year of medical-surgical nursing experience, as well as several years of psychiatric inpatient treatment experience. If the nurse has further training and experience in psychotherapy, this is an asset; however, the position description must be clear about the amount of actual psychotherapy that will be provided by the psychiatric home care nurse. In most cases, psychotherapy is not provided. The nurse must be able to delegate appropriately to other staff and supervise their performance. Working with many community agencies and resources is not uncommon, and some of these agencies may have limited knowledge and experience with psychiatric patients. The home care nurse must then provide education to them about the patient's needs.

Stulginsky discusses characteristics and requirements for the home care nurse, and many of these are also applicable to the psychiatric home care nurse.[3] Three of these are particularly important. (1) "Making do" is an essential skill for home visits. The nurse can only predict so much for a visit, because the home environment is not controlled but rather a dynamic environment. (2) The home care nurse must recognize the importance of time, which is limited for most nurses in any setting. Methods that can be used to organize work and prepare for visits are critical. (3) The nurse needs to work with and respect the system. It is also important to recognize that nurses work with many systems in addition to the home care agency: hospitals, third-party payers, the family/SOs, and community resources. Conflicts will arise with so many systems operating at one time. The nurse must understand the systems and know how to get what the patient needs with the least amount of stress for both the patient and the nurse. This is not easy to accomplish. It cannot be denied that "nurses frequently find themselves in situations where they need to work the system, e.g., documenting what needs to be documented or using the 'right' language to get reimbursement and the patient's needs met."[4(p.484)]

Home care nursing practice requires nurses who can practice independently but also know when they need to seek consultation, supervision, and further education. Pelletier suggests the following as questions that might be used to assess applicants for psychiatric home care nursing positions:[5]

- the nursing process
  1. What is the nursing process?
  2. How has the nurse used the nursing process in his or her practice?
- lethality assessment
  1. How does the nurse assess the patient's suicidal status?
  2. Does the nurse understand the difference between suicidal ideation and suicidal intent?
  3. What are interventions that might be used with the high- and low-risk suicidal patient?
- mental status exam
  1. How does the nurse perform a mental status exam?
  2. What are the elements of the exam?
- management of assaultive behavior
  1. If the nurse has had any experiences with patients who were assaultive, both physically and verbally, what was that like for the nurse?
- nurse-patient relationship
  1. What is the nurse-patient interaction?
  2. What are the phases and tasks of each phase of the nurse-patient relationship?

- collaborative relationships
    1. What is the nurse's past relationships with physicians and other staff?
    2. Describe a past conflict with a physician or other staff member.
- psychopharmacology
    1. What are the most common drugs used to treat anxiety, depression, bipolar disorder, and schizophrenia?

THE ROLE OF THE HOME CARE NURSE IN PSYCHIATRIC HOME CARE

Morgan and McCain identify elements of the registered nurse's role in home care as follows:[6]

- assurance of patient's rights and responsibilities
- initial and ongoing assessment of patient's health and psychosocial and emotional needs
- development of the plan of care
- care coordination of all services included in the plan of care with the utilization of team care conferences to facilitate communication and coordination of care/services
- provision of continuity of care 24 hours per day, 7 days per week
- consideration of legal implications and ethical issues/dilemmas
- program coordination and management
- appropriate referrals, transfers, and/or discharges
- infection control monitoring and evaluation of patients and staff; development and implementation of infection control policies and procedures; appropriate instruction to patients and staff
- assurance of quality of care through a formalized, systematic process of monitoring and evaluation; assistance in the evolution of quality assurance activities into a continuous quality improvement program
- policy/procedure development, revision, and implementation
- inservice education, orientation, and staff development
- provision of preventive, treatment, and maintenance services
- nursing management of the patient's needs and disease processes
- patient advocacy
- patient education
- supervision of environmental and personal care/support services.

Additional elements that are also important to the functioning of the nurse in psychiatric home care include the following:

- coordinating laboratory follow-up and other medical care
- obtaining medications for patients
- administering medications
- assisting the patient to organize a week's supply of medications to ensure greater compliance
- acting as a liaison between several physicians by providing a total view of the patient
- educating physicians and other home care professionals about the home and its effect on the patient and family/SOs
- identifying environmental factors affecting compliance

Discussing the nurse's role with typical professional terminology is not enough. It does not provide the complete answer to the question, "What does the nurse do with and for the patient?" A psychiatric home care nurse may use many methods for helping and teaching the patient. Some of these might be sitting quietly with the patient; talking with the patient about issues that may not be directly related to his or her problem but that help the patient learn about social conversation; developing a menu; informally having a cup of coffee as the patient reviews a homework assignment; having the patient show the nurse something that he or she has accomplished such as completion of a job application; developing a daily schedule or a clean room; demonstrating to the patient the correct method to take a medication; or walking outside to the porch to help the patient see that he or she can leave the house and still control anxiety. The list is endless and only depends on the creativity of the nurse and the needs of the patient.

PARAPROFESSIONAL STAFF

Home health aides are the most frequently used secondary service for the psychiatric patient.[7] According to Trimbath and Brestensky, "When a patient needs personal care, the MHRN (mental health registered nurse) is responsible for developing an individual plan of care with the home health aide and for providing on-site orientation, continued supervision, and evaluation of the effectiveness of the care provided."[8(pp.3-4)] As is true in most hospitals, more and more direct care is provided by paraprofessional staff. The critical difference in home care is the limited on-site supervision for these staff members. With the exception of an occasional supervisory visit, they often work independently with complex patients. As a consequence, treatment plans must be clear and concise, and open communication must exist between the home care nurse and the paraprofessional. The qualifications of paraprofessional staff should be considered carefully.

Qualifications and Training

Whenever it is possible, home health aides assigned to psychiatric patients should enjoy working with this type of patient. Forcing an aide who does not feel comfortable or who is frightened to work with this patient will not be helpful. If the aide can be supervised and taught about the illness and its care, this may help the aide overcome these negative feelings; however, for some, this will not be possible. The aide must be sensitive to others' needs; self-confident; willing to allow the patient to be independent; aware that the patient has very real problems and that it requires much effort to cope with the problems; able to communicate; and able to take direction from the nurse and yet able to express opinions and share observations.

Content that might be included in staff education for the home health aide who will be assigned to psychiatric patients includes the following topics:

- the staff-patient relationship
- confidentiality
- communication skills
- documentation of behavior and feelings
- family/SO dynamics and interventions
- psychiatric medications
- specific clinical problems (e.g., depression, anxiety, paranoia and suspiciousness, suicidality, dementia and delirium)
- emergency incidents
- substance abuse
- community resources
- the elderly and emotional problems
- use of limit setting, consistency, homework assignments, problem solving
- implementation of treatment contracts

Delegation of Responsibilities and Supervision of Paraprofessionals

For many patients, the registered nurse develops the care plan in conjunction with other health care professionals. This care plan provides the direction for the home health paraprofessionals; however, the nurse continues to be accountable for the care provided by paraprofessionals. Although supervision is extremely important, in many cases it is inadequate. It is expensive and time consuming but an important element of quality care. Nurses who have limited supervisory experience will need education about the supervisory process, delegation, communication, documentation of supervision, and adult teaching principles and process. Supervision should be done with the paraprofessional present and at the beginning of a home visit. Supervisory visits that occur five minutes before the home visit is completed are not helpful. Gilbert describes supervision guidelines that are helpful and allow for more efficient use of staff time.[9]

- The supervisory visit should coincide with the beginning of a home visit.
- The supervisory nurse asks the paraprofessional and the patient if there are any questions, problems, or issues that need to be discussed.
- The supervisory nurse asks the paraprofessional to outline a routine visit.
- The supervisory nurse then asks the paraprofessional to demonstrate skills, which can vary depending upon the needs of the patient.
- The time should be used to support, educate, and evaluate the paraprofessional.
- The plan of care and patient outcomes are also assessed.
- Specific times for supervision should be identified by the agency including after the initial placement of the paraprofessional in a home, following changes in the treatment plan, and intermittently for long-term patients.
- Documentation of the supervision must be clear and specific.
- The paraprofessional should receive feedback, both positive and negative.
- If a specific tool is used for supervision, both professional and paraprofessional need to receive training in its use. When possible, it is best to combine all the evaluation components in one tool, including staff competency evaluation, assessment of patient outcomes, supervision of the home health aides, and elements of staff performance evaluation.[10]

THE INTERDISCIPLINARY TREATMENT TEAM

According to Boling and Keenan, "The increasing acuity of illness among home care patients and complexity of the in-home service network have created a greater need for frequent communication between the various members of the interdisciplinary home care team. This will likely become an increasingly important quality-of-care issue as home care continues to expand and to incorporate advances in technology."[11(p.26)]

When a patient has a psychiatrist and other physician(s), the treatment plan must be developed and communicated to all physicians. If this is not done, there is an increased risk of conflict between the physicians and their treatment approaches and interventions. The home care nurse is the health care professional who has the overview of the plan and alerts physicians when there might be a conflict or question about the treatment. According to the ANA:

> The nurse's role as a multidisciplinary care coordinator is important in facilitating the goal of care. Since the patient often receives services from multiple providers and vendors, the home health nurse assumes

the role of care manager in coordinating and directing all involved disciplines and caregivers to optimize patient outcomes. The home health nurse shares knowledge of community health resources with the patient and caregivers. This information exchange and advocacy process is used to encourage patients, families, and caregivers to plan for and seek additional services as their needs and resources dictate. Informing, supporting, and affirming patient and caregiver determinism is an important adjunct to achieving the nursing care plan and patient goals.[12(p.6–7)]

Staff may find that, with the psychiatric patient, working with an interdisciplinary team may become more stressful. With psychiatric care there is less objectivity and more subjectivity, and some of this may be exhibited in staff behaviors during discussions about the patient's care. There is a greater potential for communication and consistency problems. There may even be a power struggle for team leadership. The team should operate with a norm of open communication, and all staff should be encouraged to share information and thoughts about the patient. The purpose of the team is to assist in providing care. Problems that interfere with this goal need to be identified and resolved. This does not mean that individual staff members should be attacked but rather that there should be a safe environment for open discussion. It is important that the team have a designated leader or it will not operate well. Staff need to help one another deal with stress, as this will improve the patient's care. The social worker on the team can be a great assistance in identifying resources that can be used to resolve patient problems, particularly for after-care, financial support, vocational issues, etc. Various therapists, such as the occupational therapist, vocational therapist, and physical therapist, may also provide services to a patient who needs these specialized services and is cooperative in receiving them.

STAFF ORIENTATION AND EDUCATION

According to Miller and Duffey, "It takes approximately three months to orient new field staff to general home care and the unique expectations of psychiatric home care. At the end of this time, one would expect that they would meet the assigned productivity standard. Unlike moving from one inpatient unit to another (which is relatively easy for most nurses and requires little transition), orienting to psychiatric home care is a two-fold process. The nurse must be oriented to home care first, then modify their traditional inpatient psychiatric nursing style to home care."[13(p.39)] Psychiatric home care nurses do not necessarily need to know how to identify complex diagnoses; however, they do need to know how to help patients and families/SOs cope with everyday problems and how to cope with behavior toward the nurse that may be difficult to handle. Examples of the latter are the angry patient, the patient who is very disorganized, the suicidal patient, or the patient who is uncooperative. In addition, it is important that the nurse has knowledge about psychopharmacology.

The nurse who works in the home will find that support and supervision are very important. There are times when the nurse will feel frustrated, particularly around the issue of success and whether the patient is improving. The nurse will at times feel overwhelmed with the patient's many problems. Acceptance of the fact that treatment will not be curative may be difficult. If the patient is very isolated, the nurse-patient relationship may become very intense. The nurse must focus on practical issues, be reality oriented, and respect the patient as an active participant in treatment. The nurse's role is in many ways determined by the patient. The nurse assists the patient in adapting to the community setting and acts as a liaison between the patient, the family/SOs, and other health care providers.

There are many methods that can be used to develop or increase nurses' knowledge about the psychiatric patient. Someone who has psychiatric experience, is a good teacher, and is willing to work with staff members who have a variety of experience is an important resource for the staff and their continuing education. Formal conferences can be scheduled to discuss patients and their problems. Telephone conference time can be established so that staff can call in and discuss their concerns. This time should be flexible enough to meet the needs of the staff, their routines, and their schedules. Important topics include the following:

- psychopharmacology
- physical assessment
- treatment planning for psychiatric problems
- legal issues
- specific diagnoses and nursing problems associated with them (e.g., anxiety, depression, suicidality, bipolar disorder, schizophrenia, escalating behavior, substance abuse)
- family/SOs as caregivers
- treatment contracts
- psychiatric rehabilitation
- community resources
- psychoeducation

NURSING STUDENTS AND PSYCHIATRIC HOME CARE

More and more nursing educational programs are including community nursing, particularly home health nursing, in their didactic and clinical experiences for nursing students. Home health agencies may find that local nursing programs are approaching them to place students in the agency for clinical experience. There are disadvantages and advantages to this trend. The disadvantages include the time that home care staff must spend with students, added complexities of assigning students to patients, determination as to what the nursing students will do, faculty supervision of students' performance, safety issues related to home visits, and staff and patients' acceptance of student visits. These are issues that hospital nurses cope with all the time when students are in the clinical facility. They can be resolved if the agency and its staff believe that it is important to have student participation. Why is it important? With shorter and shorter lengths of stay, more psychiatric care will be provided in the community requiring fewer nurses to work in the inpatient setting and more in the community. New graduates need to be prepared to fill these positions. They need to learn about home care and have some contact with home care patients. As the nursing profession learned the hard way with inpatient psychiatric nursing, if students do not have some contact with the treatment setting they are not motivated to pursue employment in the specialty area. Students also stimulate staff to teach and to pursue their own educational needs. If staff are willing to listen to them, students bring with them new ideas. According to Andresen, home health administrators and faculty "should explore how students might be used to widen the scope of community health nursing services offered by agencies. The administrator who sees the potential in students as valuable resources can expand services without additional costs. These services, although perhaps nonreimbursable, provide the agency with increased visibility in the community."[14(p.30)] Examples might be using a student to teach a patient when the patient has no coverage for this service, having a student follow up on referrals to community agencies, or having a student spend time with a sibling who is experiencing difficulty understanding an ill brother or sister's behavior and need for attention. The student learns, and the patient's needs that may not be reimbursable are met.

SUMMARY

The role of the nurse in psychiatric home care is a combination of nursing roles. The psychiatric home care role is influenced by the roles of the home care nurse and the psychiatric nurse. Medical nursing skills and responsibilities cannot be excluded, but the addition of psychiatric skills and responsibilities make the role very complex. Many nurses do not feel comfortable with the psychiatric patient in the home or with the psychiatric nursing skills required for this patient. The role that is described by the home care agency must be consistent with the treatment model that is developed by the home care agency.

NOTES

1. American Nurses Association, *A Statement on the Scope of Home Health Nursing Practice* (Washington, DC: American Nurses Publishing, 1992), 5.
2. M. Walsh, "The Challenge of Mental Health Home Care," *Caring* 5, no. 7 (1986): 17–19, at 18.
3. M. Stulginsky, "Nurses' Home Health Experience, Part II: The Unique Demands of Home Visits," *Nursing and Health Care* 14, no. 9 (1993): 476–485, at 484.
4. Stulginsky, "Nurses' Home Health Experience, Part II: The Unique Demands of Home Visits," 484.
5. L. Pelletier, "Psychiatric Home Care," *Journal of Psychosocial Nursing* 26, no. 3 (1988): 22–27, at 24.
6. K. Morgan and S. McCain, "Role of the Registered Nurse in Home Care," in *Core Curriculum for Home Health Care Nursing*, ed. K. Morgan (Gaithersburg, MD: Aspen Publishers, Inc., 1993), 7–9.
7. M. Trimbath and J. Brestensky, "The Role of the Mental Health Nurse in Home Health Care," *Journal of Home Health Care Practice* 2, no. 3 (1990): 1–8, at 2.
8. Trimbath and Brestensky, "The Role of the Mental Health Nurse in Home Health Care," 3–4.
9. N. Gilbert, "Supervision of Home Health Paraprofessionals: A Quality of Care Issue," *Caring* 11, no. 4 (1992): 10–14, at 13–14.
10. C. Twardon et al., "Home Care Aide Evaluation: Assuring Competency and Quality," *Caring* 11, no. 4 (1992): 16–20, at 17.
11. P. Boling and J. Keenan, "Communication Between Nurses and Physicians in Home Care," *Caring* 11, no. 5 (1992): 26–29, at 26.
12. American Nurses Association, *A Statement on the Scope of Home Health Nursing Practice*, 1–17, at 6–7.
13. M. Miller and J. Duffey, "Planning and Program Development for Psychiatric Home Care," *Journal of Nursing Administration* 23, no. 11 (1993): 35–41, at 39.
14. P. Andresen, "Expanding Services through Student Placements: Strategies for the Home Health Administrator," *Journal of Nursing Administration* 25, no. 6 (1995): 29–32, at 30.

SUGGESTED READING

American Nurses Association. 1992. *A statement on the scope of home health nursing practice.* Washington, DC.

Andresen, P. 1995. Expanding services through student placements: Strategies for the home health administrator. *Journal of Nursing Administration* 25, no. 6: 29–32.

Androwich, I., and P. Andresen. 1994. Student placements in home health care agencies: Boost or barrier to quality patient care? In *Handbook of home health care administration*, ed. M. Harris, Gaithersburg, MD: Aspen Publishers, Inc., 629–635.

Gibeau, J. 1993. Training paraprofessionals for psychiatric support: New supports in expanding care for the elderly. *Caring* 12, no. 4: 36–42.

Gilbert, N. 1992. Supervision of home health paraprofessionals. *Caring* 11, no. 4: 10–14.

Hansten, R., and M. Washburn, eds. 1994. *Clinical delegation skills: A handbook for nurses.* Gaithersburg, MD: Aspen Publishers, Inc.

Hinchman, A. 1986. The role of the paraprofessional in mental health home care: NAHC's home-maker-home health aide service conference 1986. *Caring* 5, no. 7: 49–50, 54.

Home Care Aide Association of America position paper: National uniformity for paraprofessional title, qualifications, and supervision. 1994. *Caring* 13, no. 4: 4–11.

Kadner, K., and K. Brandt. 1991. Homeward bound: Broadening student experience with home visits. *Journal of Psychosocial Nursing* 29, no. 9: 24–28.

Keating, S., and G. Kelmer. 1988. *Home health care nursing: Concepts and practice.* Philadelphia: J.B. Lippincott Co.

Matteoli, R. et al. 1994. Collaboration between families and university faculty: A partnership in education. *Journal of Psychosocial Nursing* 32, no. 10: 17–20.

Moore, P. et al. 1991. Collaborative model for continuing education for home health nurses. *The Journal of Continuing Education* 22, no. 2: 67–72.

Morgan, K., ed. 1993. *Core curriculum for home health care nursing.* Gaithersburg, MD: Aspen Publishers, Inc.

National Home Care Council of the Foundation for Hospice and Home Care, with the Assistance of the Administration on Aging, Department of Health and Human Services. 1990. *A model curriculum and teaching guide for the instruction of the homemaker-home health aide.* Washington, DC: Foundation for Hospice and Home Care.

Newton, N., and W. Brayer. 1989. A paraprofessional model of care: In-home mental health services. *Caring* 8, no. 6: 15–16.

Stuart, G., and S. Sundeen. 1995. *Principles and practice of psychiatric nursing.* St. Louis, MO: Mosby–Year Book.

Trimbath, M., and J. Brestensky. 1990. The role of the mental health nurse in home health care. *Journal of Home Health Care Practice* 2, no. 3: 1–8.

Twardon, C. et al. 1992. Home care aide evaluation: Assuring competency and quality. *Caring* 11, no. 4: 16–20.

Managed Behavioral Care and Psychiatric Home Care

INTRODUCTION

Managed care often arouses many negative reactions in health care providers as well as in patients and their families/significant others (SOs). According to Himali, the theory of managed care is "a good one: patients receive care through a single, 'seamless' system as they move from wellness to sickness back to wellness again. Continuity of care, prevention and early intervention are stressed. It's providing exactly the type of primary health care services nurses do best."[1(p.1)] However, this statement represents the ideal, and it is not yet found in most managed care providers.

As managed care began to evolve, it became clear in the 1980s that psychiatric patients required different knowledge and skills from medical patients. Separate companies began to form that focused only on the psychiatric population, and this is now referred to as *managed behavioral care*. The development of managed care has brought with it complex new organizations with their own language that often confuses the public as well as other health care professionals and organizations. For health care providers to survive and help patients use their insurance coverage in the most effective way, it has become increasingly important for providers to understand this new world of managed care and how it can be used in psychiatric home care. The home care nurse must take an active patient advocate role, and this role will also be affected by managed care. The home care administrator and home care nurses should become very familiar with new information about managed care and begin to develop plans to cope with the inevitable changes. Why is this important? Many home care patients are in managed care plans of some type, and reimbursement for their psychiatric home care comes from these sources. Home care staff should understand these plans, their benefits, documentation requirements, and specific criteria for receiving specific care. Psychiatric home care agencies will need to market their services to these plans, but in order to succeed agency staff must be knowledgeable about the plans. It may be necessary to convince some managed care plans that providing psychiatric home care is to their benefit and to the benefit of their patients.

Managed care has been suggested as the major method for alleviating health care problems. In 1992, an editorial in *Hospital and Community Psychiatry* described managed care as

> the latest in a long series of attempts to slow the steep rise of health and mental health care costs. For individual mental health practitioners, managed care is often an annoying interference with their clinical judgment. For hospitals it may be a threat to investments in staffed beds and to accustomed sources of revenue. For insurers and employers it offers hope that wildly growing mental health costs can be brought to heel. For patients it can mean an interruption of helpful relationships, or more positively, an earlier return to normal functioning. Whatever else it means, managed care for mental illness is clearly a strong stimulus for innovation in the private sector, where private providers are busy developing alternatives to inpatient treatment such as partial hospitalization, rehabilitation programs, case management, and even supported housing.[2(p.205)]

In addition, this editorial comments that public sector psychiatry has been moving toward a managed care approach that focuses only on the care the patient needs and no more, within a system that allows for flexibility and reduced barriers. The hope is that the private and public sectors will merge and that there will no longer be a two-tiered system of psychiatric care. This, however, will be very difficult to achieve.

FACTORS AFFECTING HEALTH CARE COSTS

Rising health care costs has been a topic for many years, and despite all the discussions, costs continue to rise. In all of these discussions about the suggested sources of this inflation, the central theme is the lack of cost-consciousness and the many complex, inappropriate incentives within the health care system. The American Academy of Nursing identified several factors affecting health care costs. They are listed below, along with additional discussion of their applicability to psychiatric home care.[3]

- *High costs of pharmaceuticals.* The high costs of pharmaceuticals has certainly been a problem in psychiatric care. Many patients must take long-term medications, and many of these medications are expensive. The most recent complaint about excessive cost focused on clozapine, an atypical neuroleptic used to treat schizophrenia. Pharmaceutical companies argue that the cost of medications is due to high research and development costs. They also point out that using medications can be less expensive than other forms of treatment. Certainly, it is often less expensive to treat a patient with schizophrenia in the home or as an outpatient with medications rather than long-term hospitalization; however, the cost of the medication should be reasonable.

- *Expensive technologies.* Expensive technologies is not as applicable to psychiatric care, an area of care that uses these technologies minimally. It does, however, apply to psychiatric patients in the home who also have medical problems that require medical equipment and supplies.
- *Administrative costs.* Inefficiency in insurance functions as well as in the delivery of care are cited as reasons for high administrative costs. Inherent within documentation are considerable costs (e.g., staff training, paper and printing, changes in form design, systems to manage documentation and supervision, and maintaining records over a long period of time).
- *Provider income.* The growth of physician income as well as hospital income has driven up health care costs. It is not uncommon for physicians to make hospital visits that consist of five minutes with the patient and then to charge for an hour session. Another problem is limited consideration of the most appropriate and least expensive method of treatment. Many other examples could be cited, and managed care is clearly directed at eliminating these expensive practices.
- *Defensive medicine.* Defensive medicine is used to minimize the risk of malpractice suits. Psychiatry does not have as many problems with excessive, inappropriate testing; however, psychiatrists may select more extreme interventions due to concerns about malpractice. For example, a patient who is suicidal might be placed on suicide precaution in the hospital; this is an expensive, labor-intensive intervention that uses one-to-one observation. Another example is, instead of trying less restrictive interventions for a patient whose behavior is escalating, the patient is placed in seclusion or restraints in the hospital (requiring more intensive nursing care). Defensive medicine may lead the physician to hospitalize a patient rather than use a less restrictive treatment alternative such as partial hospitalization or psychiatric home care.
- *Physician-induced demand.* The increased number of physicians is decreasing physicians' income. Psychiatry has a greater number of different types of providers, such as nurse psychotherapists, psychologists, and social work-

ers. This increases the potential number of providers who need patients, and competition increases. Marketing costs to build census have increased. It is not clear that this has driven up the costs for psychiatric care, but it may affect them. Marketing costs also increase overall health care costs.

- *Medicare.* Medicare and care for the aging population has increased costs, particularly for hospitals that must cover expenses that are not paid by Medicare.
- *Private insurance.* Private insurance has grown and has had a great impact on health care costs. As is commonly known, private insurance has not provided sufficient coverage for psychiatric care, particularly in such settings as the home, partial hospitalization, and psychiatric rehabilitation programs.
- *Aging population.* The aging population has been increasing, and health care for this population has greatly affected health care costs in general. Its effect on psychiatric costs is unclear. With the increasing number of patients with Alzheimer's disease, there is an increasing number of such patients in psychiatric care. Elderly patients who are admitted to a psychiatric unit inevitably have complex discharge problems that often result in a longer length of stay than is typically required, even though their length of stay is decreasing due to pressures to discharge quickly. Elderly patients come to psychiatric units with multiple medical problems. This increases costs, which may be greater than if such patients were treated on a medical unit. When these elderly patients are discharged, they go home with complex problems and continue to need treatment that may not be recognized by third-party payers. Family/SOs are often left to be the sole caregivers.
- *Extreme measures.* Extreme measures to maintain the lives of critically ill patients has not been an important factor in the rising cost of psychiatric care, but it has affected the overall cost of health care.
- *Social problems.* Social problems have had a major effect on the cost of psychiatric care. Drugs and alcohol; urban violence; divorce; single parenting; problems in schools; and economic problems that have resulted in unemployment, inadequate insurance coverage, and poor living situations all can lead to increased stress and mental illness. Some patients do not seek care until there is a crisis and, consequently, longer-term treatment may be required. Many of these patients do not have insurance and consequently end up in public psychiatric facilities and programs, which are overburdened with seriously ill patients and often have inadequate treatment resources. These complex problems, which are difficult to solve, make it difficult to assist the patient and prepare the patient for discharge. The patient is sent home with many problems. More time is spent with little result. Since psychiatry is labor intensive, staff time is the most expensive resource used.

COMMUNITY MENTAL HEALTH AND MANAGED BEHAVIORAL CARE: PARALLELS

There is a connection between community mental health and managed behavioral health care. As noted in the introduction, the public sector has attempted to provide a system whose goals are similar to those of managed care. Managed behavioral care will be unsuccessful if alternative treatments for psychiatric patients are limited. Simply providing outpatient psychotherapy and inpatient treatment will not be helpful. A continuum of services is required that, at a minimum, provides the following services:[4]

- self-help groups
- weekly outpatient psychotherapies
- more intensive outpatient interventions
- home- and community-based health care
- partial hospitalization, both day and evening
- halfway houses
- residential care in group homes
- acute inpatient hospitalization
- long-term residential care

This continuum is clearly idealistic and, in many communities, the health care system is a long way from providing all of these services. However, these services are needed to meet the many needs of patients at various points in their psychiatric illnesses. Community mental health and managed care also share many of the same values, including the following:[5(pp.9–10)]

- facilitating easy access to care
- taking responsibility for a defined patient population
- triaging patients into the least restrictive care that is most effective for the patient
- providing care within a well-coordinated and complete continuum of care system
- using multidisciplinary treatment providers and teams

MANAGED CARE METHODS

Managed care methods for containing costs have evolved from managing benefits, to managing care, to managing health.

- *Managing benefits.*[6] Managing benefits focuses on annual and lifetime maximums, deductibles, outpatient copayments, and inpatient coinsurances. Some plans exclude specific illnesses from coverage. Others use gatekeeping, which requires patients to see a designated staff member before they can see a specialist, and requires authorization by managed care staff prior to treatment. Retrospective denial is another method that is used, which can cause great problems as payment is frequently denied after the care is provided.

- *Managing care.*[7] Managing care focuses on the management of care rather than manipulation of benefits. The goal is to limit authorization for care, in order to reimburse only for care that is necessary and appropriately delivered in the least-restrictive, and least-intrusive treatment setting, by qualified providers. Methods used to accomplish this include providing a complete continuum of care; prior authorization; concurrent review of ongoing care management; medical necessity determinations; development of and supervision of a network of behavioral health care providers; and standardized pretreatment assessment and treatment planning supported by forms, practice pattern analysis, and outcomes management. The provider is assessed continuously to determine if identified goals are met.
- *Managing health.*[8] The focus of managing health is on disease state management, demand reduction, and behavioral health promotion and wellness. The employee assistance programs have been influential in promoting health among workers, but they have primarily focused on substance abuse. Other methods are individual health risk assessments, health education programs, financial incentives for meeting personal health management goals, self-help groups, crisis debriefing services, and outreach programs to high utilizers of health care services. Some of these methods work well with the seriously mentally ill; others do not, due to the fact that many of these patients have poor employment histories. If the method is part of an employment health plan, it will miss many seriously mentally ill patients.

MODELS OF MANAGED CARE

Managed care is a term that refers to a variety of "prepayment arrangements, negotiated discounts, and agreements for prior authorizations and audits of performance."[9(p.250)] There are many methods of providing managed care; however, there are similarities among all of them. They all have restrictions on traditional fee-for-service, unlimited access to providers, and they have a binding contract arrangement. These restrictions are used to change the provider's and consumer's behaviors by using financial penalties and rewards. Methods for controlling delivery of care are used to improve efficiency and thus gain maximum value for the resources used.[10] Some health care experts believe that the managed care approach will not be enough to control costs. They support the need for greater competition. Managed competition is an approach to health care reform that "attempts to foster genuine price competition among plans through standard benefit packages, providing information on quality and services to consumers to enhance their ability to assess value, monitoring health maintenance organizations (HMOs) for selection practices, and setting premium contributions at or near the low-cost plan, thus giving consumers the incentive to shop for value among plans."[11(p.14)]

TYPES OF MANAGED CARE SYSTEMS

As there is no one definition that applies to managed care, there are many different types or systems in which managed care is used. Some of the more common ones include the following:

- *Health maintenance organization (HMO).*[12] Most nurses are familiar with the HMO. This is the most structured and controlling of the managed care organizations; however, there are many different organizational structures that might be used for an HMO. All of these structures have five common characteristics:
  1. There is a contractual responsibility to provide specific health care services.
  2. The HMO provides care for an enrolled, defined population of patients/ clients (the subscribers).
  3. Subscribers and providers voluntarily participate or work in the plan.
  4. There is a capitation rate per enrollee that is independent of services actually rendered.
  5. All financial risk for the contracted services is held by the HMO.
- *Preferred provider organization (PPO).*[13] PPO is a generic term, and there are several different methods for organizing PPOs. A major difference between the PPO and the HMO is that the PPO uses financial incentives rather than controls. The incentives are used to encourage enrolled members to use a provider from a specific panel of health care providers, and usually the incentives are in the form of a waiver of deductibles and decreased coinsurance requirements. The providers selected by the PPO must demonstrate cost-efficient care, quality care, and effective practice management. The PPO providers do not assume the insurance risk, but they do assume a business risk by agreeing to accept a negotiated fee. If there are a reduced number of patients, the provider's income will be less. Most PPOs continue to operate on a fee-for-service basis, even if discounted; consequently, there is little financial incentive for providers to control the use of services. The PPO must use some form of utilization review to contain excessive use of inappropriate services.

- *Point-of-service option.* Some HMOs allow enrollees to select non-HMO providers for a specific service. The enrollee or member must pay higher premiums, deductibles, and coinsurance for this specific service. This provides members with more freedom of choice, and this is important to many members.
- *Managed behavioral carve-out program.* In this type of program, mental health services are taken out of or carved out of the larger health plan. A selective independent organization is used to provide the services under contract. The important factor in this program is that "the care and the decision making about what care is provided are turned over to a subcontractor so that utilization review becomes entirely internal."[14(p.325)] "HMOs have suffered dramatic market share losses as managed behavioral carve-out vendors grew."[15(p.8)] In some parts of the country, home health staff encounter this type of program for their psychiatric patients rather than HMOs, because businesses have become dissatisfied with services provided to psychiatric patients by HMOs. Some HMOs have responded to this loss of business by developing their own behavioral health care carve-out benefits.

MANAGED CARE TECHNIQUES

The techniques for managing care focus on the utilization of health care services. Incentives and restrictions are placed on the provider's and consumer's decisions. The single entry point is a critical technique that limits or, in many plans, eliminates the possibility of entering the health care system through more than one provider. That provider then determines if the patient needs to be seen by another provider. For psychiatric problems this may mean that a patient will first be seen by a nonpsychiatric provider for referral to a psychiatric provider. These techniques lead to a risk of problems with the quality of care, particularly with the need for specialized assessment and diagnosis and with patient compliance. After seeing the initial provider, the patient may not be willing to see a psychiatric health care provider. Careful monitoring and evaluation of the quality of care is necessary. Generally the controls or techniques for managing care are focused on financial incentives, utilization controls, medical management practices, and quality improvement tools.

- *Financial incentives*[16] focus on modifying the consumer's and the providers' behaviors that increase costs. Cost-reducing methods used with the consumer include reducing or eliminating deductibles and coinsurance when the enrollee uses a preferred or designated provider; requiring that the enrollee use the services of a designated provider in the HMO; ensuring that the most appropriate, least costly setting is used for services; requiring that the enrollee pay a percentage of the costs if the more costly setting is chosen; and utilizing second opinions, preadmission certification, and preauthorization. Cost-reducing methods used with the provider include penalizing inefficient use of resources, payment per admission, and capitation.

- *Utilization controls*[17] focus on the efficient management of patient care. Utilization review is not unknown to hospitals, and the same methods are used in managed care. Utilization control methods include the following:

  1. *Prospective utilization review* for inpatient care has primarily been done by using preadmission certification, screening before admission to determine the medical necessity of the admission. This practice is very common for psychiatric hospitalization. In ambulatory care services, it is done by requiring prior authorization before the patient may see a specialist. Second opinions are also used in prospective review.

  2. *Concurrent review* focuses on three areas. (1) The admission review reexamines the appropriateness of the hospitalization or treatment. The types of services and procedures may also be reviewed to ensure that only preauthorized services are provided. (2) The length-of-stay or treatment review is done to ensure the shortest possible stay or treatment for the patient's needs. Continued stay must be approved. (3) Discharge review focuses on discharge planning from the time of admission and, in some cases, before the actual admission.

  3. *Retrospective review* focuses on the care or service after it is provided. In this case, payment may be denied for services already provided.

- *Medical management practices* focus on the behavior of the provider with the goal of decreasing behaviors that increase costs. The two most frequently used methods are education and discipline through an identification of specific problems, corrective behavior, and identification of the consequences of failure to change practice.

- *Quality improvement tools.* Quality has always been difficult to define and to determine. Monitoring and evaluation of performance are critical in a system such as managed care that may have greater risks for problems with quality care. If providers are encouraged to provide care at lower costs, they must ensure that care is appropriate for the patient's needs. This monitoring must be ongoing and comprehensive. The following utilization control objectives have been identified for PPOs:[18(pp.103–104)]

  1. to provide the data necessary for identifying areas of underutilization, overutilization, and inefficient utilization of resources

  2. to assist providers in identifying and eliminating medically unnecessary services

  3. to measure the aspects of quality assessment that relate to efficiency, effectiveness, timeliness, appropriateness, accessibility, and acceptability of services

4. to provide the tools necessary to evaluate the impact of cost-containment activities on the quality of care and to determine the point at which quality may be compromised
5. to provide the technical expertise necessary to evaluate diagnostic and/or treatment protocols to ensure that both quality and cost-effectiveness issues are addressed in the evaluations
6. to create an environment of cooperation among hospitals, physicians, and other providers as common goals and objectives are identified and addressed
7. to provide the necessary mechanisms by which structure and process can be objectively evaluated and change can be instituted
8. to provide a mechanism for responding to questions related to cost or quality raised by payers
9. to provide the information necessary to document performance and to provide information to patients, regulators, and others as appropriate

Many of these techniques have developed into policing rather than facilitating, and this is problematic for health care providers, as well as for patients and their families/SOs.

THE HOME CARE NURSE AND MANAGED CARE

Home care nursing has been and will continue to be affected by managed care. Patients will be admitted to home care in more acute conditions than in the past, due to the influence of managed care on the length of stay in hospitals and on the denial of hospitalization. Adaptation of nursing care to these changes will be critical. Nursing assessments and nursing interventions must be developed to respond quickly to the psychiatric patient. If patients have a limited number of home care visits approved by their managed care plans, discharge planning from home care will become even more critical. To prepare patients and families/SOs for earlier home care discharge, education will be an important component of care. There will be a greater need for coordinated care and for documentation of outcomes. The nursing process is consistent with the process of care used by managed care and should help nurses adapt to managed care demands.

Ethical Concerns[19]

Ethical concerns related to managed care and health care reform cannot be ignored. Some of the positive ethical considerations related to these changes include more emphasis on the basic right to care, equity, benign cost-consciousness, efficiency, informed consumer involvement, and required sharing of quality review and outcomes. There are also negative ethical concerns, such as the possibility of undertreatment through inappropriate utilization to decrease costs; excessive profit motives; loss of choice regarding the provider and treatment options; cost-benefit analysis making it difficult to make trade-offs in treatment; and rationing. These are not new ethical concerns for health care providers; however, they may become more important. With managed care intervening in the care process, the home care nurse may find that the role of patient advocate is more complex.

Effects of Managed Care on Clinical Practice

Psychiatric care is complex. Definitions of diagnoses, descriptions of treatments, and determinations of outcomes are difficult to describe, and it is difficult to gain a professional consensus about these issues. There are the additional difficulties of predicting lengths of stay and costs and, in many cases, determining the success of a specific treatment. Although these issues existed before managed care and will continue, new problems may arise due to the managed care approach.[20] Clinical decisions may be based on the benefits package alone. The relationship between health care provider and patient has becomes a triangle, with the third-party payer playing a pivotal role. The treatment focus is each individual episode of illness rather than the illness over time. For patients with chronic problems, such as schizophrenia, this approach limits the care that they require. It limits clinical decisions to short-term interventions rather than consideration of information about the effectiveness of short-term and long-term interventions. If additional treatment in a particular setting (such as an inpatient unit) is denied and yet the patient still requires care, managed care often offers no alternatives; managed care fails to take advantage of such alternatives as partial hospitalization, intensive outpatient therapy, home care, psychiatric rehabilitation programs, halfway houses, etc. Another problem may occur with patients who are prone to manipulate and increase staff conflicts; when the third-party payer becomes involved in treatment decisions and there is disagreement with staff about those decisions, this may only feed into the patient's psychopathology.

To be successful, managed care must provide appropriate, quality care at the lowest possible cost. Health care providers need to identify possible effects on clinical practice and to develop plans to cope with these potential problems positively, or they will affect outcomes negatively. Access, underutilization, and denial of care will be frequent problems as the nurse works with managed care to get the best care for the psychiatric client. Fiscal management of services has often led to the failure "to recognize that chronicity and recidivism in psychiatric illness are inevitable aspects of the disorders and not simply the by-product of the patient's weakness or the clinician's ineptitude and greed."[21(p.326)]

As patient advocates, nurses have responsibilities to protect patients' rights and interests related to their treatment, and this is especially important in the managed care process. Home care agencies help to do this by developing and implementing policies that do the following:[22]

- Provide accurate and current documentation describing the reason for home care treatment, why continued treatment is required, and why specific modalities are being used. Homebound status must be supported with data.
- Develop treatment plans that are realistic and based on patients' needs with short- and long-term goals for specific treatment with appropriate time frames. Patients and their families/SOs should be included in the planning.
- Prepare objective information to support clinical decisions, especially those that might be questioned. Such sources might be research data, legal cases, and outcome studies.
- Develop a communication system for contact between the home care agency staff and the managed care staff.
- Provide proper release of information when required.
- Appeal any refusals to certify for treatment when deemed inappropriate; inform patients that they may seek legal counsel if appeal denied.

SUMMARY

Some authors argue that managed care in psychiatry is reinventing the wheel, because managed care has been done in public sector psychiatry. Although this is not a totally fair assessment, it does make one important point. Public sector psychiatry has tried to develop alternatives for hospitalization and manage the patient's treatment. In some communities, this has been more successful than others. According to Shore: "The aim in the most sophisticated public systems has been to titrate care so that patients receive all the care they need and no more. Achieving this goal requires a system of care that permits patients to move easily among services as determined by clinical needs rather than financial criteria. Operating such systems requires skilled clinical judgment and reduced barriers between service components in areas related to records, confidentiality, and admission and discharge procedures."[23(p.205)] This is a legitimate goal for all managed care, and one that has not been reached. It is this goal that home care staff will find themselves constantly battling to support as they provide care for the psychiatric patient in the home.

NOTES

1. U. Himali, "Managed Care: Does the Promise Meet the Potential?" *The American Nurse* 27, no. 4 (1995): 1–20, at 1.
2. M. Shore, "Managed Care: Reinventing the Wheel," *Hospital and Community Psychiatry* 43, no. 3 (1992): 202–207, at 205.
3. American Academy of Nursing, *Managed Care and National Health Care Reform: Nurses Can Make It Work, Working Paper* (Washington, DC: 1993), 29–33.
4. R. Schreter, "Ten Trends in Managed Care and Their Impact on the Biopsychosocial Model," *Hospital and Community Psychiatry* 44, no. 4 (1993): 325–327, at 327.
5. M. Freeman et al., *Managed Behavioral Healthcare: History, Models, Key Issues, and Future Course* (Washington, DC: U.S. Department of Health and Human Services, U.S. Center for Mental Health Services, October 5, 1994), 1–48, at 9–10.
6. Freeman, *Managed Behavioral Healthcare*, 1–2.
7. Freeman, *Managed Behavioral Healthcare*, 2.
8. Freeman, *Managed Behavioral Healthcare*, 1–2.
9. D. Madison and T. Konrad, "Large Medical Group-Practice Organizations and Employed Physicians: A Relationship Transition," *Milbank Memorial Quarterly* 66, no. 2 (1988): 250.
10. L. Hicks et al., *Role of the Nurse in Managed Care* (Washington, DC: American Nurses Association, 1993), 1.
11. American Academy of Nursing, *Managed Care and National Health Care Reform*, 14.
12. Hicks et al., *Role of the Nurse in Managed Care*.
13. Hicks et al., *Role of the Nurse in Managed Care*.
14. Schreter, "Ten Trends in Managed Care," 325.
15. Freeman, *Managed Behavioral Healthcare*, 8.
16. Hicks et al., *Role of the Nurse in Managed Care*, 24–28.
17. Hicks et al., *Role of the Nurse in Managed Care*, 29–33.
18. D. Cobbs, ed., *Preferred Provider Organizations: Strategies for Sponsors and Network Providers* (Chicago: American Hospital Publishing, 1989), 103–104.
19. American Academy of Nursing, *Managed Care and National Health Care Reform*, 21–22.
20. Schreter, "Ten Trends in Managed Care," 326–327.
21. Schreter, "Ten Trends in Managed Care," 326.
22. M. Weingart, "Community Managed Healthcare: An Experience," *Nursing Management* 22, no. 1 (1991): 40–41.
23. Shore, "Managed Care: Reinventing the Wheel," 205.

SUGGESTED READING

Christianson, J., and F. Osher. 1994. Health maintenance organizations, health care reform, and persons with serious mental illness. *Hospital and Community Psychiatry* 45, no. 9: 898–905.
Fishel, L. et al. 1993. A preliminary study of recidivism under managed mental health care. *Hospital and Community Psychiatry* 44, no. 10: 919–920.

Hanston, R., and M. Washburn. 1994. *Clinical delegation skills: A handbook for nurses.* Gaithersburg, MD: Aspen Publishers, Inc.

Hood, L., and S. Sharfstein. 1992. Managed care for patients who are treatment resistant. *Hospital and Community Psychiatry* 43, no. 8: 774–775.

Lazarus, A. 1995. The role of primary care physicians in managed mental health care. *Psychiatric Services* 46, no. 4: 343–345.

Olsen, D. 1994. Ethical considerations of managed care in mental health treatment. *Journal of Psychosocial Nursing* 32, no. 3: 25–28.

Pomerantz, J. 1995. A managed care ethical credo: For clinicians only? *Psychiatric Services* 46, no. 4: 329–330.

Sabin, J. 1994. A credo for ethical managed care in mental health practice. *Hospital and Community Psychiatric* 45, no. 9: 859–860.

Shore, M., and A. Biegel. 1996. The challenges posed by managed behavioral health care. *New England Journal of Medicine* 334, no. 2: 116–118.

Case Management: Beyond the Walls

INTRODUCTION

Case management is still a very new system in health care. How it will develop and the effects it will have on other systems continue to be unclear, and there is great diversity in case management programs. According to Redford, "Although the components of the case management process, e.g., assessment, care or service planning, and the arrangement, monitoring, reassessment and evaluation of services, are defined similarly across programs, disciplines, and specialty fields, the ways in which these components are implemented are highly diverse."[1(p.5)]

PURPOSE OF CASE MANAGEMENT FOR THE PSYCHIATRIC PATIENT

Case management helps patients who have "substantial deficits in their social skills, judgment, and initiative that interfere with successful community functioning. Thus as case managers help patients negotiate with a complex social environment, their role can be conceptualized more accurately as one of 'travel agent.'"[2(p.362)] Cohen and Cesta report that "In general, case management has been associated with reduced total costs per patient case, decreased patient length of hospital stay, increased patient turnover, and potential increase in hospital-generated revenues."[3(p.166)] In this age of health care reform and cost containment, these are good words to hear; however, as case management programs develop, further research is required. Because there is no single right way to implement case management, it may not be easy to compare costs and cost-effectiveness between programs. Development of case management and its initial implementation is expensive, and staff time is required. As costs for the program are identified, management should analyze the budgetary effects of case management on other aspects of home care delivery. Because case management does not exist in isolation, it should never be analyzed in isolation.

DESCRIPTION OF CASE MANAGEMENT

There is no single definition of case management; however, most definitions identify the characteristics of continuity of care, individualization, comprehensiveness of services, and longitudinality or providing services over time.[4] Some definitions focus on brokering case management, which emphasizes providing patients with appropriate environmental supports. Others emphasize clinical case management, in which the case manager assumes some clinical responsibilities. This type of case manager is most like the home care nurse. Between these two types of case management are many variations. According to Bachrach, "There is great uncertainty within the mental health field about whether case management should be regarded as an administrative task, a nonclinical direct service, or a clinical specialty."[5(p.467)] This uncertainty may carry over into psychiatric home care. It is important that home care staff understand the concept of case management, because they may be interacting with case managers from psychiatric inpatient programs, other psychiatric facilities, and managed care organizations.

Kanter describes clinical case management as "a modality of mental health practice that, in coordination with the traditional psychiatric focus on biological and psychological functioning, addresses the overall maintenance of the mentally ill person's physical and social environment with the goals of facilitating his or her physical survival, personal growth, community participation, and recovery from or adaptation to mental illness."[6(p.361)] Clinical case management is not simply an administrative system for coordinating services, which is probably the most common view of its purpose. Kanter's description emphasizes the many components of case management. The following principles should be considered as a case management program is developed, implemented, and monitored:[7]

- Continuity of care emphasizes the patient's need for support and treatment over an extended period of time. This requires an ongoing relationship with the case manager who understands the patient's past and present illness, functioning, and social resources.
- The case management relationship is very important in developing a collaborative relationship with the patient, family, and other caregivers.
- Titrating support and structure is a critical part of case management, and it is more than brokering services for the patient. The case manager collaborates with patients and social networks in titrating the levels of environmental support and structure needed to facilitate survival, personal development, and

adaptation. The case manager is concerned with both inadequate and excessive interventions.

- Flexibility is part of case management, or case management will fail when the patient changes.
- Facilitating patient resourcefulness necessitates helping the patient manage his or her own life.

Bower's description of case management includes the following elements:[8]

- Case management is a *system* that focuses on achievement of patient outcomes for the episode of the illness within all treatment settings for that episode. Its critical elements are assessment and problem identification; planning; procurement, delivery, and coordination of services; and monitoring to ensure that needs are met.
- Case management is a *role* in that the patient has a health care provider who coordinates his or her care.
- As a *technology*, case management generates tools and techniques to assist in organizing care.
- The case management *process* expands on all of the components of the nursing process.
- As a *service*, it provides facilitating and gatekeeping functions for the patient.

To be successful, the case management program should have the following characteristics:[9]

- is episode-based
- is longitudinally based (across the continuum of illness)
- is targeted at selected patient populations
- offers coordination of services
- is quality-outcome driven
- is fiscally aware and responsive
- is focused on patients and families/significant others (SOs)
- is collaborative
- provides accessible services
- is proactive

The agency's decision to develop and implement case management requires careful thought and planning for its implementation. It will affect the home care delivery system, and this requires careful analysis. Home care nurses will often be required to work with case managers from managed care organization or the patient's third-party payer.

CASE MANAGEMENT FUNCTIONS

Generally case managers are gatekeepers and facilitators of the health care system. They also help patients make informed decisions.[10] The American Nurses Association (ANA) has identified primary functions of a nurse case manager that are important. Others may be added as required for a specific home care program. These functions are as follows:[11(p.21)]

- coordinating care and services, including coordination of care and service providers responsible for furnishing services needed by a given patient and, in many models, of all payment sources that reimburse providers for those services
- case-finding and screening to identify appropriate patients for case management
- assessing comprehensively the patient's goals, as well as his or her physical, functional, psychological, social, environmental, and financial status
- assessing the patient's informal and formal support systems
- analyzing and synthesizing all data to formulate appropriate nursing diagnoses and/or interdisciplinary problem statements
- developing, implementing, monitoring, and modifying a plan of care through an interdisciplinary and collaborative team process, in conjunction with the client and his or her caregivers
- linking the patient with the most appropriate institutional or community resources, advocating on behalf of the patient for scarce resources, and developing new resources if gaps exist in the service continuum
- procuring services, including eligibility decisions and authorizing hospitalization and home care, which is essential in some programs
- problem solving with the patient, family/SOs, other health care professionals, and home care staff
- facilitating access
- providing direct patient care (in some programs)
- providing liaison services to other agencies and resources
- educating the patient, the family, and community support services; facilitating the goal of self-care for the patient and his or her family
- facilitating communication with all concerned with the patient's care
- documenting planning, interventions, and results
- monitoring the patient's progress toward goal achievement and periodically reassessing changes in health status
- monitoring the plan to ensure the quality, quantity, timeliness, and effectiveness of services; providing periodic reassessment to assure that services are appropriate, cost-effective, and not increasing the patient's dependence

- monitoring activities to ensure that services are actually being delivered and meet the needs of the patient
- evaluating patient and program outcomes to determine whether the patient should be discharged or assigned inactive status

This is a long list of functions, most of which are done by a home care nurse. Thus, in many cases, the home care nurse holds a dual position of care provider and case manager, even if the position is not identified as such. Home care agencies that use case management must develop a position description that outlines these functions and an appropriate performance appraisal form for the case manager.

CASE MANAGEMENT DOCUMENTATION

Documentation requirements for a case management system vary from home care agency to home care agency.[12] If the agency is directly associated with a hospital, the case management documentation system should be coordinated with the hospital's system, as many of the referrals will come from the hospital.

Two types of documentation that relate directly to the clinical process are critical paths and case management plans. These forms of documentation are similar to standard care plans and protocols. These methods are used in most case management programs. The *case management plan* is a plan that "articulates particular clinical problems which patients and families are likely to encounter, along with interventions expected to resolve these problems. These are outlined within specific time frames."[13(p.53)] The case management plan is interdisciplinary and includes expected outcomes for each of the disciplines that might be involved in the care. Nursing problems or diagnoses must still be addressed and clear in the documentation. A *critical path* defines the critical or key events that may happen for a particular time period during the treatment of the episode of illness with appropriate interventions. The timeline might be based on hours, days, weeks, or months. The critical path provides a sequencing of interventions. It is an abbreviated form of the case management plan. Variances from the case management plan require analysis by the case manager. A variance is when something does not happen when it is expected to happen; the case management plan should specify what constitutes a variance. For example, if the plan indicates that the patient assessment should be completed during the first home visit, the leeway might be identified as "During Visit 1." Delays may be categorized in the following ways:[14]

- *operational delays*—delay in receiving messages, laboratory report lost, inadequate staffing, inadequate information received regarding appointment cancellation

- *health care provider delays*—physician preference or practice pattern difference; occupational therapist not available for assessment
- *patient delays*—patient refusal of medication, patient complication/suicidal ideation, patient refusal to see home care staff
- *unmet clinical indicator delays*—when the clinical indicator (such as "by the third home visit the patient will identify the following about his or her medications: name, purpose, side effects and interventions that might be taken, dosage and frequency, and how the patient will obtain prescription and medication") is not met. The analysis of these variances is documented, and plans are changed as required. When health care provider variances occur, discretion must be used in documenting these variances due to increased risk of liability. Stating facts is critical, and subjective information should not be included.

Each home care agency has many documentation requirements. During the planning stages for case management, all documentation that is relevant should be reviewed to determine how case management might affect it. One change in documentation often means that other aspects must be changed or are obsolete. Duplication must be avoided.

Case management is monitored by the home care quality assessment (QA) program. Monitors need to be developed to assess the effectiveness of the program. Indicators might focus on improved patient outcome, patient and family/SO satisfaction, staff satisfaction, referral source satisfaction, physician satisfaction, communication and collaboration, and costs.

PATIENT SELECTION CRITERIA

Determining which patients would benefit from case management is one step in the planning process. Most programs focus on patients who are high risk, high volume, and/or high cost. Possible candidates for case management include patients diagnosed with schizophrenia, major depression, or dual diagnosis; patients with multiple relapses and a history of noncompliance; patients with complex medical problems and psychiatric diagnoses; and patients with complex or fragile support systems. Case management is particularly helpful for patients who have difficulty negotiating the service system and managing their own care. In the past, when psychiatric inpatient stays were longer, patients learned more compliant behavior that prepared them to accept services.[15] This preparation made adjustment to a case management program easier. Today, patients who stay in the hospital for short periods of time or who are not hospitalized may be less compliant. This characteristic is not necessarily negative; however, it must be considered as the case management relationship is developed.

THE HOME CARE CASE MANAGER FOR THE PSYCHIATRIC PATIENT

What Are the Characteristics and Qualifications of the Case Manager?

The case manager is a staff member who is committed to the program and willing to take risks. Collaboration is critical and, thus, a staff member who is able to collaborate will be more successful. Keeping lines of communication open supports the process and ultimately helps the patient. A conflict can easily arise between the case management role and the strategies for promoting the patient's self-care potential.[16] Case management provides support and direct guidance to the patient, and this can deny the patient some responsibility for self-care. The case manager must be very aware of this potential conflict and make all efforts to balance the two.

What Training Is Required?[17]

Considering the extensive roles of the case manager, most home care staff require training for this new position. Training is based on the knowledge base that is required to fulfill case manager functions. The following seven training content areas are recommended:

1. in-depth psychiatric clinical knowledge and skills
2. care resources both in the hospital and the community (such as partial hospitalization programs, outpatient clinics, self-help groups, family support groups, assistance with housing, psychiatric home care, long-term care facilities, and training programs)
3. teaching skills
4. discharge planning
5. health care financial information including third-party payer systems and government payment systems
6. management skills
7. quality assessment and improvement

Orientation and ongoing education is important. Many educational programs are being offered that provide opportunities for staff to learn about case management. These programs can be excellent sources of ongoing education; however, as is true for all information gained from an outside educational program, it must be assessed in conjunction with the setting in which it will be applied. Ongoing educational opportunities within the home care agency must also be offered to meet the educational needs of individual case managers.

What Is the Case Management Process?[18]

The case management process, which is very similar to the nursing process, is composed of several steps. A multidimensional, functional assessment is the first step in the process. Data from this assessment are then used to develop the written service plan, which must be done in collaboration with the patient and the family/SOs. The case manager uses brokering, negotiation, conflict resolution, and creative persuasion during all phases of the process. To implement the plan, the case manager must identify the client's formal and informal support network and the willingness of those resources to help the patient. Awareness of the costs of services is critical when choosing services to meet the patient's needs. The case manager must monitor the care, following up to ensure that it is implemented appropriately, adequately, and effectively. Throughout the case management process, reassessment must be done. The patient will change, and needs will change.

To Whom Does the Case Manager Report?

It is important to identify clearly to whom the case manager reports. This may vary from one home care agency to another. However, the case manager should report to one person, who is clearly identified in the position description for the case manager.

SUMMARY

According to Williams, "Case management is fast becoming one of the health care buzz words of the 90s. Despite its popularity, everyone has a different view about what it is, who should do it, how it should be used, whether it is cost effective, and how eventual outcomes can be measured. Nevertheless, case management is here to stay, and many questions arise as various disciplines scramble to claim ownership of the process."[19(p.33)] Dvoskin and Steadman state that "Intensive case management is not a panacea. It will fail if appropriate treatment and human services are not available in the community."[20(p.684)] In the home care setting, case management may have a direct and indirect influence on the patient's care. When the roles of the home care nurse and the case manager are compared, it is difficult to see the differences in the two roles. The home care nurse often interacts, usually by telephone, with the patient's third-party payer case manager. Thus, it is important for the home care nurse to understand the role of the case manager in the patient's treatment.

NOTES

1. L. Redford, "Case Management: The Wave of the Future," *Journal of Case Management* 1, no. 1 (1992): 5–8, at 5.

2. J. Kanter, "Clinical Case Management: Definition, Principles, and Components," *Hospital and Community Psychiatry* 40, no. 4 (1989): 361–368, at 362.

3. E. Cohen and T. Cesta, *Nursing Case Management: From Concept to Evaluation* (St. Louis, MO: Mosby–Year Book, 1993), 166.

4. L. Bachrach, "Continuity of Care and Approaches to Case Management for Long-Term Mentally Ill Patients," *Hospital and Community Psychiatry* 44, no. 5 (1993): 465–468, at 465.

5. Bachrach, "Continuity of Care and Approaches to Case Management," 467.

6. Kanter, "Clinical Case Management," 361.

7. Kanter, "Clinical Case Management," 363.

8. K. Bower, *Case Management by Nurses* (Washington, DC: American Nurses Association, 1992), 4.

9. Bower, *Case Management by Nurses*, 12.

10. D. Pittman, "Nursing Case Management: Holistic Care for the Deinstitutionalized Chronically Mentally Ill," *Journal of Psychosocial Nursing* 27, no. 11 (1989): 23–26, at 23.

11. Bower, *Case Management by Nurses*, 21.

12. A. Finkelman, *Psychiatric Nursing Administration Manual* (Gaithersburg, MD: Aspen Publishers, Inc., 1995), 5–3:6–5–3:7.

13. K. Giuliano and C. Poirer, "Nursing Case Management: Critical Pathways to Desirable Outcomes," *Nursing Management* 22, no. 3 (1991): 52–55, at 53.

14. Cohen and Cesta, *Nursing Case Management*, 122.

15. J. Dvoskin and H. Steadman, "Using Intensive Case Management to Reduce Violence by Mentally Ill Persons in the Community," *Hospital and Community Psychiatry* 45, no. 7 (1994): 679–684, at 681.

16. Redford, "Case Management: The Wave of the Future," 6.

17. Finkelman, *Psychiatric Nursing Administration Manual*, 5–3:6.

18. Redford, "Case Management: The Wave of the Future," 6–8.

19. R. Williams, "Nurse Case Management: Working with the Community," *Nursing Management* 23, no. 12 (1992): 33–34.

20. Dvoskin and Steadman, "Using Intensive Care Management to Reduce Violence by Mentally Ill Persons in the Community," 684.

SUGGESTED READING

Bower, K. 1992. *Case management by nurses*. Washington, DC: American Nurses Association.

Brennan, J., and C. Kaplan. 1993. Setting new standards for social work case management. *Hospital and Community Psychiatry* 44, no. 3: 219–222.

Case Management Society of America. 1995. *Standards of practice for case management*. Little Rock, AR.

Cohen, E., and T. Cesta. 1993. *Nursing case management: From concept to evaluation.* St. Louis, MO: Mosby–Year Book.

Dongen, C., and J. Jambunathan. 1992. Pilot study results: The psychiatric RN case manager. *Journal of Psychosocial Nursing* 30, no. 11: 11–14.

Dubler, N. 1992. Individual advocacy as a governing principle. *Journal of Case Management* 1, no. 3: 82–86.

Dvoskin, J., and H. Steadman. 1994. Using intensive case management to reduce violence by mentally ill persons in the community. *Hospital and Community Psychiatry* 45, no. 7: 679–684.

Ethridge, P., and Lamb, G. 1989. Professional nursing case management improves quality, access, and cost. *Nursing Management* 20, no. 3: 30–35.

Giron, S., and D. Chassler. 1994. The quest of uniform guidelines for long-term care case management. *Journal of Case Management* 3, no. 3: 91–97.

LaPierre, E., and J. Padget. 1992. What does a nurse need to know and do to maintain effective level of case management? *Journal of Psychosocial Nursing* 30, no. 3: 35–39.

Maurin, J. 1990. Case management: Caring for psychiatric clients. *Journal of Psychosocial Nursing* 28, no. 7: 7–12.

McGurrin, M., and M. Worley. 1983. Evaluation of intensive case management for seriously and persistently mentally ill persons. *Journal of Case Management* 2, no. 2: 59–65.

Mound, B. et al. 1991. The expanded role of nurse case managers. *Journal of Psychosocial Nursing* 29, no. 6: 18–22.

Mullahy, C. 1995. *The case manager's handbook.* Gaithersburg, MD: Aspen Publishers, Inc.

Pitman, D. 1989. Nursing case management: Holistic care for the deinstitutionalized chronically mentally ill. *Journal of Psychosocial Nursing* 27, no. 11: 23–27.

Seuntjens, A. 1995. Case management/care management. In *Advanced nursing practice*, ed. M. Snyder and M. Michaelene, 135–152. New York: Springer.

Willenbring, M. 1994. Case management applications in substance abuse disorders. *Journal of Case Management* 3, no. 4: 150–157.

Zander, K. 1994. Nurses and case management: To control or to collaborate? In *Current Issues in Nursing*, ed. J. McCloskey and H. Grace, 254–260. St. Louis, MO: Mosby.

Application of the Nursing Care Process to the Psychiatric Home Care Patient

CHAPTER

10

Psychiatric Assessment and Diagnosis

INTRODUCTION

When a patient returns home from the hospital, he or she experiences many feelings about the hospitalization and the reason for the hospitalization. The patient may feel responsible for the problems that led to the hospitalization. Family or significant others (SOs) may say or imply that the patient could have done better. It is a sensitive time for the patient, filled with fears of failure and concern for the future. In most cases, the patient's first encounter with the home care nurse is for the home care admission assessment. This sets the stage for home care and provides the initial information for the treatment plan; however, reassessment during the period of home care is required to determine whether changes have occurred in the patient that indicate the need for adjustments in the treatment plan. The assessment is the essential first step in the treatment process with a psychiatric home care patient. According to Mosher and Burti, "The ability to implement a psychosocial intervention depends on a shared understanding of the patient's current situation, of the life experiences involved in its development, and of the resources available for dealing with the problem, as defined by the patient."[1(p.52)] All psychiatric home care patients have some difficulties with relationships with others. It is one of the reasons that they need help. The treatment process itself, beginning with the assessment, places the patient directly in a situation in which the patient is asked to work in a relationship with the home care staff. Thus, the assessment process cannot really be considered as a process that is separate from the treatment process. Although these two components are separated when the nursing process is described, it is important to recognize that assessment provides information for treatment decisions and that obtaining this information is also a part of the patient's treatment.

HOSPITALIZATION VERSUS COMMUNITY CARE

Psychiatric observation in the hospital and in the home are different. Exhibit 10–1 identifies some of these differences that are important in providing care to psychiatric patients in the home, especially new patients. The home care nurse must recognize the differences and understand both the strengths and limitations of assessing the patient in the home. In the home the nurse can focus on one patient at a time, but in the home there are fewer immediate resources and support for the nurse.

Mosher and Burti have written about community mental health; this information is applicable to the psychiatric home care setting, which is part of community mental health. According to these authors, hospital-based care is not required for most disturbed patients if [2(p.31)]

- in-home family crisis intervention is available
- a properly organized intentional social environment is available to those who cannot be maintained in the family environment or do not have a social network that can be organized to act as a temporary caregiver; and
- the identified patient is not a battle scarred veteran of the mental health wars ("chronic") who is so attached to (the idea of) hospitals that he/she or the family is unwilling to accept treatment that does not include hospitalization

There are times, however, when hospitalization should be used for patients, such as when they require the following:[3(p.37)]

- complex, technologically sophisticated, diagnostic processes that require frequent observation by specially trained personnel available only in hospitals

---

Exhibit 10–1 Hospital and Home Observation

Hospital	*Home*
Narrow focus	Broader agenda
Direct technical data	Direct personal data
Extensive resources	Limited resources
Professional team	Family team
"Generic" care	Patient-specific care

Source: Reproduced by permission of the National Association for Home Care, from *CARING* Magazine XI, no. 5 (May 1992).

- initiation of a treatment process with risks that need to be monitored over a period of time by specially trained personnel, e.g., preplanned drug detoxification, beginning lithium or neuroleptic drugs in persons with complicated medical problems
- medical treatment of a person sufficiently disturbed, suicidal, or homicidal so as to render care elsewhere too difficult for the staff, other patients, families, or significant others
- treatment of acute intoxicated states, e.g., alcohol, PCP, cocaine
- management of agitated, overactive, acutely psychotic persons who leave open settings and are a serious danger to themselves because of confusion and disorganization

Access to an emergency department that offers psychiatric evaluation is important in psychiatric home care to assist in determining when a patient might benefit from more intensive treatment. It is an important resource for the home care nurse. All home care agencies that provide psychiatric home care should establish a relationship with the staff of the local emergency departments and crisis intervention clinics. When a psychiatric assessment is done on admission to home care, the nurse must always consider whether the patient requires more intensive care. There are also times when, as a result of reassessment, the nurse must consider a change in the patient's status that might indicate a need for more intensive treatment, such as partial hospitalization or hospitalization. Local psychiatric emergency resources are very important in the decision-making process. The nurse must also consider past experiences that the patient and the family/SOs have had with emergency resources, as these will affect their willingness to seek emergency assistance. Chapter 29 discusses crises and emergencies in the home in more detail.

THE ASSESSMENT IN THE HOME ENVIRONMENT

As each assessment is conducted, the nurse considers three critical issues: potential duplication of services, the focus of nursing interventions, and service benefits for the patient.[4] The assessment in the home is conducted in the patient's territory. The home care nurse has less control than the nurse in a hospital or outpatient setting over interruptions, noise, and—more importantly—the patient. The assessment process includes the following:

- preparation (e.g., setting up the initial appointment, contacting the patient's physician(s), contacting the referral source, reviewing any available medical records, preparing any forms required for the initial assessment)
- greeting the patient and family/SOs

- determining where in the patient's home to conduct the assessment
- setting the interview guidelines (e.g., explaining the purpose of the interview to the patient, emphasizing confidentiality and who will review the information, discussing the importance of the family's/SOs' participation, asking the patient to participate in the assessment and treatment process)
- collecting the data (e.g., asking the necessary questions, encouraging the patient to share as much information as possible during the assessment)
- terminating the interview (e.g., asking if the patient has any questions or concerns; developing the plan with the patient and, when appropriate, with the family/SOs)
- setting up the next appointment, determining with whom and for what purpose
- documenting the assessment (e.g., completing the assessment/admission forms and other required documentation)
- initiating nursing care (e.g., communicating with other home care staff, establishing the time schedule for nursing care, initiating interventions)

Goals of Psychiatric Assessment

The Joint Commission on Accreditation of Healthcare Organizations (Joint Commission) identifies the overall goal of the assessment function as the determination of "the care and services to be provided by the organization through the assessment of the patient's needs."[5(p.5)] Jernigan identifies overall goals for psychiatric treatment that should be considered prior to identifying the specific assessment goals for an individual patient. These are as follows:[6(p.7)]

- to determine the maladjustment or coping dysfunction, e.g., nursing diagnosis
- to interrupt any repetitive, destructive mental patterns, and assist patient/family/SOs to
  1. become aware of their destructive patterning/mind set
  2. assess/correct over-exaggerations, and misconceptions or faulty interpretations of their surroundings
  3. see the benefit of overcoming this patterning
  4. believe the risk of trying is worth the effort
  5. gain some understanding of the cause, e.g., results from their stress
  6. believe they can gain some control; that effort will produce results
- to assist patient/family/SOs in restorative mental health:
  1. strengthen adaptive responses and capabilities
  2. reduce actual potential impact from stressor
  3. assist in alleviating knowledge deficits regarding home care
  4. maximize available support systems
  5. utilize stressful situation as potential for inner growth and family strength.

When the goals for the psychiatric assessment are met, treatment goals are developed and implemented. The overall goals for the assessment are as follows:

- to gather pertinent data about the patient, strengths and limitations, significant others, and resources
- to begin to establish a collaborative working relationship with the patient
- to determine the direction that treatment will take
- to decrease the patient's anxiety about home care
- to develop an evolving and compassionate understanding of the patient.

The assessment is "the systematic process of collecting relevant patient data for the purpose of determining actual or potential health problems and functional status."[7(p.42)] The assessment or database is completed during the admission, and reassessment is conducted throughout the home care process.

The assessment process communicates to the patient that the nurse is interested in the patient. Why does the patient stay up all night drinking coffee and listening to music? Is the patient just being stubborn? Sleeping too much during the day? Experiencing a medication side effect? Staying up because he or she does not care? Or is the patient experiencing auditory hallucinations that are interrupting sleep? Simply collecting data is not assessment. The process includes gathering data to assess the patient's needs and analyzing those data to create the information necessary to develop the interventions to meet the patient's needs. Interpretation of data must be done in order to make decisions about patient care.

Components of the Nursing Assessment

The Joint Commission home care standards identify the following psychiatric and nonpsychiatric components of the assessment:[8]

- physical status
- nutritional status
- functional status
- discharge planning needs
- identification of possible victims of abuse
- emotional, behavioral, and psychosocial assessments

Gerace has identified two levels of a psychiatric home care nursing assessment, the macrolevel and the microlevel assessment. These are described in Exhibit 10–2. The macrolevel assessment, which provides data about the circumstances in which the patient lives that will help to identify potential or actual daily problems, focuses on three major areas. The first is the community and its resources for the patient and family/SO (such as mental health services, pharmacy, and support and advocacy groups). Familiarity with these and other resources

Exhibit 10–2 Macrolevel and Microlevel Assessment Plan

Macrolevel Assessment	Microlevel Assessment
Community	Patient's level of functioning
Atmosphere	Mental status
Facilities	Management of illness
Mental health resources	Medication compliance
	Activities of daily living
Home environment	Psychosocial stressors
Physical features	Situational
Privacy	Illness-induced
Family response	Family caregiver burden
Conceptualization of illness	Objective
Relationship with mental health care providers	Subjective
Family-patient interaction	

Source: Reprinted from L. Gerace, "Nursing Assessment in Psychiatric Home Health Care," *Journal of Home Health Care Practice,* Vol. 2, No. 3, p. 10, © 1990, Aspen Publishers, Inc.

will expedite interventions. Other community assessment factors might include safety of the neighborhood, accessibility of alcohol and other drugs, and transportation accessibility. Each of these may make it difficult for the patient to obtain long-term community care or may prevent progress. The second area is the home environment, particularly the physical environment and the availability of privacy for both the patient and the family/SOs. The third macrolevel assessment area is the family's response to the patient in the home, their understanding of the illness, their relationship with health care providers, and the family-patient interaction. The microlevel assessment focuses on specific data about the patient's status, including psychosocial, physical, and functional data. It also provides data about the family/caregiver burden, which is discussed in more detail in Chapter 3. Microlevel data combined with data from the macrolevel assessment will help to identify the patient's stressors.

Assessment Questions[9]

Each home care agency's assessment will be different in some of the content areas, format, and phrasing of specific questions. Questions that are usually covered in some manner include the following:

- What symptoms of mental illness is the patient experiencing? (Consider both thought patterns and affect.)
- What areas of functioning are impaired, and to what degree?
- Is the patient's behavior being influenced by delusions or hallucinations; and if so, to what degree?
- What is the patient's participation in activities of daily living, such as personal hygiene, household chores, and socializing?
- Does the patient acknowledge the presence of mental illness?
- What does the patient know about his or her illness?
- To what degree does the patient participate in the management of the illness (e.g., developing personal treatment goals, setting clinic appointments, taking medications)?
- Can the patient identify changes that signal potential relapse?

At the conclusion of the assessment, the nurse should be able to comment about each of these areas based on an analysis of the assessment data.

Functional Assessment

The functional assessment is the assessment of the patient's behavioral assets and deficits. It is very important for patients with serious mental illness and for those who lack social skills, which includes many psychiatric home care patients. According to Liberman, this assessment provides information about the following:[10]

- stressors that may overwhelm the individual's coping skills and competencies in social and instrumental roles, thereby evoking an exacerbation or relapse of symptoms;
- presence or absence of premorbid and current coping skills and competencies that may serve as buffers against stress; and
- the reasons for deficits in an individual's coping and problem-solving skills, such as disuse, reinforcement of the sick role, or loss of motivation

In order to plan care that addresses the patient's problems in living in the community, it is important to understand the patient's coping skills, competencies, deficits, and stressors.

During the functional assessment process, the nurse considers the following:[11]

- behavior deficits, particularly behaviors that need to be initiated, increased in frequency, or strengthened in form
- behavior excesses, particularly behaviors that need to be terminated, decreased in frequency, or altered in form

- behavior assets, particularly strengths in such areas as social skills, activities of daily living, affects, and cognitions
- assessment of symptoms or side effects to determine if they can be better controlled through pharmacotherapy

These are all major nursing concerns. These data help to identify the most common areas in which patients require interventions. When a treatment plan is reviewed, these issues should be addressed: strengths and limitations, learning new coping skills and new behaviors, symptom monitoring, and medication side effects. Because it is difficult to complete the assessment during the admission visit, this analysis will be ongoing. In addition, the patient will change. As the nurse observes patient interactions with others, the nurse will develop a clearer view of the patient's motivations and the antecedents and consequences of the patient's problems.

Klebanoff identifies the following assessment categories as important in the initial assessment, during reassessment, and at the time of discharge from home care:[12(p.762)]

- physical, emotional, intellectual, psychological, social, cultural, religious, spiritual, community, and environmental history; support systems; lifestyle factors; and stressors
- patient and family's growth and development, dynamics, perceptions, vulnerabilities, risk factors, and current and past coping strengths or mechanisms
- sleep, rest, and activity patterns; appetite and nutritional-metabolic patterns; elimination patterns; other patterns and habits affecting health, knowledge, and motivation
- self and role-relationship enactments and patterns, including sexuality-reproductive patterns
- mental and emotional status, including thought processes, perceptual patterns, and cognitive functioning
- understanding of and receptivity to home care, expectations of the psychosocial home care program

In the literature there are many suggestions about what items and questions should be included in the assessment. These suggestions provide guidance as the home care agency develops its own psychiatric home care assessment.

Eisen, Dill, and Grob conducted a research project on the use of a brief patient-report assessment from the patient's perspective to be used for outcome assessment with most psychiatric inpatients.[13] The research focused on inpatients; however, the items in the assessment scale have relevance for psychiatric home care patients. The following items were included in this project to evaluate the outcome of treatment:

- close feelings with others
- recognition and expression of emotions
- relationships outside family
- realistic attitude about self and others
- lack of self-confidence
- goals and direction in life
- relationships with family
- management of day-to-day life
- role functioning
- satisfaction with life
- leisure time and recreation
- apathy or lack of interest in things
- confusion, concentration, memory problem
- independence and autonomy
- suicidal feelings and behavior
- depression and hopelessness
- physical symptoms
- isolation and loneliness
- fear, anxiety, or panic
- adjustment to major life stresses
- impulsive or illegal behavior
- use of illegal drugs or misuse of drugs
- use of alcoholic beverages
- uncontrolled temper, anger, violence
- mood swings, unstable moods
- unreal thoughts or beliefs
- manic or bizarre behavior
- hearing voices or seeing things
- sexual activity or preoccupation

These items might be included in the assessment completed by the nurse as well as in self-assessments completed by the patient.

Assessment Methods

The critical components of data collection include subjective verbal data, objective nonverbal data, symptoms, etiology, risk factors, and critical indicators. The nurse should know what these are in order to identify them in an individual patient. Data will be obtained from the patient, family/SOs, medical records, the physician, and other referral sources. Much of the assessment data can be obtained by conversing with the patient and family/SOs and observing interactions. It is not necessary to obtain all data in a structured interview. As the home care nurse becomes more experienced with the data required, it will become easier to gather the data in a nonstructured way.

Self-report questionnaires, interviews, self-monitoring, behavioral observation, behavioral outcomes, biological measures such as heart rate or biofeedback, drug-behavior interactions, sociocultural measures such as a recent change in relationships or social support are all assessment methods.[14]

The assessment assists staff in understanding the patient by assessing the status of the patient and the patient's family/SO status at the time of admission, previous health care status, and response to previous treatment. This helps to identify potential problems that may occur during home care and after discharge from home care. The nurse wants to understand the patient's view of the world and his or her problems. The assessment notes significant changes in the patient's behavior in such areas as sleep, appetite, hygiene, energy, motivation, self-image, self-esteem, sexual drive, and competence or the patient's understanding of the consequences of his or her behavior. To collect data and ultimately to formulate nursing diagnoses from the data, several assessment methods may be used depending upon the patient, the nurse, and the home environment. Typical data resources are the patient, family/SOs, the home environment, physicians and other health care providers, and past medical records. Common assessment methods that can be used in the home include the following:

- *Interviewing.* Interviewing occurs during the structured admission assessment and throughout home care. Exhibit 10–3 provides sample interview questions.
- *Direct observation.* Direct observation is ongoing; however, there may be times when it should be more conscious, and the nurse should plan what will be observed or guide paraprofessional staff in their observation.
- *History and physical examination.* The history and physical examination must be included in each admission. The extent of the exam varies, depending upon the date of the patient's last exam and the availability of this data, agency policy, and condition of the patient. It should never be assumed that the psychiatric patient does not have physical problems. In addition, many medications may cause physical problems, and many physical problems may cause psychiatric problems. A baseline of vital signs is important when using psychotropic medications that may cause alterations in vital signs.
- *Self-observation.* It is important to help the patient "translate vague and general problem descriptions into more specific or concrete terms."[15] When a

Exhibit 10–3 Assessment Questions and Statements

The following are some examples of questions and statements that might be used by a nurse who interviews a patient for an assessment. These are not intended to be memorized to repeat back to a patient, but rather to offer some examples. Each nurse develops his or her own style. Assessment questions should feel comfortable to the nurse in order to be effective with the patient.

- What led up to the problem?
- What have you done to stop your symptoms?
- Is there anything else you'd like to tell me?
- Have you taken any drugs not prescribed by a doctor? Which drug(s)? How much? When was the last time taken? How long have you been taking the drug(s)?
- Have you ever taken more medication than the doctor prescribed? What medication? What happened when you did this?
- How much do you drink? When did you drink last? What happens when you drink? Have you ever had treatment for drinking?
- Do you smoke? How much? Have you ever tried to stop? What happened?
- Do you feel you have to take drugs or alcohol?
- Have you ever had seizures? Blacked out? How often? When did this last occur?
- How does your mood affect your work? School work? Relationships? Eating? Sleeping?
- Has your appetite changed? In what way?
- It sounds like . . . .
- Can you tell me a little about your (wife, husband, boss, mother, father, etc., as needed)?
- How is your appetite?
- How is your job?
- Share with me some of your thoughts about . . . .
- What made you decide to come to the hospital today?
- You seem . . . .
- When did the problem begin?
- Describe the problem for me.
- I'd like to understand more about . . . .
- Has something happened recently to upset you?
- Have you been under a lot of stress? What kind of stress? When did it begin? How do you react to the stress?
- How are you sleeping? Eating? Working? Is this a change?
- Tell me a little about your close relationships. How are these relationships going?
- Have you been physically sick? In what way?

continues

Exhibit 10–3 continued

- Have you been in a hospital for emotional problems? What was that like for you? When? Where? How long? What do you think that hospitalization did for you?
- Have you seen a professional for your emotional problems in the past? Who? Where? How long? What kind of treatment did you receive? Describe for me the results.
- Do you ever hear or see things that others don't hear or see? What is that like for you? Is it happening now? How often does it happen? Does it happen at any special time? What do you do when it happens? Do the voices tell you to hurt yourself or someone else? Have you ever done what the voices told you to do? What was that like?
- Do you take medications? What? What is the medication for? What does the medication do for you? How much do you take? When?
- What are some of your thoughts about . . . ?
- Does your mood ever change rapidly?
- How would you assess your reaction to anxiety?
- Do you have thoughts that you cannot get out of your mind and that keep repeating? What are these thoughts?
- Do you feel compelled to do something? Can you describe it to me?
- Do things easily upset you?
- What do you do when you get upset?
- Do you have any fears? What?
- What is your energy level lately?
- How do you adapt to change?
- Tell me about that.
- Explain to me what you mean by . . . .
- It would be helpful to understand more about . . . .
- You look . . . .
- That was helpful, now will you tell me about . . . .
- I realize how stressful this time is for you.
- This information is to help us help you.
- How long has this problem been bothering you?
- Whom do you go to for support? Is this person available to you now?
- Tell me about your typical day. What do you do?
- Have you ever felt like striking out at someone else? What happened?
- How would you describe yourself?
- What are your goals for this hospitalization?
- What have been some of your accomplishments?
- What would you describe as some of your limitations?
- If you feel you have experienced some failures in your life, how would you describe these? How did you cope with them?
- How do you feel others see you (or view you)?
- What has it been like for you to come into the hospital?

patient says he or she feels worthless, depressed, confused, what does this really mean to the patient? Because the patient's perspective is critical, the patient should not be told what these feelings might mean. What is the patient thinking, feeling, and doing? Self-observation can be done with rating scales, diaries, journals, logs, wearing a wrist counter (e.g., golfer's counter), grocery price tabulator, or making checkmarks on a piece of paper. Self-observation emphasizes patient commitment, recognizes the patient's strengths, and increases feedback and communication. Learning self-monitoring takes time and guidance, but it is a very worthwhile skill for the patient to learn. It will become even more important after discharge from home care, when the patient will be responsible for monitoring symptoms and self-management.

- *Rating scales.* Rating scales or standardized psychosocial assessments represent another, more standard assessment method. There are many scales that can be used, some requiring more staff training than others. Rating scales can save time, decrease costs, and provide more data about the patient's needs. If the home care agency has many psychiatric patients, it would be helpful for staff to learn more about these scales. The agency may decide that it is important to include rating scales in its psychiatric home care treatment model and use them during patient assessment. O'Conner and Eggert have reviewed many of these tools by identifying their focus.[16]

   1. *Focus on symptoms.* Some scales focus on symptoms or behaviors, cognitions, and/or emotions that assist in identifying mild to severe psychosocial impairment. The two most common ones are the Scale for the Assessment of Negative Symptoms (SANS),[17] which is used to assess the symptoms of schizophrenia, and the Brief Psychiatric Rating Scale (BPRS),[18] a more comprehensive measurement of mental illness. The BPRS consists of four factors, each with symptom clusters. These are factor 1 (withdrawal-retardation), which includes emotional withdrawal, conceptual disorganization, blunt affect, hallucinatory behavior, mannerisms and posturing, motor retardation, and tension; factor 2 (anxious depression), which includes anxiety, depressive mood, guilt feelings, and somatic concerns; factor 3 (hostile-suspiciousness), which includes hostility, suspiciousness, and uncooperativeness; and factor 4 (thinking disturbance), which includes grandiosity and unusual thought content.[19]

   2. *Focus on functional performance.* Scales may focus on the ability to manage life and roles. Examples are the Quality of Life Scale (QLS),[20] the Social Adjustment Scale (SAS),[21] and the Global Assessment of Functioning Scale (GAF).[22]

3. *Focus on personal efficacy.* This type of scale focuses on the patient's view of self or events, communication ability, or coping styles. Examples are the Self-Esteem Scale[23] and the Interpersonal Communication Inventory (ICI).[24]
4. *Focus on family.* Other scales assess the family environment, for example the Family Environment Scale (FES).[25]

Rating scales can be used during the admission assessment and to assist in assessing progress and outcomes. Many such scales are available. Some of these scales are used by the nurse and some can be used by the patient/family/SOs. Scales may focus on symptoms, functional performance, personal efficacy, family, and interpersonal and social resources.

- *Homework assignments.* Homework assignments can be used in many ways with patients and their families/SOs. They help to reinforce the patient's responsibilities and the need for the patient's active participation in the home care treatment process. A passive patient will not progress. Assignments can be as simple as asking the patient to maintain a log of the number of times the patient said hello, answered the telephone, or brushed his or her teeth; or they can be as complex as asking the patient to take on a new task at home and to assess its success (such as cooking dinner with the family/SOs). The use of homework does not relieve the home care nurse and other home care staff of their responsibilities. Plans must be made to develop homework assignments that will be helpful, to review homework assignments during each visit, and to check progress regularly. Success in one area helps support the patient as he or she tries new skills. Breaking tasks into smaller components, especially if a patient is depressed or confused, is helpful. It is important for the patient to feel success, not more despair. In addition, assessment data can be obtained as the nurse observes how the patient copes with a homework assignment and the results of the assignment.

For some home care patients, staff members from several health care disciplines may participate in the assessment. Staff target data required for each discipline's specific interventions, such as data for the nurse, the physician, the social worker, or the occupational therapist. Usually, all clinical staff feel they need to ask every question. The assessment, however, should be focused and correlated with other assessments to prevent repetition. Repetitive assessments will only frustrate the patient and family/SOs. Staff members from each discipline need to ask what information is required at what time, and how assessment can be made easier for the patient and yet meet the needs of the different disciplines. Each discipline does not need to cover all of the possible assessment content areas or components; however, it is necessary to be aware of all components to understand each patient.

Typical Components of a Complete Psychiatric Assessment

The typical components of a complete psychiatric assessment are as follows:

- *Identifying data.* Identifying data are usually collected during the admission process completed at the time of the patient's referral to home care. These data include such items as name, diagnosis, age, race, marital status, occupation, insurance coverage, referral source, psychiatrist, medical physician, address, telephone, and family/SOs contact.
- *Presenting problem or chief complaint.* The first step in the assessment is to ascertain the patient's view of the reasons for home care or the chief complaint stated in the patient's own words. Often the first words the patient uses to describe his or her problems and reactions to home care provide the most revealing information about the patient. A verbatim quote is most helpful.
- *History of the present illness.* The history of the present illness focuses on data related to the chronological development of the symptoms. How is the problem perceived by the patient? Is it interpersonal, somatic, and/or sociological? When was the problem first noticed (onset)? How long has it lasted (duration)? Does the patient have any ideas about the possible causes of the problem(s)? Has it become worse or better? If so, when did the change occur? Describe the change and its effect on the patient. Has the patient found any solution or ways to feel better? Has the patient had any treatment for the present problem, and what were the results?
- *Past psychiatric history.* This component includes past mental health problems, treatment, and the results of treatment including outpatient psychotherapy, hospitalization, medications, electroconvulsive therapy, partial hospitalization, residential treatment, and home care. Substance abuse history, both drugs and alcohol, should always be assessed.
- *Medical history.* The medical history includes medical illnesses and surgery; congenital, biological, chemical, or physical injury to nervous system, particularly head injuries; current medical treatment; allergies; medications; current physicians and other health care providers. A related assessment is the physical exam, which may be included in the patient's medical records that are sent to the agency. The nurse completes a physical assessment based on the agency's policy.
- *Social history.* The social history includes interpersonal and environmental information. Included are chronological events (education, marriage, divorce or death of spouse, childbirth, family deaths, etc.), significant relationships, sexual relationships, marital issues, parenting issues, school, employment, economic status, and availability of food and housing. The patient's current and past stresses are identified, including strengths and coping methods. The patient is asked to describe his or her daily activities.

- *Family history.* This component includes psychiatric and other medical illnesses in the patient's family, and data regarding family/SO relationships and communication. If the nurse cannot get the information from the patient, the patient is asked for permission to talk with the family/SOs. If the patient is a child or adolescent, this permission is not required; however, it is important to tell the patient that the nurse will be speaking with family/SOs.
- *Suicidal/homicidal potential.* This is a very important component of the assessment and is never omitted. Data are collected related to present and past feelings and behavior. Direct and specific questions communicate to the patient that the nurse is interested and gives the patient permission to discuss these very frightening feelings. Critical questions include the following:
  1. Are you thinking about killing yourself (others, hurting self)? Right now? In the past?
  2. Do you have a plan?
  3. What is the plan?
  4. Do you have what you need to carry out the plan?
  5. Do you trust yourself to keep these feelings under control?
  6. Are you hearing voices that tell you to hurt yourself or someone else?
  The nurse must then determine if the plan is lethal; if the method is reasonable and accessible; if the plan is reasonable as to time and place; and if the patient is experiencing auditory hallucinations related to these feelings. All of the assessment data are documented, and it is very important to provide details.
- *Military history.* This component is not always done but may be relevant for some patients, particularly patients with posttraumatic stress disorder or a substance abuse problem. Data that might be included are the branch of service and dates of service, drafted or volunteered, highest rank, duties, wounds or injuries, combat experience, any disciplinary actions, service-connected conditions, special commendations, and type of discharge.
- *Legal history.* For some patients, legal history and current problems may greatly affect the treatment. It may even be the motivation for treatment. This history would include current charges, past history of legal charges and/or imprisonment, and problems or legal charges during childhood and adolescence.
- *Developmental and psychogenetic history.* This component focuses on the development of the patient from birth to the present including birth trauma, developmental milestones, toilet training, education, and early relationships. There is controversy as to relevance of delving into the past in such detail, even for inpatient treatment with its decreasing length of stay. The routine use of these data for psychiatric home care is even more questionable. The home care agency may receive a psychiatric assessment from the patient's

psychiatrist and/or hospital that includes this information and, consequently, it is important for the staff to understand that it might be included in a comprehensive psychiatric assessment.

- *Mental status exam.* The mental status exam is one of the only methods that the nurse uses during the assessment in which the patient is observed directly solving problems and coping with situations of potential anxiety. If the patient expresses concern about concentration or memory or if the nurse identifies these difficulties during the interview, it is easy then to suggest that the nurse and the patient talk more about these problems. This is one way to assess mental status. A typical neurological exam consists of the following elements:[26]
  1. cerebral function
  2. state of consciousness (alert or comatose)
  3. emotional state (affect, mood, responsiveness)
  4. intellect (memory; orientation to person, place, and time; simple calculations; recognition of familiar objects and words; oral and written comprehension; judgment)
  5. behaviors (appearance, expressions, gestures, attentiveness, expression of ideas and thoughts, perceptions)
  6. speech (quality, quantity, ability to form words)
  7. cranial nerves (particularly important are pupil size, equality, and reaction)
  8. cerebellar function (balance and coordination)
  9. motor system (muscle atrophy, asymmetry; strength/weakness; involuntary movements)
  10. sensory systems (light touch, pain, vibration)
  11. reflexes (tendon and plantar reflexes)

The broad areas covered in a mental status exam are appearance and behavior; speech and language; thought process and content; mood and affect; cognitive functioning including orientation, concentration, memory, and intellectual functioning. Much of this is assessed throughout the assessment interview. Specific assessment of cognitive mental status (such as orientation, attention span, memory functions, and general intellect) is usually part of a discrete exam. Exhibit 10–4 provides an overview of specific mental status exam components.

The Assessment Process

The initial contact with a psychiatric home patient may begin in several ways. If the patient is in the hospital and the hospital has a relationship with the home care agency, there may be an established method for contact, such as attendance at a discharge planning meeting or telephone conference with the patient's physi-

Exhibit 10–4 Mental Status Exam

- *Patient's general appearance.* Describe the patient's grooming, dress, physical deformities, eye contact, and how the patient relates to the interviewer. Note any unusual physical characteristics. Describe the patient's posture. Are tardive dyskinesia symptoms present? Is there evidence of self-mutilation (e.g., scarring, needle marks)?
- *Affect.* Describe the patient's ability to express emotions (appropriate or inappropriate? changes or remains the same?). Observe facial expression for anxiety, depression, anger, bizarreness. Is affect masklike indicating possible drug toxicity?
- *Mood.* Describe the primary emotional tone (such as angry, anxious, depressed). Is it appropriate?
- *Psychomotor activity.* Describe the patient's psychomotor activity and the rate of observable mental and physical behavior?
- *Thought.* Describe the patient's thought process (rational or illogical) and content (what the patient thinks about).
- *Speech.* Describe the patient's speech quality (e.g., loud, monotone, pressured, whisper), quantity, and content.
- *Sensorium.* Describe the following:
  1. orientation (time, place, person, situation)
  2. attention (internal, external)
  3. memory (immediate recall, short-term, long-term)
  4. concentration
  5. perceptions (evidence of auditory and/or visual hallucinations, delusional thinking, illusions)
  6. abstracting (word similarities, proverb interpretation)
  7. general knowledge (specific questions such as "Who is the president?")
  8. judgment (ability to use information from interview and past; ability to make reasonable life decisions and manage activities of daily living)
  9. insight (patient's awareness of his or her problem)

---

cian and nurse. If the nurse meets the patient briefly, this allows the patient to see a connection between hospitalization and after-care in the home. If this cannot be done, then the home care nurse should call the patient and discuss the initial home care visit. Koren and Schrague have noted that referring staff often have a single question or reason in mind when making the referral for home care. Listening carefully during these contacts may provide important information about the patient, the family/SOs, reasons for home care referral, and previous experience the patient has had with other health care providers. After a discussion with the referral source, other issues often arise.[27] Review of any available records is critical, particularly the results of laboratory and diagnostic studies for comparison later in treatment. If records are not available, the referral source should be contacted to discuss significant results and the problems that require follow-up. Of course, the nurse will be given a diagnosis by the patient's physician; however, it is dangerous for any health care professional to assume that the diagnosis provides the most important information about the patient. The best approach should be to assume that one does not know the patient.[28]

If the patient has been recently discharged from an inpatient or partial hospital setting, it is best to schedule the first visit within 24 to 48 hours after discharge. The patient should have a home care appointment before leaving the hospital and the telephone number for the home care agency. The home care nurse should follow up after discharge to confirm the appointment. Discharge is a stressful time, and information can easily be forgotten.

THE INTERVIEW

The Interview Environment

The ideal setting for an interview offers privacy, quiet, comfort, and minimum distractions, all of which may be difficult to obtain in the home setting. The nurse communicates confidentiality verbally and by attitude. It is important for the patient to feel that what he or she is saying is important and that it will be shared only with those who need to know the information.

Attitude and Behavior

Often the family/SOs and the patient will not understand why the patient is being sent home sick from the hospital requiring psychiatric home care. There will be many misconceptions about what will happen. The telephone call to set up the appointment must be made with these factors in mind. The nurse must identify himself or herself, the name of the home care agency, the referral source, and reason for the referral. The nurse should sound interested and concerned. This can be done by communicating some understanding of the patient's problem (e.g., "I understand that you have just been discharged from the hospital after a stay of one week. It is often difficult to adjust to being home and remembering to take your medication"). An appointment time must then be established. At the conclusion of the call, the patient and family/SOs are given the necessary telephone numbers to use if they have questions or require help. This written information is provided again at the initial visit.

Interview Guidelines

Throughout the interview, the nurse must assess the patient's tolerance to the interview. The nurse may need to stop the interview and complete it on the next visit. The decision to postpone completing the assessment should be documented in the medical record. The patient should be told that the nurse and the patient will complete the interview at the next visit. Even if the assessment is not completed on the first visit, the nurse must implement an initial treatment plan based on available information. As the interview is conducted, the following guidelines may help the nurse:

- The patient should be treated as an individual, even if the patient appears to be unaware of the nurse or the surroundings. Flexibility is required to make adjustments for the patient's needs and moods. The initial impression of the nurse is important. Most patients are afraid that the home care nurse will not understand them. From the very beginning, decreasing the patient's anxiety is part of the assessment and any interview with the patient. The patient is a unique individual, not just another admission. One way of communicating individuality to the patient is to ask after the introduction, "Before we go on, do you have any questions?" Most patients are trying to figure out if it is okay to share personal information, which information to share, and telling their story "right"; but it may be difficult for them to do this in their home.
- To establish rapport, it is necessary to understand that the patient feels threatened. A warm and concerned approach will help establish rapport, addressing the patient by name, introducing self, and explaining the role of home care staff and home care. Home care staff introduce themselves with first and last names. Patients may use either name when they refer to staff; however, staff should initially address the patient as Ms. or Mr. _____ and ask the patient what he or she likes to be called. The patient is told that the purpose of the interview is to obtain information about the patient that will help the staff provide care for the patient and to work with the patient to identify the best methods for helping the patient. The emphasis is on the patient's participation in the treatment planning and treatment.
- The nurse is a participant-observer, meaning the nurse both participates and observes the patient and family/SOs to collect relevant data for home care.
- The interview will be greatly influenced by empathy, which Shea defines as "the ability to accurately recognize the immediate emotional perspective of another person while maintaining one's own perspective. . . . Most patients are not searching for a person who feels as they do; they are searching for someone who is trying to understand what they feel."[29(p.14)] Empathy is frequently communicated nonverbally. The home care nurse can overuse or

underuse empathetic comments. An empathetic statement often begins with, "It sounds like. . . ."

- Anxiety is contagious, so it is important to avoid a tense, hurried approach. There should be as few interruptions as possible. This is more difficult to control in a home environment with telephone calls, television, family activities, etc. The nurse may need to be direct about the importance of no interruptions with the patient and the family/SOs.
- Facial expressions should show interest and concern.
- Styles of communicating are highly individualized from nurse to nurse; however, there are some general guides that can be used in interviews. Listening to the patient and identifying hidden needs is a part of every interview. When the patient is invited to share a personal experience, it is helpful to use a gentle tone of voice with phrases such as "Tell me about . . ." or "Describe for me. . . ." This offers support to the patient during a potentially traumatic discussion. Encouraging the patient to describe personal thoughts might be introduced with, "What are some of your thoughts about . . . ?" Some health care professionals feel that the use of "why" should be avoided as it is judgmental and it implies there is only one answer. It might help to rephrase, using "what." During the interview, asking two questions at once confuses the patient.
- Attentive listening requires continuous introspection. The nurse focuses on what is heard and seen.
- It is critical to remember what is said and what is not said. Making assumptions without enough facts can be counterproductive. The most important thing that is said is what is not said. Look for the holes in the data, such as when a married patient does not mention the spouse.
- Listen for themes, such as "I fail at everything I do."
- Observe the patient's nonverbal behavior (e.g., the patient is talking about a topic that may be sad, but the patient is smiling).
- Vague questions are not helpful. The patient is anxious and experiencing decreased problem-solving ability. The nurse may need to repeat a question due to the patient's decreased concentration; however, the nurse should not sound frustrated with the need for repetition.
- The patient is asked if he or she has had home care in the past. What was this like for the patient? This may help understand the patient's response to home care. Previous experiences may also affect the patient's family/SOs.
- When care is provided in the home, consideration of the patient's cultural beliefs and values is even more important than in the hospital setting.
- The patient may bring up topics that do not fit in the nurse's moral system; however, the nurse must not communicate personal beliefs to the patient. These beliefs and conflicts should be dealt with in supervision or in a peer

group. The nurse is inviting the patient to share highly personal information to a stranger; the patient does not need a judgmental attitude but does need help with problem solving and learning new coping skills.

Assessment as an Interactive Process

The nurse conducting the assessment must be able to communicate, observe carefully, listen, remain objective, identify interaction patterns, and communicate the data to others verbally and in written format. The interview is an interactive process between the nurse interviewer and the patient. How the patient and the nurse respond to each other will affect the results of the assessment interview. The interview is usually fairly structured with a form to complete. This form should be clear and concise and organized in a manner that facilitates the interview process. An example of a psychiatric home care assessment is found in Exhibit 10–5.

The nurse is a participant observer—asking questions and observing. It is particularly important to observe the patient for increasing anxiety and escalating behaviors. Sitting very close to the patient may increase the patient's anxiety. No one likes this with a stranger. The nurse allows the patient space and avoids touching. This is important since there has not been opportunity to assess the patient's response to touch and the patient's need for space. For safety, the nurse should avoid blocking the doorway or exit. The patient may see this as someone blocking his or her escape. If the patient is very upset, a family/SO member may be present or the door may be left open. If there is concern about escalating behavior or a history of escalation, it is best not to do the assessment in an isolated area. If the patient is unable to sit for an extended period of time, the nurse might provide short breaks, sit and have a cup of coffee with the patient, or walk in the yard to relieve some of the tension.

Effective Interview Techniques

Mosher and Burti, who have worked with many psychiatric patients in community settings, have described effective interviewing techniques that can also be used in the home.[30] Assessment interviewing includes two major focuses, the history and mental status of the patient and the relationship between the interviewer and the patient. The greater emphasis is usually placed on the history and mental status, which is a serious mistake. Mosher and Burti state: "[We view the] initial contact, building rapport, and establishing a collaborative working relationship as central to the work. In addition, we believe that our problem-focused, relationally oriented, contextualizing approach to the story the user brings, preserves and

Exhibit 10–5 Sample Psychiatric Home Care Nursing Assessment

Patient's Name _____
Address _____
Telephone _____
Patient Number _____

PSYCHIATRIC HOME CARE ADMISSION ASSESSMENT
(Must be completed by an RN)

Date _____ Time _____
Admission diagnoses _____
Information obtained from: Patient _____ Other _____
Patient's language _____
Hearing impairment _____ Speech impairment _____
Transport mode: Ambulatory _____ Walker _____ Wheelchair _____
BP _____ Pulse _____ Resp _____ Temp _____ Ht _____ Wt _____

Patient's view of home care and willingness to cooperate and participate: _____
_____
_____

Patient's goals for home care:
_____

Current medications (Include nonprescription drugs):

Medication	Dose	Frequency	Date Began	Comments

Patient using safety caps? _____ If not, why not? _____

Allergies?

continues

Exhibit 10–5 continued

Hospitalization for medical problems:

Dates	Hospital	Reason

Past health history:

	Yes	No	Comments
Diabetes			
High blood pressure			
Heart attack			
Heart disease			
Seizures			
Ulcers			
Jaundice/hepatitis			
Asthma			
Emphysema			
Tuberculosis			
Kidney/bladder			

Date of last physical exam _____ By whom _____

Do you have a problem with the following:

	Yes	No	Comments
Shortness of breath			
Cough			
Sputum			
Blood			
Cardiac problems			
Gastrointestinal problems			
Bowel problems			

Exhibit 10–5 continued

	Yes	No	Comments
Increased weight			
Decreased weight			
Unusual eating patterns			
Inadequate fluid intake			
Somatic complaints			
Physical limitations			
Menstrual problems			
Last period			
Last exam			
Increased sleep			
Decreased sleep			
Early awaking			

Diet:

	Yes	No	Comments
Are you on a special diet?			
Do you have likes?			
Do you have dislikes?			

Do you need any of the following:

	Yes	No	Comments
Eyeglasses			
Contact lenses			
Dentures			
Hearing aid(s)			
Other			

continues

Exhibit 10–5 continued

History of dangerous behavior:

	Yes	No	Comments
Suicidal thoughts			
Suicidal behavior			
Suicidal plan			
Family history/suicide			
Homicidal thoughts			
Homicidal behavior			
Destruction of property			

Substance abuse history:

	Yes	No	Amount	Frequency	Comments
Caffeine					
Tobacco					
Alcohol					
Sleeping pills					
Tranquilizers					
Barbiturates					
Stimulants					
Marijuana					
PCP					
Hallucinogens					
Cocaine					
Heroin					

	Yes	No	Comments
Withdrawal symptoms			
Memory loss			
Blackouts			
Seizures			

Exhibit 10–5 continued

Relationships and activities:

What is the patient's view of self? _____

What strengths does the patient describe?

_____
_____

What limitations does the patient describe?

_____
_____

How does the patient handle:
  Stress: _____
  Anger: _____

DAILY ROUTINE/SCHEDULE

Time	Activity	Time	Activity

continues

Exhibit 10–5 continued

Attitude and behavior during interview:

	Y	N		Y	N		Y	N
Cooperative			Trustful			Seeks support		
Passive			Hostile			Suspicious		
Manipulative			Mute			Loud Speech		
Soft speech			Rapid speech			Slowed speech		
Hypoactivity			Hyperactivity			Flat affect		
Inappropriate affect			Labile			Depressed		
Anxious			Fearful			Elevated mood		
Loose			Flight of ideas			Delusions		
Answers reluctantly			Unable to comprehend					
Disoriented:	Time:		Place:			Person:		
Hallucinations:	Auditory:					Visual:		

Summary and Analysis:

The following have been completed:
___ Initial patient orientation
___ Consents signed
___ Patient and family/SOs provided with written information about home care
     including emergency number to call
___ Patient/family/SO informed that next visit will be _____
___ Names and times for other home care staff to visit _____
___ Appropriate equipment and supplies available for patient
___ Have been ordered
___ Patient has appropriate medications
___ Informed about administration of medications

Completed by: _____
                                              Date   Time

enhances patient self-control and power. Thus, the critical therapeutic process of remoralization is begun immediately."[31] Problematic attitudes that the nurse may bring to the interview include "What can I quickly get out of the patient" and/or "I can rescue the patient." The nurse can communicate these attitudes to the patient, and they are both detrimental and contradict the approach suggested by Mosler and Burti.

The following interview techniques and pointers are helpful:

- The nurse and the patient should be as comfortable as possible in the interview setting. Factors such as seating, temperature, noise, and interruptions are important.
- The nurse should understand that the patient may be anxious, hesitant, confused about the purpose of the home visit, and fearful of rejection.
- The nurse should understand that this may be the first time the patient has had a health care professional in his or her home. Some patients may wonder if home care staff should be treated as a guest (e.g., serve food, clean up for the home care visit). Other patients will not care.
- The nurse should introduce himself or herself with full name and ask the patient for his or her name. The patient's first name should not be used until the patient says what he or she would like to be called. If the patient asks questions, the nurse should be as direct as possible with answers; however, if the question is too personal, it is best to remind the patient gently that the nurse is in the home to talk with the patient. It is the patient's time.
- When the appointment is made and upon arrival, the time frame for the visit should be stated.
- Upon arrival, the nurse should ask the patient what is the best place in the home to talk quietly. This will help to assess the patient's ability to observe and make decisions. If the place is not appropriate and can be improved, the nurse should gently suggest this to the patient.
- During the visit, the nurse should observe the patient's eye contact and how it changes. It may communicate that the patient is immediately involved, becomes more involved as the visit progresses, or becomes less involved. Many patients appear passive on the initial visit. Much of this may due to unclear expectations, fear, medication, or lack of sleep.
- The nurse should observe the patient's physical presentation. How does the patient move and hold his or her body? It is particularly important to assess how side effects from medication are affecting motor behavior. Side effects are uncomfortable for the patient and may make it more difficult for the patient to socialize. It is important for the nurse to recognize this as he or she works with the patient to participate more in the family and the community.

- The nurse should assess the patient's attitudes and behaviors during the interview. Exhibit 10–6 identifies attitudes and behaviors that are important to assess.
- The nurse should respect the patient's need for distance and allow some space between them.
- It is easy for the nurse to appear to have the attitude of the "helper knows best." The patient will be very familiar with this attitude. It is not productive, nor does it communicate to the patient that this will be a participative experience. On the other hand, the patient will be nervous about involvement.
- During the interview, it is important to ask the patient about his or her understanding of the need for home care and his or her expectations. The nurse shares with the patient the reasons the patient was referred for home care. This can stimulate a discussion about differences in expectations and encourage collaborative decisions about the expectations for home care. The nurse should communicate honesty and openness.

Exhibit 10–6 Patient Attitudes and Behaviors during Interview

ATTITUDE	PHYSICAL BEHAVIOR	SPEECH
• cooperative	• hypoactive	• rapid
• seeks support	• hyperactive	• slowed
• passive	• abnormal movements	• loud
• suspicious		• soft
• manipulative		• monotonic
• answers reluctantly		• mute
• hostile		
• trustful		

MOOD AND AFFECT	COGNITIVE PROCESSES
• inappropriate affect	• loose
• flat affect	• flight of ideas
• labile	• disoriented (time, place, person)
• depressed	• hallucinations (auditory, visual)
• elevated mood	• delusions
• manic	
• anxious	
• fearful	
• cyclothymic	

- As the interview progresses, the nurse should consider three variables: the relationship by assessing distance; verbal output by assessing cognition; and body activity by assessing affect. According to Mosher and Burti, "Greater structuring of the interview will result in greater organization and control but can also have the effect of dampening overall responsiveness and frightening patients who fear being controlled."[32(p.64)]

HOME ENVIRONMENT ASSESSMENT

The patient's home environment will affect treatment and response to treatment. It has always been important to discuss the patient's home environment when someone is hospitalized. When the care is provided in the home, this is even more important, both at the time of admission and throughout treatment. Not all aspects of the home environment are important to every patient. Exhibit 10–7 provides an example of a home environment assessment.

DIAGNOSTIC PROCESS

At the conclusion of the assessment, the nurse documents a narrative summary that provides a picture of the patient's functional status. It must be clear and support the need for psychiatric home care services and it must be based on an analysis of the assessment data. Diagnosis is the recognition and identification of patterns of response to actual or potential psychiatric illnesses and mental health problems.[33] Another definition is "a clinical judgment about individual, family, or community responses to actual and potential health problems/life processes. Nursing diagnoses provide direction for the selection of nursing interventions to achieve outcomes for which the nurse is accountable."[34(p.71)] According to the American Nurses Association, the psychiatric-mental health nursing phenomena of concern provide a framework for the nursing diagnosis. Exhibit 10–8 identifies these phenomena.

Liberman has identified problem and asset categories that are important in the psychiatric rehabilitation assessment, and these are complementary to nursing diagnoses/problems.[35] In addition to Liberman's categories, the following assessment methodologies are suggested:

- *cognitive problems:* difficulty in processing incoming information; use of rating scales such as the Brief Psychiatric Rating Scale for assessment
- *affective problems:* emotions or feelings; use of target complaint scale for patient self-ratings
- *social-interpersonal problems:* relationships with others; use of observation and patient/family/SOs assessment

Exhibit 10–7 Home Environment Assessment

Element	Observed	Comments
Type of housing		
Number of rooms		
General condition (cleanliness, orderliness)		
Furnishings		
Privacy		
Sleeping arrangements		
Adequacy of bathrooms		
Adequacy of food preparation area		
Availability of food		
Alcohol, smoking, other drugs		
Adequacy of:		
Water supply		
Waste/garbage disposal		
Lighting		
Heating, cooling, ventilation		
Laundry facilities		
Telephone		
Safety factors:		
Smoke alarms		
Locks on doors		
Storage of medicines; poisons		
Loose rugs; clutter		
Stairs with railing		
Crime prevention methods		
Swimming pool		
Pets		
Neighborhood		
Transportation availability		
Other family/SO/neighbors nearby		
Are they helpful?		
Hours patient is alone		
How do the patient/family/SOs feel about the living environment?		
Do patient/family/SOs feel safe?		
Availability of emergency numbers		
What are the strengths and limitations of the home environment?		
Can the limitations be improved?		

Exhibit 10–8 Psychiatric-Mental Health Nursing: Phenomena of Concern

---

Actual or potential mental health problems of clients pertaining to:

- the maintenance of optimal health and well-being and the prevention of psycho-biological illness
- self-care limitations or impaired functioning related to mental and emotional distress
- deficits in the functioning of significant biological, emotional, and cognitive systems
- emotional stress or crisis components of illness, pain, and disability
- self-concept changes, developmental issues, and life process changes
- problems related to emotions such as anxiety, anger, sadness, loneliness, and grief
- physical symptoms that occur along with altered psychological functioning
- alterations in thinking, perceiving, symbolizing, communicating, and decision making
- difficulties in relating to others
- behaviors and mental states that indicate the client is a danger to self or others or has a severe disability
- interpersonal, systemic, sociocultural, spiritual, or environmental circumstances or events which affect the mental and emotional well-being of the individual, family, or community
- symptom management, side effects/toxicities associated with psychopharmaco-logic intervention and other aspects of the treatment regimen

Source: Reprinted with permission from American Nurses Association, *A Statement on Psychiatric-Mental Health Clinical Nursing Practice and Standards of Psychiatric-Mental Health Clinical Nursing Practice*, p. 8, © 1994, American Nurses Association.

- *independent living skills:* how much is the patient able to do for self; use of observation and patient/family/SOs assessment
- *behavioral excesses:* frequency, intensity, or duration are too high (e.g., spends too much time alone); urinates in pants; has difficulty falling asleep; has nightmares; spends too much time listening to music; is fatigued all the time; fantasizes strange thoughts; has auditory hallucination with depreciatory content; use of observation and patient/family/SOs assessment
- *behavioral deficits:* certain behaviors occur at insufficient frequency, inadequate intensity, or inappropriate form, referred to as negative symptoms (e.g., poorly sustained concentration, not completing tasks, unable to make or maintain friendships, not eating, diminished self-care skills, lack of social

or instrumental activities, unresponsive to questions, poverty of speech, lack of affect, mute); use of observation and assessment of patient/family/SOs
- *behavioral assets:* social competence, coping efforts, social supports (Patients with poor premorbid histories have few of these assets. In some cases, it is best to set goals based on assets rather than symptoms. Strengthening assets may indirectly displace or reduce psychopathology and symptomatology, and this is very important.)

As these problems and asset categories are assessed, questions that might be considered when data are collected and analyzed include the following:[36]

- What are the areas in which the patient functions well (now or in the past)?
- What are the patient's interpersonal resources and social support network?
- What agencies and helping professionals can be mobilized for participation in a treatment plan?
- How aversive are the patient's current impairments to the patient and his or her family/SOs, and can this serve as a source of motivation for change?
- How responsive is the patient to the therapeutic alliance and setting?

Treatment will be more successful if based on existing strengths with less focus on problems.

As the nurse analyzes each of the patient's problems, it is helpful to identify and assess the antecedents and consequences of a problem or behavior for the patient. Liberman suggests that the functional or behavioral analysis of conditions should include antecedents and consequences of problems as well as the patient's motivations.[37] Antecedents of problems are important. Analysis of antecedents focuses on where, when, and with whom the problems occur; what life events and stressors, both episodic and ambient, may be triggering or influencing problems or relapse; whether symptoms, side effects of drugs, or cognitive impairments are interfering with functions. Consequences of problem behaviors are also analyzed, including what would happen if the problem is ignored. Particularly important to consider are the roles of sympathy, nurturance, attention, anger, and coercion by others. What reinforcers or benefits would the patient gain or lose if problems were decreased? In addition to analysis of antecedents and consequences, the patient's motivation is always important and means the difference between success and failure. Does the patient acknowledge problems and desire change? Does verbal behavior match follow-through in participation?

To begin a functional or behavioral analysis, the nurse might ask the patient and family/SOs to describe a typical day in detail. It may be necessary to use active questioning, focusing on the following:[38]

- *Setting.* In what situations does the problem behavior occur? At home, at work, in public places, when you are alone? Who is usually with you when the problem is present or maximal? How does the person respond to you? At what time during the day does this happen? What else are you likely to be doing at the time?
- *Antecedents.* Typically antecedents follow this pattern: "Depressed person's withdrawing from a social event: (1) The person anticipates awkwardness and rejection (cognitive). (2) The person feels especially low that day (affect). (3) The person observes a person in the setting who previously has been critical and rude (interpersonal). (4) The person fantasizes humiliation (imagery). (5) The person enters a room that has been the scene of an unpleasant experience (situational). (6) The person did not sleep well the night before (biological)."[39] There are many disturbed areas for this patient. Questions that might be asked to identify the antecedents include the following:
  1. What typically happens right before the problem anxiety behavior occurs?
  2. Does anything in particular seem to start this behavior?
  3. Is there a particular place or situation that is associated with the onset of the problem behavior (e.g., in schizophrenia, overstimulating or understimulating social environments can lead to symptoms and their worsening)?
  4. What combination of multimodal levels of behavioral experience appear to contribute to the maladaptive behavior?
  5. Might the maladaptive behavior be prevented by blocking the occurrence of one or more of the multimodal levels of behavior (e.g., cognitive, affect, interpersonal, imagery, situational, and biological)?
  6. What cognitive response or labeling appears to be functional as a mediating step in maintaining the clinical problem? (An example might be the patient who says, "I'm a loser and can't succeed." This increases the patient's anxiety when asked to do something, and the patient fails again.)
  7. Does modeling, which is observing and learning from others, influence the form or occurrence of the problem behavior?
- *Consequences.* What usually happens right after the problem behavior? How do you feel when that happens? Does anyone respond or interact with you at that time? The nurse should also be concerned with the consequences or reinforcers of behavior as they can either strengthen, increase, weaken, or decrease the frequency, duration, and intensity of behaviors that precede them. Reinforcers are "environmental consequences that increase the probability that a preceding behavior will occur in the future or be learned."[40(p.85)] The time between the behavior and the consequence is important. If the nurse can identify reinforcers that provide motivation for treatment and for maintain-

ing the improved behaviors, this can be very helpful and can be taught to the family/SOs. Medications may also help the patient respond more positively to reinforcers. Some reinforcers are tangible and others are more natural such as praise and attention. The nurse identifies reinforcers by observing and asking the patient and family/SOs to identify reinforcers. It is important to remember that there may be discrepancies between what the patient sees as antecedents and consequences and what the nurse actually observes. Feedback from family/SOs can assist in clarifying observations about the patient.

Diagnostic Classification Systems

In psychiatry and psychiatric nursing, diagnoses can be confusing. The source of psychiatric diagnoses is the *Diagnostic and Statistical Manual of Mental Disorders,* referred to as *DSM-IV*.[41] This is the source for medical diagnoses (e.g., schizophrenia, major depression, and panic disorder). Because the *DSM-IV* is used to identify the psychiatric diagnosis for a psychiatric home care patient, it is important that home care nursing staff are familiar with the manual and have a copy of it as a reference resource.

The *DSM-IV* medical classification system is a multiaxial system including an assessment of five axes:

1. *Axis I—clinical disorders.* These syndromes represent the primary psychiatric diagnosis. An example of an axis I diagnosis is schizophrenia. In addition, *V* codes are identified and used for conditions not attributable to a mental disorder that are a focus of attention or treatment. Examples of *V* codes are noncompliance with treatment, occupational problems, or marital problems.
2. *Axis II—personality disorders and mental retardation.* These disorders, long-term interpersonal dysfunction, usually begin in childhood or adolescence and continue into adulthood in stable form. Mental retardation is also included in this axis. An example of an axis II diagnosis would be an axis I of depression with an axis II of borderline personality disorder.
3. *Axis III—general medical conditions.* Axis III represents any current physical condition or disorder that is potentially relevant to understanding or clinical management. This axis emphasizes the critical importance of every patient's physical health and the need for an evaluation of that health status.
4. *Axis IV—psychosocial and environmental problems.* This axis identifies psychosocial and environmental problems that may affect diagnosis, treatment, and prognosis. What are the reality-based problems the patient faces? Typically these fall into the categories of problems with primary support group, the social environment, education, occupation or employment, hous-

ing, finances, access to health care services, interaction with the legal system/crime, and other relevant problems.[42]

5. *Axis V—global assessment of functioning.* Assessment for this axis focuses on a rating scale, Global Assessment of Functioning Scale, that provides information related to the patient's psychological, social, and occupational functioning in the past year and currently. This scale is found in the *DSM-IV* manual.

Concerns about using psychiatric diagnoses include the overuse of labels and the stigma that is attached to certain diagnoses. Health care professionals tend to label patients, referring to them as "borderlines" or "schizophrenics" rather than as "patients with schizophrenia." Medical diagnoses are used to help determine treatment, including medication and other types of treatment. Medical diagnoses provide consistent language to describe patient problems for communication, documentation, and reimbursement purposes; however, they are not the end point. It is difficult to determine a diagnosis for a psychiatric patient objectively, because there are no laboratory tests; signs and symptoms are nonspecific and can be mimicked by other conditions; and the use of drugs/alcohol affects symptoms. It is very important to reevaluate the diagnosis, especially if it was made during an acute crisis. Because there is a high percentage of substance abuse among patients who have serious mental illness, and a smaller percentage of patients with mental illness also have mental retardation, dual diagnosis must also be considered. Dual diagnosis will affect interventions chosen for the patient and the outcomes of care.

As a profession, nursing has been actively working on a diagnosis classification system since the early 1970s through the North American Nursing Diagnosis Association (NANDA). A diagnostic classification system offers a common language for communication about nursing care problems. Many psychiatric nurses believe that the work done by NANDA is very limiting for psychiatric nursing; however, these diagnoses can be used with psychiatric patients. Problems or diagnoses that have been used in psychiatric nursing are similar to the type of problem identification that is found in psychiatric rehabilitation. These problems must be operationalized into behavioral terms, considering frequency or how often behavior occurs, intensity or the magnitude or severity of the symptom, and duration or the amount of time spent behaving in a specific way. Behavior can be a problem because it occurs at inappropriate times or under inappropriate conditions with the patient having inadequate skills. Instead of describing the patient as "socially withdrawn," it is clearer to say that the patient "does not initiate conversation; does not eat meals with others; spends more than 80 percent of time alone." This is very important in documentation, and it is much more helpful for reimbursement.

Why does psychiatric nursing need another diagnostic category when *DSM-IV* provides a diagnostic system? Many psychiatric nurses believe that a psychiatric nursing diagnostic system will ensure that nursing issues are addressed. To provide nursing care, however, nurses in the practice setting should know how to work with the *DSM-IV* and how it is used with their patients. *DSM-IV* diagnoses are used by the physician in the admission to home care, for the medical treatment plan, for discharge diagnosis, and for reimbursement.

ASSESSMENT SUMMARY

What information should be included in the summary or analysis at the end of the nursing assessment? This a frequently asked question. It is recommended that the nurse do the following:[43(p.29)]

- briefly summarize the patient's behavior and responses during the interview
- briefly describe the initial plan for nursing interventions, especially those related to safety
- identify the nursing diagnoses/problems (the medical diagnosis, such as depression, is not used in the nursing summary, but rather specific nursing problems or diagnoses)

The summary describes how the nurse views the patient at the time of the admission assessment, as well as the patient's usual behavior patterns and the changes that have occurred in these patterns. There are four possible assessment conclusions:

1. no problem evident at this time; no health promotion activities or patient education indicated
2. no problem evident at this time; health promotion activities or patient education indicated
3. actual, potential, possible clinical problem or medical problem
4. actual, potential, possible nursing problem

POSTDISCHARGE PROBLEMS

Wells described the management of early postdischarge adjustment reactions following psychiatric hospitalization that has relevance for psychiatric home care.[44] The most common postdischarge symptoms are anxiety, depression, insomnia, hypersomnia, changes in appetite, phobias, increased addictive cravings, and outbursts of anger. Some patients try to cover up their symptoms by appearing cheerful; increasing activity; or experiencing euphoria, irritability, impatience, or a lack of affect. During the time of discharge from the hospital, some patients try to postpone discharge, regress, feel suicidal, or rush out without saying good-bye. It is not uncommon during the initial postdischarge period for the patients at home to experience a reoccurrence of symptoms that led to hospitalization; however, these usually disappear within one to two weeks. Wells explored whether these postdischarge reactions were an adjustment reaction rather than an exacerbation of the patient's primary illness. Hospitalization leads to dependency and security, even if the patient has a short length of stay. Patients can easily feel disappointment after discharge; most patients return to the environment in which they feel they failed, and they are anxious about failing again. For patients who are psychotic, expectation and rewards are less clear in the community, and thus they experience more anxiety. Increased stimulation and less structure can also be problems after discharge, particularly for patients with organic brain syndrome. Patients may also be embarrassed about their hospitalization, and this may make it difficult for them to reenter their community. It is difficult to assess whether these postdischarge symptoms are a prodromal sign of recurrence of illness or a normal reaction to the stressful situation of discharge. It is necessary for the home care nurse to assess postdischarge symptoms carefully.

At the conclusion of the study, Wells recommended several preventive measures.[45]

- During hospitalization, potential problems that might occur during the postdischarge period should be openly discussed with the patient and family/SOs. With shorter stays, this must also be done soon after admission to home care, with the home care nurse helping the patient and family/SOs identify potential problems and teaching them coping skills. Wells did not discuss home care, but clearly this discussion needs to continue in home care, and home care staff needs to provide support to the patient and family/SOs during the critical postdischarge stage. This is particularly important for patients who have had repeated problems following discharge that have led to rehospitalization.
- During discussions with the patient and family/SOs both in the hospital and in the home, this phenomenon should be called "postdischarge adjustment reaction."
- Staff need to identify community support resources for the patient and family/SOs.
- After-care planning must be increased; passes home before discharge are helpful and provide the patient and family/SOs an opportunity to discuss the experience.
- At the time of discharge, postdischarge adjustment reaction should be discussed again. Some hospitals offer return visit programs and opportunity for telephone contact with hospital staff. For some patients, this may be helpful.

Many patients who are in psychiatric home care do not make use of such programs and receive their support from home care staff or other resources.

- The first home care appointment should occur within three days after discharge, when there is a greater likelihood of the patient participating in the visit. An earlier visit is always better.

McIntosh and Worley also conducted a study to identify the most frequent postdischarge problems.[46] They interviewed 127 patients by telephone. The average length of stay was 14 days, and the patients had a variety of diagnoses. These authors identified the following problems, which are more specific than the postdischarge problems identified by Wells:[47]

- medications: forgetting to take, side effects, lack of funds to purchase, misuse, and substitution
- symptomatology: actual recurrence, anxiety about recurrence
- follow-up appointments: forgetting, canceling, expressing feelings of lack of need for treatment, transportation problems
- structuring time: inability to transfer structure learned in hospital to home situation, frequent daily viewing of television of up to 10 to 12 hours to fill time, inability to think of alternative activities
- sleeping: inability to develop healthy sleeping patterns, inability to use or remember relaxation techniques taught during hospital stay
- eating: inability to follow food plan, inability to organize time for meal preparation, decrease in appetite, lack of sufficient intake, eating at inappropriate times
- family relationships: discord in the family, inability to work with feelings, inability to negotiate with family, resentment of family vigilance
- support groups: lack of incentive or perceived value of support group, difficulty with transportation to groups, inability to organize time

Each of these problems has relevance for psychiatric home care. They indicate areas to assess and typical areas in which patients need help from psychiatric home care staff. The home care nurse must be aware of potential problems in order to prevent them.

Validating assessment data before determining the nursing diagnoses is important but not required for all data. Some data will appear to be incomplete or confusing. The home care nurse clarifies these data. In addition, the assessment data may initially appear to be overwhelming; however, grouping and analyzing the data will help to identify data that are relevant to the patient's current health problem(s). The data are then sorted into categories that relate to each other. As the data are compared to norms, analysis begins. It is always easier to identify problems than to identify strengths; however, it is the strengths that will help the patient reach outcomes. Analysis must include an identification of patient strengths whenever problems are described.

REASSESSMENT

A major concern in psychiatric care is the "revolving door" or frequent readmission to the hospital. For some patients, psychiatric home care may prevent this from happening by ensuring that patients take medication, attend medical appointments, and learn the skills necessary to function in the home.

During each home care visit, staff should reassess the patient. To assist paraprofessional staff, a simple checklist might serve as a reminder. A sample checklist is provided in Exhibit 10–9.

Reassessment is critical to determine patient responses to treatment, to determine the need to adjust treatment, and to identify the potential for relapse. Re-

---

Exhibit 10–9 Reassessment Checklist

Patient Name	Patient Number	Date	Time	Staff
Assessment Parameter		Yes	No	Comments
Anxious				
Sad				
Crying				
Fearful				
Angry				
Confused (time, date, person, place)				
Pacing or increased physical activity				
Inactivity				
Unwilling to cooperate or participate				
Complaining of physical problems				
Noncommunicative				
Problems interacting with family/SOs				
States that feels like harming self or others				
Mute				
Other				

lapse is common in patients with serious mental illness. It is demoralizing, is painful, and disrupts progress. The nurse must avoid feeling hopeless during these times. Preparing the patient and family/SOs and teaching them how to watch for relapse will make them feel more in control. Symptoms of relapse can be monitored and often information can be used to prevent further deterioration. Reassessment should always be done when there is a change in the patient's condition, a need to determine response to treatment, or a question about a change in diagnosis.

What are the early symptoms that indicate a relapse may be occurring?[48] For most patients, symptoms begin at least two weeks prior to relapse, but patients vary. Typically the earliest symptoms are associated with anxiety and/or depression (e.g., sleep disturbance, agitation, anger/hostility, somatic concerns, preoccupation with one or two things, social withdrawal, discouragement, loss of interest). Low-level psychotic symptoms may also occur, but usually they appear later than affective symptoms. If staff can intervene with medication and psychosocial support, there may be an 80 percent success rate of preventing a relapse. For this reason, it is very important for the nurse to recognize that these symptoms can be identified by patient, family/SOs, and the home care staff. Many of these symptoms are always present, so it is important to establish the patient's baseline to determine more easily when changes are occurring. Listening to the patient and the family/SOs is the most important step. Assessing symptoms can be done by using one of the standard rating scales or by targeting symptoms with the patient and family/SOs. The patient helps to identify important symptoms and to assess how much the symptoms bother the patient at the time. Exhibit 10–10 describes one tool for patient self-monitoring or self-assessment.

In addition to assessment, it is important to develop an intervention plan with the patient and family/SOs to be used if there is a negative change in the patient. Specific strategies need to be identified. This should be included in the patient's treatment plan and communicated to relevant family/SOs.

Paraprofessionals who care for the patient play an important role in reassessment. For many patients, they provide much of the care and interact with the patient more frequently. The following questions can be used to guide paraprofessionals as they care for psychiatric patients as well as the nurse who supervises paraprofessionals:

- What do you notice about the patient?
- Is the patient more able to cope with problems? Less able?
- Has the patient's mood changed? What is the change?
- Is the patient talking more or less, making sense, or confused?
- Is the patient interacting with family/SOs? In what ways?

Exhibit 10–10 Target Complaint Scale

Target complaint to be monitored: _____

Description	Date	Date	Date	Date	Date	Date	Date	Comments
Could not be worse								
Very much								
Pretty much								
A little								
Not at all								

Source: Adapted with permission from R. Liberman, ed., *Psychiatric Rehabilitation of Chronic Mental Illness*, p. 70, © 1988, American Psychiatric Press, Inc.

- How does the patient react to your visit?
- Is the patient having problems following rules or guidelines?
- Is the patient eating? Too little? Too much? Is the patient eating only certain foods? Does the patient have rituals? Is the patient following diet?
- Is the patient drinking fluids? Too much? Too little?
- Is the patient losing or gaining weight?
- What are the patient's vital signs?
- Is the patient sleeping? Too much? Too little? When is the patient sleeping?
- Does the patient appear to be hallucinating?
- Is the patient talking about hurting self or others?
- Is the patient talking positively or negatively about progress?
- Can the patient solve simple problems such as taking a shower, washing hair, doing the laundry, making the bed, or preparing a cup of coffee?
- Is the patient able to ask for help? How does the patient ask for help?
- What are the patient's usual activities?
- Does the patient need pressure to participate in activities?
- Does the patient seem to understand what you are saying?
- Does the patient recognize that he or she has problems that need resolving?
- Does the patient feel that these problems can be resolved?
- What are the topics the patient usually discusses with you?
- Does the patient ask questions? What are some of these questions?
- Is the patient taking his or her medications as prescribed?

- Is the patient drinking alcohol or using nonprescription drugs?
- Does the patient maintain his or her personal hygiene? If not, what are the problems in this area?

The paraprofessional can provide critical information about the patient and should be asked to communicate it verbally and through documentation.

SUMMARY

According to Carpenito, "Each patient is an autonomous and precious person who interacts in a unique manner with his or her environment and must be assessed within the context of this uniqueness. Because nursing diagnoses are derived from these assessments and because people are continually interacting with their environment, the nurse must apply the process in a continuous round of assessment, planning, implementing, and evaluating."[49] Assessment begins on admission and is never complete until discharge. Assessment data provide the information for making treatment decisions by identifying problems/diagnoses, strengths, resources, limitations, and educational needs.

NOTES

1. L. Mosher and L. Burti, *Community Mental Health: Principles and Practice* (New York: W.W. Norton & Company, 1989), 52.
2. Mosher and Burti, *Community Mental Health*, 31.
3. Mosher and Burti, *Community Mental Health*, 37.
4. M. Miller and J. Duffey, "Planning and Program Development for Psychiatric Home Care," *Journal of Nursing Administration* 23, no. 11 (1993): 35–41, at 38.
5. Joint Commission on Accreditation of Healthcare Organizations, *1995 Accreditation Manual for Home Care*, Vol. 1 (Oakbrook Terrace, IL: 1994), 5.
6. D. Jernigan, "Mental Health Assessment and Intervention: An Integral Part of Nursing Service," *Caring* 5, no. 7 (1986): 5–10, at 7.
7. American Nurses Association, *A Statement on Psychiatric-Mental Health Clinical Nursing Practice and Standards of Psychiatric-Mental Health Clinical Nursing Practice* (Washington, DC: 1994), 42.
8. Joint Commission on Accreditation of Healthcare Organizations, *1995 Accreditation Manual for Home Care*, 5–6.
9. L. Gerace, "Nursing Assessment in Psychiatric Home Health Care," *Journal of Home Health Care Practice* 2, no. 3 (1990): 9–15, at 12–13.
10. R. Liberman, ed., *Psychiatric Rehabilitation of Chronic Mental Patients* (Washington, DC: American Psychiatric Press, Inc., 1988), 60.
11. Liberman, *Psychiatric Rehabilitation of Chronic Mental Patients*, 62.

12. N. Klebanoff, "Psychosocial Home Care," in *Psychiatric-Mental Health Nursing: Adaptation and Growth*, ed. B. Johnson (Philadelphia: J.B. Lippincott Co., 1993), 757–774, at 762.

13. S. Eisen et al., "Reliability and Validity of a Brief Patient-Report Instrument for Psychiatric Outcome Evaluation," *Hospital and Community Psychiatry* 45, no. 3 (1994): 242–247.

14. Liberman, *Psychiatric Rehabilitation of Chronic Mental Patients*, 63.

15. Liberman, *Psychiatric Rehabilitation of Chronic Mental Patients*, 90.

16. F. O'Conner and L. Eggert, "Psychosocial Assessment for Treatment Planning and Evaluation," *Journal of Psychosocial Nursing* 32, no. 5 (1994): 31–42.

17. N. Andreasen, "Scale for the Assessment of Negative Symptoms," *British Journal of Psychiatry Supplement* 155, no. 7 (1989): 53–58.

18. D. Lukuff et al., "Manual for the Expanded Brief Psychiatric Rating Scale (BPRS)," *Schizophrenia Bulletin* 12, no. 4 (1986): 594–602.

19. S. Acorn, "Use of the Brief Psychiatric Rating Scale by Nurses," *Journal of Psychosocial Nursing* 32, no. 5 (1993): 9–12, at 11.

20. D. Heinrichs et al., "The Quality of Life Scale: An Instrument for Rating the Schizophrenic Deficit Syndrome," *Schizophrenia Bulletin* 10, no. 3 (1984): 388–398.

21. National Institute of Mental Health, "SAS-FAMILY, SAS-PATIENT," *Treatment Strategies in Schizophrenia Cooperative Agreement Program* (Rockville, MD: 1985).

22. American Psychiatric Association, *Diagnostic and Statistical Manual of Mental Disorders*, 4th ed. (Washington, DC: 1994), 758.

23. M. Rosenberg, *The Measurement of Self-Esteem* (Princeton, NJ: Princeton University, 1965).

24. M. Bienvenu, "An Interpersonal Communication Inventory," *Journal of Communication* 21 (1971): 381–383.

25. R. Moos and B. Moos, *Family Environment Scale Manual* (Palo Alto, CA: Consulting Psychologists, 1981).

26. D. Jernigan, "Mental Health Assessment and Intervention: An Integral Part of Nursing Service," *Caring* 5, no. 7 (1986): 5.

27. M. Koren and H. Schrague, "Psychiatric Home Care," *Caring* 5, no. 7 (1986): 29–35, at 31.

28. S. Godschalx, "Experiencing Life with a Psychiatric Disability," in *Chronic Mental Illness: Coping Strategies*, ed. J. Maurin (Thorofare, NJ: SLACK, Inc., 1989), 3–29, at 23.

29. S. Shea, *Psychiatric Interviewing: The Art of Understanding* (Philadelphia: W.B. Saunders Company, 1988), 14.

30. Mosher and Burti, *Community Mental Health*, 51–75.

31. Mosher and Burti, *Community Mental Health*, 51.

32. Mosher and Burti, *Community Mental Health*, 64.

33. American Nurses Association, *A Statement on Psychiatric-Mental Health Clinical Nursing Practice and Standards of Psychiatic-Mental Health Clinical Nursing Practice*, 26.

34. North American Nursing Diagnosis Association, *Nursing Diagnoses: Definitions and Classification* (Philadelphia: 1994), 7.

35. Liberman, *Psychiatric Rehabilitation of Chronic Mental Patients*, 78–79.

36. Liberman, *Psychiatric Rehabilitation of Chronic Mental Patients*, 79.

37. Liberman, *Psychiatric Rehabilitation of Chronic Mental Patients*, 63.

38. Liberman, *Psychiatric Rehabilitation of Chronic Mental Patients*, 83–85.

39. Liberman, *Psychiatric Rehabilitation of Chronic Mental Patients*, 83.

40. Liberman, *Psychiatric Rehabilitation of Chronic Mental Patients*, 85.

41. American Psychiatric Association, *Diagnostic and Statistical Manual of Mental Disorders*, 29–30.

42. American Psychiatric Association, *Diagnostic and Statistical Manual of Mental Disorders*, 29–30.

43. L. Carpenito, *Nursing Diagnosis: Application to Clinical Practice* (Philadelphia: J.B. Lippincott Co., 1983), 29.

44. D. Wells, "Management of Early Post-Discharge Adjustment Reactions Following Psychiatric Hospitalization," *Hospital and Community Psychiatry* 43, no. 10 (1992): 1000–1004.

45. Wells, "Management of Early Post-Discharge Adjustment Reactions Following Psychiatric Hospitalization," 1003.

46. J. McIntosh and N. Worley, "Beyond Discharge: Telephone Follow-Up and Aftercare," *Journal of Psychosocial Nursing* 32, no. 10 (1994): 21–27.

47. McIntosh and Worley, "Beyond Discharge: Telephone Follow-Up and Aftercare," 25.

48. F. O'Conner et al., "Psychosocial Assessment for Treatment Planning and Evaluation," *Journal of Psychosocial Nursing* 32, no. 5 (1994): 31–42, at 38.

49. Carpenito, *Nursing Diagnosis: Application to Clinical Practice*, 24.

SUGGESTED READING

Acorn, S. 1993. Use of the brief psychiatric rating scale by nurses. *Journal of Psychosocial Nursing* 31, no. 5: 9–12.

American Nurses Association. 1994. *A statement on psychiatric-mental health clinical nursing practice and standards for psychiatric-mental health clinical nursing practice*. Washington, DC.

American Psychiatric Association. 1994. *Diagnostic and statistical manual of mental disorders*. 4th ed. Washington, DC.

Berthot, B.D. et al. 1989. What does it mean? A new scale for rating patients' behavior. *Journal of Psychosocial Nursing* 27, no. 10: 25–28, 37–38.

Bostrom, A. 1988. Assessment scales for tardive dyskinesia. *Journal of Psychosocial Nursing* 26, no. 6: 9–12.

Braverman, B. 1990. Eliciting assessment data from the patient who is difficult to interview. *Nursing Clinics of North America* 25, no. 4: 743–750.

Carmin, C., and R. Ownby. 1994. The relationship between discharge readiness, inventory scales and the Brief Psychiatric Rating Scale. *Hospital and Community Psychiatry* 45, no. 3: 248–252.

Catherman, A. 1990. Biopsychosocial nursing assessment: A way to enhance care plans. *Journal of Psychosocial Nursing* 28, no. 6: 31–35.

Duffey, J. et al. 1993. Psychiatric home care: A framework for assessment and intervention. *Home Healthcare Nurse* 11, no. 2: 22–28.

Forchuk, C. et al. 1989. Establishing a nurse-client relationship. *Journal of Psychosocial Nursing* 27, no. 2: 30–34.

Gerace, L. 1990. Nursing assessment in psychiatric home care. *Journal of Home Health Care Practice* 3, no. 9: 9–15.

Jackson, J., and M. Neighbors. 1990. *Home care client assessment handbook*. Gaithersburg, MD: Aspen Publishers, Inc.

Jernigan, D. 1986. Mental health assessment and intervention: An integral part of nursing service. *Caring* 5, no. 7: 5–10.

Johnson, B., ed. 1993. *Psychiatric-mental health nursing: Adaptation and growth.* Philadelphia: J.B. Lippincott Co.

Keating, S., and G. Kelmer. 1988. *Home health care nursing: Concepts and practice.* Philadelphia: J.B. Lippincott Co.

McGorry, P.D. et al. 1988. The development, use and reliability of the Brief Psychiatric Rating Scale (Nursing Modification)—and assessment procedure for the nursing team in clinical and research settings. *Comprehensive Psychiatry* 29, no. 6: 575–587.

Merker, M. 1986. Psychiatric emergency evaluation. *Nursing Clinics of North America* 21, no. 3: 387–396.

Michaels, R.A. et al. 1989. Identifying akinesia and akathisia: The relationship between patient's self-report and nurse's assessment. *Archives of Psychiatric Nursing* 3, no. 3: 97–101.

Nathenson, P., and C. Johnson. 1992. The psychiatric treatment plan. *Perspectives in Psychiatric Care* 28, no. 3: 32–36.

O'Conner, F. et al. 1994. Psychosocial assessment for treatment planning and evaluation. *Journal of Psychosocial Nursing* 32, no. 5: 31–42.

Seifert, P., and C. Beck. 1989. Psychiatric assessment tool. In *Clinical assessment tools for use with nursing diagnosis*, eds. C. Guzzeetta et al., 161–171. St. Louis, MO: C.V. Mosby.

Shea, S. 1988. *Psychiatric interviewing: The art of understanding.* Philadelphia: W.B. Saunders Company.

Soreff, S. 1985. Indications for home treatment. *Psychiatric Clinics of North America* 8, no. 3: 563–575.

Stuart, G., and S. Sundeen. 1995. *Principles and practice of psychiatric nursing.* St. Louis, MO: C.V. Mosby.

Wilson, H., and A. Skodol. 1994. Special report: DSM-IV: Overview and examination of major changes. *Archives of Psychiatric Nursing* 8, no. 6: 340–347.

11

Patient-Centered, Outcome-Based Treatment Plan

INTRODUCTION

Treatment planning for the psychiatric home care patient is critical. It is, however, important to remember that "process has no value in itself; it must be tied to an intention to benefit the patient."[1(p.173)] Outcomes are the focus of treatment for each patient. It is easy to lose sight of this, as staff struggle to develop the best treatment plan for the patient. According to Mosher and Burti, "Treatment is not something that is 'done'; rather, it is a functional characteristic of the approach to the patient's needs. The therapeutic intervention does not exist; no intervention is by itself therapeutic or not. It is the sum of all interventions that has to be 'therapeutic,' and the service has to be organized in a way to make this possible."[2(p.28)] Becoming too involved in the process of treatment planning and losing sight of the patient and outcomes will ultimately interfere with the patient's care. There are additional problems with treatment planning for the psychiatric patient. Physical illness exists in an objective sense whereas mental illness is more subjective. This makes it more difficult to analyze assessment data, to identify problems and desired outcomes, and to identify interventions to reach the outcomes. Each home care nurse focuses on outcomes and interventions that can be used to encourage normalization for the psychiatric patient in the home.

COMPLIANCE AND RELAPSE

Compliance is a term that has mixed messages. It is easy to associate it with coercion or adherence. This approach is not helpful for patients and may have something to do with the problems that staff and patients encounter with compliance. It is difficult to talk about noncompliance without discussing recidivism or seriously mentally ill patients who use services on a revolving-door basis. These patients may have multiple crises within a brief period. "Although each patient is

231

different, these crises are all precipitated by the same underlying problem, namely the uncontrolled psychiatric illness."[3(p.31)] Typically the patient is blamed for non-compliance and recidivism when staff, family/SOs, and even the patient should see them as part of the illness. This negative labeling leads to self-fulfilling proph-ecies, low self-esteem, and noncompliance.[4] Effective treatment considers these factors; when home care staff reframe how they view recidivism and noncompli-ance, they can help the patient and the family/SOs cope more positively.

Noncompliance usually relates to medication, which is a critical intervention for the psychiatric home care patient. Noncompliance with medications also leads to noncompliance with other treatment interventions. Typically the reasons for medication noncompliance fall into five areas: (1) side effects, (2) unrealistic fears about medications, (3) lack of information, (4) trust and control issues, and (5) environmental factors. Examples of reasons for noncompliance that the home care nurse may experience with patients include the following:[5]

- The patient experiences uncomfortable and disabling side effects.
- The patient does not fully understand the illness or its seriousness or that it may be necessary to take the medication indefinitely.
- Medication reminds the patient that he or she is sick and lowers self-esteem.
- Most patients leave the hospital before symptoms are controlled and may be too sick to take medications correctly.
- The patient may not understand the delayed connection between stopping medication and experiencing relapse, because often weeks or even months pass between when the body metabolizes the medication and when the re-lapse occurs.
- The patient may feel that street drugs help more.
- It is difficult for the patient to remember to take medications.

The home care nurse can try some interventions to prevent noncompliance, relapse, and recidivism; however, it is important to remember that patient compli-ance will be influenced by the home environment and family/significant others (SOs). The home care nurse might consider the following interventions.[6]

- The medication selected should be one that is acceptable to the patient with the fewest side effects and lowest effective dose.
- If the patient is not reliable in taking the medication, long-acting depot medi-cation might be helpful. If relapse occurs while taking this type of medica-tion, staff will know that the relapse is not due to poor compliance with medications.
- Drug holidays (e.g., one weekend a month without medication) may decrease side effects and provide the patient with hope. This must be done with a physician's order and careful consideration of the patient's clinical status.

- The patient must be told if the medication will need to be taken long-term and given time to discuss his or her reaction to this news.
- Home care staff should develop specific methods to help the patient remember to take medications, and these need to be reviewed carefully with the patient.
- The home care nurse should provide complete education about all of the patient's medications for the patient and family/SOs; and often repetition is necessary.
- Medication self-assessment forms, checksheets for side effects, information pamphlets, information about when the patient can tolerate medication, and medication maintenance groups can be useful for the patient.
- It may be necessary to monitor blood levels for medications for which testing is available. This testing should be explained to the patient, and the results reviewed with the patient.
- Polypharmacy (the practice of administering more than one medicine) increases the risk of medication problems.
- Positive attitudes about the use of medications and the benefits of their use for the patient should be discussed with the patient/family/SOs.
- The patient needs to know how to appropriately negotiate changes in medications.
- Home care staff should develop interventions that will help the patient cope with medication side effects.
- Dietary requirements related to specific medications should be reviewed periodically.
- The patient must be taught to recognize symptoms that need to be reported to home care staff and the physician.

All interventions must focus on preparing the patient to be more independent and preparing the patient for discharge from home care.

TREATMENT PLANNING

After assessment data are obtained, treatment planning becomes the focus; however, it must be done quickly in order to focus on the care that the patient requires. The Joint Commission on Accreditation of Healthcare Organizations (Joint Commission) standards on home care state: "Care planning is performed to ensure that care and services are appropriate to each patient's specific needs and problems and the severity of his or her problems and needs."[7(p.10)] The care planning process must include the patient's individual problems and needs, goals, specific care and services to be provided, and actions or interventions to be taken.

Both the Joint Commission standards and Medicare require the following items in the plan of care:[8]

- pertinent diagnoses
- mental status
- types of services and equipment
- frequency of visits
- prognosis
- rehabilitation potential
- functional limitations
- activities permitted
- nutritional requirements
- medications and treatments
- safety measures
- instructions for timely discharge

The American Nurses Association (ANA) *Standards of Home Health Nursing Practice* and *Standards of Psychiatric-Mental Health Clinical Nursing Practice* both indicate the need for a treatment plan and goals or outcomes.[9,10] Appendixes B and C provide details about these standards. It is critical to include the patient in the planning as soon as the process begins. Exhibit 11–1 describes one tool that can be used to emphasize the need for active participation to the patient.

Exhibit 11–1 Activities and Support Interventions Log

What types of activities and support have been helpful to you in decreasing your depression?

Activity or Support	Have Tried Successfully	Should Use More Often	Would Like To Try

Source: Reprinted with permission from M. Copeland, *The Depression Workbook*, p. 81, © 1992, New Harbinger Publications, Inc.

CRITICAL PATHWAYS

Many health care providers have struggled for some time to develop methods for expediting the development of the treatment plan. The focus today is on critical pathways, clinical pathways, and disease management pathways. These methods are similar and all have definitions that continue to change. Several of these definitions are as follows:

- "A clinical pathway is a proactive multidisciplinary set of daily prescriptions and outcomes for the care of a specified patient population from pre-admission to post-discharge."[11(p.42)]
- "A critical pathway is a map or track of the patient's treatment."[12(p.53)]
- "The critical pathway method as it relates to the planning process is simply a diagram of a sequence of events leading to a desired outcome."[13(p.35)]

Critical pathways serve many purposes for the patient, home care staff, family/SOs, and the home care agency:[14–16]

- target the treatment focus
- sequence interventions predictably and avoid last-minute problems
- serve as orientation tool for staff
- specify expected outcomes with timelines
- provide guidelines for documentation
- minimize unnecessary documentation
- provide standards of care
- support cost-effective care
- provide tool to evaluate care provided
- provide reimbursement sources with information about home care delivered
- ensure the provision of patient/family/SO education

When the home care agency develops its own critical pathways, it may be difficult to know where to begin. According to Homan, "Psychiatric care is abstract and deals with behaviors, so it can be difficult to write a psychiatric critical path."[17(p.135)] The place to begin is with those diagnoses that have a high volume. An audit of past patients provides information about these diagnoses, typical interventions, and frequency of visits. As the home care staff assess the present pattern of care for the patient, three questions may guide this analysis.[18]

- At what points during the patient's home care do key interventions occur?
- What are the barriers to providing these interventions?
- What measurable clinical outcomes are the patient/family/SOs expected to achieve per visit?

Responses to these questions will provide data about the usual care provided to patients.

After the current practice is described, staff must then determine the optimal patterns and outcomes to include in the agency's critical pathways. Questions that can be used to guide this part of the analysis are:[19(p.43)]

- What clinical outcomes must be achieved for each home care visit to meet the expected outcomes by discharge?
- How should key interventions be sequenced to achieve the outcomes by discharge from home care?
- How should the work of each discipline be processed to provide the key interventions?
- What barriers exist to achievement of ideal clinical outcomes?

Exhibit 11–2 provides a format for critical pathways.

When critical pathways are implemented, home care staff must then focus on outcomes and variances. Was the care provided as described in the critical pathway? If not, why did a variance occur? Reasons usually can be categorized into staff, system, equipment, and cost. It may be that the pathway was not developed correctly. Staff will need to use the pathway for a reasonable period of time before changing it.

TREATMENT FOCUS AREAS

There are many approaches to organizing the treatment focus areas or determining how to categorize patient problems and treatment requirements. One system identifies seven areas: (1) psychological impairment, (2) social skills, (3) dangerousness, (4) activities of daily living/occupational skills, (5) medical problems, (6) substance abuse, and (7) ancillary problems (e.g., financial, housing, employment, legal, transportation).[20] Most home care patient problems can be assigned to one of these categories. These categories remind the home care staff of important areas to assess in determining whether the patient requires assistance.

PATIENT OUTCOMES

An expected patient outcome is a desired change in the patient. The most important characteristic of a desired patient outcome is that it should state "the *patient* will" rather than "*staff* will." In addition, expected outcomes should be clear and concise; realistic, observable, and measurable; and time oriented. They must be described in order to evaluate interventions. The patient participates in identi-

Exhibit 11–2 Example of a Critical Pathway Format

Each critical pathway covers the number of expected visits for a specific diagnosis (e.g., depression, schizophrenia, anxiety disorder). Each visit includes relevant assessment, laboratory tests, medications, specific interventions, teaching, and family/SO interventions.

Visit Number	Actions To Be Taken	Completed	Reasons Not Completed
	Assessment:		
	Laboratory tests:		
	Medications:		
	Specific interventions:		
	Teaching:		
	Family/SO interventions:		

fying desired outcomes for his or her care. Outcomes that are formulated by the home care staff or in conjunction with the family/SOs excluding the patient will fail. As outcomes are developed, they should be solution-focused; to ensure that they are, staff can consider the following:[21]

- Identify what is already working for the patient/family/SOs; often they already have knowledge and may simply need increased confidence about their observations.
- Recognize and use existing patient/family/SO strengths. Strengths can always be identified, but they often are less obvious than weaknesses. Reframing is a new perspective brought to a situation by considering alternative, equally possible, interpretations of events or the context of events.
- Write outcomes so that they are understandable and practical.
- Change occurs with change in behavior in the patient's real world with family/SOs participation as much as possible.

- The patient is the most important expert about his or her life.
- Ask thoughtful questions that help the patient recognize and value his or her own answers. Interventions are not what home care staff do to a patient but rather something they do *with* a patient.
- Use the patient's language and values; this respects the patient's worldview and facilitates culturally sensitive counseling.
- Use right-brain thinking; humor, music, images, and stories can increase patient learning.

As desired outcomes are developed, staff should consider time frames as they discuss outcomes with the patient. Klebanoff states: "Because home care services are provided on an episodic, intermittent basis, very long-term or enduring goals usually will not be met for months or years after discharge from psychosocial home care services."[22(p.764)] It is often easier to make grandiose plans rather than to focus on what can realistically be accomplished in a specified time period. Home care staff should not establish outcomes that lead to patient failure and a loss of self-esteem. The patient has had enough of these experiences. Priorities are set, and safety should always be first. Safety is the first consideration during the initial visit to the home, and it must be assessed at each visit. Exhibit 11–3 provides examples of expected patient outcomes.

As the patient's expected outcomes are developed, the home care nurse may need to work with the family/SO to develop outcomes for the family/SOs. Klebanoff recommends considering the following general outcomes when developing specific patient outcomes:[23]

- Maximize the patient's level of independence through health promotion, maintenance, and restoration.
- Prevent complications in the home through health teaching, education about psychoactive medication, and sharing information about community resources.
- Avert or minimize a psychiatric crisis through anticipation and planning.
- Delay an admission to a long-term care facility.

INTERVENTIONS

Generally, interventions for the psychiatric home care patient fall into the following categories:[24]

- crisis intervention
- medication administration, monitoring, and teaching
- individual, couple, family, and group counseling and psychotherapy
- verbal and written contracts with the patient

Exhibit 11–3 Examples of Patient Outcomes

- The patient will not attempt to harm self in any way until the nurse returns in 24 hours.
- The patient will call the hotline if he/she feels suicidal.
- The patient and family/SOs will identify two times that they make a positive statement to each other during the next two days.
- The patient will get up by 7:30 AM; be dressed each morning by 8:30 AM, and go to bed by 11 PM.
- The patient will identify three symptoms that indicate he or she is becoming anxious.
- The patient will identify how he or she can reduce anxiety.
- The patient will identify three side effects from his or her medication.
- The patient will follow the method designated for remembering to take his or her medication.
- The patient will identify the diet restrictions related to his or her medications.
- The family/SOs will attend a National Alliance for the Mentally Ill (NAMI) meeting every week.
- The family/SOs will allow the patient to assist in preparing one meal a day by giving him/her a specific task to do for the meal. If the patient is successful for three consecutive meals, he or she may then be given a choice as to which task to complete.
- The patient will identify two harmful effects of his or her anger.
- The patient will express anger appropriately every day.
- The patient will participate in the family discussion about _____.
- The patient will participate in planning care by identifying an outcome and ways to arrive at that outcome by the next home visit.
- The patient will participate in self-care by _____ for the next three days.
- The patient will take medications as ordered every day.
- The patient will ask for help when _____.
- The patient will demonstrate knowledge about _____ (e.g., illness, medications, specific intervention).
- The patient will identify three situations that lead to his or her anxiety.
- The patient will identify two methods to relieve his or her anxiety.
- The patient will apply the following methods to relieve anxiety: _____.
- The patient will differentiate between realistic and unrealistic fears.
- The patient will describe information or where to locate information needed to get emergency help.
- The patient will recognize his or her denial.
- The patient will use problem-solving techniques.
- The patient will share his or her feelings appropriately with family/SOs.

continues

Exhibit 11–3 continued

- The patient will share his or her feelings appropriately with home care staff.
- The patient will participate in activities of daily living.
- The patient will write and follow a schedule.
- The patient will sleep _____ hours per night.
- The patient will not sleep during the day.
- The patient will take a quiet time every day at _____.
- The patient will engage in social interactions at least _____ times per day.
- The patient will develop two interventions for _____ (problem behavior) with family/SOs.
- The patient will accept responsibilities for actions.
- The patient will tolerate a home visit.
- The patient will attend _____ (e.g., physician's appointment, AA group).
- The patient will abstain from use of alcohol (drugs).
- The patient will accept positive feedback from family/SOs and home care staff.
- The patient will accept negative feedback from family/SOs and home care staff.
- The patient will show concern for family/SOs by listening to them and respecting their rights.
- The patient will participate in family life by _____.
- The patient will discuss reasons for noncompliance.
- The patient will report side effects from medications to home care staff.
- The patient will monitor symptoms by keeping a daily log.
- The patient will use relaxation techniques once a day.
- The patient will develop a plan to increase activities.
- The patient will describe how he or she will obtain the prescription.
- The patient will describe how to use the bus (subway, cab).
- The patient will identify two of his or her strengths.
- The patient will be oriented to time, place, and person.
- The patient will remove self from disturbing stimuli or environment.
- The patient will interpret stimuli correctly.
- The patient will decrease social isolation by _____.

- health guidance and referral
- patient advocacy
- case management activities
- mental, emotional, physical, and spiritual observation, interpretation, and evaluation
- home care team coordination
- liaison activities
- communication with the physician and other health care providers

- role modeling/social skills education
- psychoeducation

The chapters of this book that focus on specific clinical problems discuss extensive specific interventions that can be used with patients. The focus here is on those interventions that can be used with a variety of patients and interventions that focus primarily on psychiatric rehabilitation. These interventions emphasize improving interpersonal and independent living skills, behavioral and cognitive skills, and social skills.

Self-Care Skills

Interventions related to social skills vary greatly from one patient to another. Patients with serious mental illness such as schizophrenia or severe depression or those with Alzheimer's may require interventions in the following additional areas:

- taking a bath or shower
- brushing teeth
- shampooing hair
- shaving
- feminine hygiene
- applying makeup and styling hair
- changing clothes and wearing appropriate clothes
- eating and drinking
- menu planning
- shopping
- preparing meals safely
- paying bills and banking
- using the telephone
- using public transportation

Self-care skills help the patient feel in control. They are a very important part of renormalization. Some patients need to learn how to do these skills, some just require guidance, and others need to have another person do them. The latter group of patients must be considered carefully; they must always be encouraged to participate in self-care when it is reasonable. Dependency can be reinforced when self-care activities are done for and to the patient. This, of course, is not the goal of psychiatric rehabilitation or psychiatric home care. Home care staff should concentrate on what the patient can do for himself or herself and respond with positive feedback. It often is easier to respond to limitations and negative behavior, neither of which is helpful.

Social Skills Training

Some patients have never developed social skills; for others, the illness may have affected these skills negatively. The patient may also have problems expressing feelings or expressing them appropriately, and this affects social skills and interactions with others. To develop social skills, the patient will need to use accurate perception and cognitive processing, and to send appropriate responses. Home care staff may observe poor eye contact, inappropriate facial expression, poor gestures and posture, poor response time, poor interpersonal judgment, and inadequate recognition of emotions. In order to assess or develop the patient's social skills, the home care nurse can ask the patient to practice verbally accepting a compliment or a criticism, to problem solve and carry on a negotiation, to assert himself or herself, and to use recreational or leisure time appropriately.[25]

The social skills training process includes the following steps and activities:[26]

- *Problem definition*—The home care nurse and the patient identify deficits of socially acceptable behavior.
- *Inventory of assets*—The home care nurse and the patient identify strengths and capabilities in social relations (e.g., Has the patient maintained a friendship? Does the patient know how to greet people? Does the patient know how to sustain a conversation?).
- *Therapeutic alliance*—The home care nurse and the patient develop a relationship and agree to work on the patient's problems together with the nurse respecting the patient's participation and rights.
- *Goal setting*—The home care nurse and the patient should move quickly from problems to establishing positive goals rather than reinforcing problems by dwelling on them. These goals should be specific and concrete, and relate to interpersonal skills. Activities that might be used to meet these goals include behavioral rehearsal, positive reinforcement, shaping, prompting, and modeling.
- *Behavioral rehearsal*—The home care nurse through role play simulates situations that approximate the patient's real-life circumstances. After a role play, the nurse asks questions such as "Who were you talking with? What did the other person want? How was the other person feeling? What was your short-term goal in the situation? What alternatives could you have used to deal with the situation?"
- *Positive reinforcement*—Staff will use verbal and nonverbal praise or a high-frequency reinforcer. This is any behavior that occurs at high frequency that will reinforce other more adaptive behaviors that are not occurring enough.
- *Shaping*—Shaping is used to make a large task easier to learn. When staff break down the large task into smaller components, the process is less overwhelming for the patient. The patient can then experience success when

smaller components are accomplished rather than failure when he or she cannot complete another, larger task.

- *Prompting*—Staff may not always be able to wait for desirable behavior to provide positive feedback or reinforcement. They may need to prompt or cue the patient to use the skill.
- *Modeling*—Staff may demonstrate a particular skill or component of a skill for the patient.

Homework

Assigning homework for the patient to do is an intervention that can be used very successfully. It communicates directly to the patient that he or she must participate. It establishes expectations and provides concrete activities for the patient to do between home care visits. Homework can provide a link to specific activities that the patient and family/SOs must do together. Assignments are also an excellent method for evaluating progress and providing opportunity to give positive feedback to the patient; however, it is important for home care staff to always find something positive to say about the homework assignment. If staff approach homework with an authoritarian attitude and "a red pencil," the therapeutic alliance will be damaged. Some patients are more sensitive to criticism, and others want criticism to support their low self-esteem. Home care staff should assess the patient's response to criticism or feedback and consider this response when caring for the patient. Family/SOs may also need help in understanding the patient's responses. The following are examples of homework assignments that might be used:

- Set goals for week with home care staff.
- Sleep eight hours during the night.
- Keep a log of times when patient felt _____ (e.g., happy, anger, confused, hallucinating, etc.).
- Problem solve with family/SOs about _____ (add specific problem).
- Eat three meals a day.
- Take a shower every morning by 9 AM.
- Take medication as ordered.
- Brush teeth two times a day (morning and night).
- Change clothes every day by 9 AM.
- Make bed every morning by _____ AM.
- Get out of bed by _____.
- Go to bed by _____.
- Do a specific household task _____ a specific number of times _____.
- Initiate a conversation with _____ about_____.

- Express anger appropriately by _____.
- Eat at the table with the family/SOs.
- Telephone a friend or relative.
- Make an appointment with _____.
- Develop the shopping list.
- Attend medication maintenance group.
- Use the bus to get to_____.
- Visit a neighbor.
- Use relaxation technique once a day; write in your log how you felt before and after.
- Clean room and change bed linens on _____ (specific day).

Examples of tools that may be used for homework are found in Exhibits 11–4, 11–5, 11–6, 11–7, 11–8, and 11–9.

Treatment Contract: Coping with Inappropriate Behavior

When treatment contracts are made with the patient, it is assumed that the patient has rights regarding his or her care and that the home care nurse is a responsible professional who is competent to negotiate a contract with the pa-

---

Exhibit 11–4 Homework Record

Name: _____

Date assignment given: _____ Date due: _____

Goal: _____

Homework assignment:

Home care staff name: _____

Assignment completed: _____ Yes _____ No

Reason not completed:

Exhibit 11–5 Target Complaint Scale

Describe the specific target complaint (e.g., audio hallucination, crying, sleeping during the day). Fill in date columns. For each date, the patient rates the target complaint by checking the appropriate horizontal columns. The patient may make any comments about the target symptom in the comment column.

Patient's Name: Date Begun:

Specific Complaint:

Description	Dates							Comments
Did not experience								
Experienced only during the day (6 AM–5 PM)								
Experienced only during the night (5 PM–6 AM)								
Did not interfere with my activities								
Was overwhelming								

Source: Adapted with permission from R. Liberman, ed., *Psychiatric Rehabilitation of Chronic Mental Illness*, p. 70, © 1988, American Psychiatric Press, Inc.

tient. Contracts help the patient try new behaviors and responses and learn new coping techniques. The contract includes a written set of the home care staff's and the patient's expectations or desired outcomes and responsibilities. Contracts are openly negotiated and clearly stated. Both home care staff and the patient have a copy of the contract. The contract can be used to evaluate progress with the

Exhibit 11–6 Warning Signs Checklist

> *The patient and the home care staff should identify the patient's early warning signs in the appropriate column. The patient will then check off the days in which the patient experiences these signs that might indicate the patient is experiencing more problems and possible relapse.*

Week: _____

Early Warning Sign	Monday	Tuesday	Wednesday	Thursday	Friday	Saturday	Sunday

Source: Reprinted with permission from M. Copeland, *The Depression Workbook*, p. 109, © 1992, New Harbinger Publications, Inc.

Exhibit 11–7 Homework Log: Interactions with Others

Day	Person involved	What did he/she say or do?	What did you say or do?
Monday			
Tuesday			
Wednesday			
Thursday			
Friday			
Saturday			
Sunday			

Exhibit 11–8 Symptom Management Worksheet

1. Identify a symptom.

2. How does this symptom affect your overall stability?

3. In the past how did you respond to this symptom?

4. What could be a more productive way of handling this symptom?

5. Who could you use for more support to deal with this symptom?

Source: David L. Favreau, LMHC, LCSW, Assertive Communications, 24 Hoover Street, Dracut, MA 01826.

patient. A contract is renegotiated or terminated and should never continue indefinitely. Prior to negotiating the contract with the patient, the home care nurse should have some ideas as to possible content and expectations. The patient needs to understand the purpose of the process. The home care agency should have a standardized form for the contract, such as the one found in Exhibit 11–10.

The goal of the treatment contract is to help the patient. Throughout the process of developing and implementing the contract, the patient needs positive feedback, both verbal and nonverbal. Staff should let the patient know that the patient can take responsibility for himself or herself. The contract is part of the patient's record; it documents interventions, patient participation, and progress. A treatment contract can help to focus the work that is being done with a patient, particularly when the staff or the patient feel that it is difficult to know what is going on in the care process. Contracts can also be developed between the patient and

Exhibit 11–9 Daily Schedule

Time	Planned Activities and Expectations	Actual Activity	How It Felt
7–8 AM			
8–9 AM			
9–10 AM			
10–11 AM			
11–12 noon			
12–1 PM			
1–2 PM			
2–3 PM			
3–4 PM			
4–5 PM			
5–6 PM			
6–7 PM			
7–8 PM			
8–9 PM			
9–10 PM			

Source: Reprinted with permission from M. Copeland, *The Depression Workbook*, p. 63, © 1992, New Harbinger Publications, Inc.

the family/SOs as a method to clarify interventions that they will use together. Home care staff should explain the process and help them develop contracts. This is an intervention method that family/SOs can continue to use after the patient is discharged from home care.

The patient's family/SOs must find ways to cope with inappropriate behavior. Esser and Lacey recommend the following interventions for some common behaviors that cause problems; however, the interventions must be individualized for each patient.[27]

- *Violent outbursts.* First, get a safe distance away from the ill person. Yell, "STOP!" once. Do not repeat the yelling and arguing, as it will only make matters worse. If your effort for getting attention works, keep your distance and calmly talk to the person; ask what has upset him or her. If the person

Exhibit 11–10 Treatment Contract

The contract is between _____ and _____, RN

Date Begun _____ Evaluation Dates _____ Date Terminated _____

Problem Behavior	Outcome	Date	Patient Responsibilities	Home Care Staff/Family/SO Responsibilities

does not talk, try to figure out what might have caused the outburst. Was a routine changed? Was the person unsuccessful at performing a task? Was the person in a social or crowded situation that was overwhelming? Did a movie or television show precede the event? Is there undue stress among members of the household?

- *Inappropriate manners.* Ignore inappropriate manners as much as possible. Try using positive reinforcement for the behaviors done correctly or start a conversation about something the recovering person enjoys.
- *Excessive smoking.* Develop rules on where a person can smoke. In the beginning, it is not advisable to let the recovering individual smoke in the bedroom unless this activity is under control. This means that you may need to write a schedule or make a contract to ensure that the individual knows when and where smoking is allowed, how to use ashtrays, how to make sure that nothing is left burning when there is an interruption, etc.
- *Refusal to get out of bed.* Check with the ill family member's schedule, saying, "This schedule says that the time to get up is 8 o'clock. Are you up yet?" You cannot give a check mark if the task has not been completed.
- *Refusal to bathe.* Refer to and read the schedule with the ill family member; always ask questions; do not make demands. Reinforce any actions taken toward bathing.
- *Refusal to change clothes.* Check with the schedule again. Give the ill family member clean clothing, saying, "I'll be happy to wash the favorite clothes you have on if you will give them to me. I know that you like the feel and smell of your favorite clothes being clean." Another approach might be, "As soon as you put on these clothes, we will go out."
- *Refusal to speak when spoken to.* Sometimes, the recovering person just does not have anything to say, or maybe the statements were misunderstood. If it is important for the recovering person to answer you, just wait until later to talk.
- *Running away or wandering away.* This is one of the saddest events that can occur. Sometimes, the ill person believes his or her voices are saying to go somewhere else. The response to the voices can be devastating. Make sure the person always has vital information, such as address and telephone, in his or her possession. A medic alert necklace or bracelet may be worn. Name tags and telephone number should be on articles of clothing. Hide a small amount of money in some article of clothing, such as shoes, and tell the ill family member that this is for emergencies. Practice with the ill family member what to do in case he or she ever becomes lost. For example, look for a person in a uniform and show that person the medic alert necklace or bracelet; ask for a telephone; call home; stay in the place or outside the door where the telephone call was made.

- *Leaving the ill person alone.* Sometimes this is a difficult situation, especially when the ill family member may not be entirely trustworthy. If you must leave him or her alone at times, start by leaving the person for very short intervals, then slightly longer intervals, then gradually stay away for longer lengths of time. Tell the recovering person where you will be, when you will return, and your expectations of him or her. You can also start teaching some basic house rules.
- *Family meals.* Do not insist that the ill person eat with the family or share in conversation at first if this is not the person's chosen activity. Invite the ill family member to join you, but do not make a big deal out of it if you are refused. You must, however, tell the recovering person where he/she can eat. Remember that you are in charge of the household.

Problem Solving

Problem solving is a limitation for all psychiatric patients and often for their families/SOs. Home care staff will need to work with patients and their families/SOs to improve these skills. The home care nurse can assess their problem-solving ability by meeting with them and asking them to solve a specific problem in 5 to 10 minutes. The nurse should not participate but rather observes their interactions and the results, entering into the conversation only if required to control escalating emotions. This should be made clear to the family/SOs prior to the request to problem solve. As a result of this experience, the nurse may obtain more information about their problem-solving skills and limitations. This will provide a place to begin to help them. Many patients who have limited problem-solving skills initially define the problem too broadly, making it difficult to solve (e.g., I am too messy). The problem needs to be described more specifically; this will help guide the choice of the intervention to solve the problem (e.g., I leave my dirty dishes all over the house; never wash my laundry; leave dirty ashtrays, etc.). Selecting the best solution will require a specific description of the problem that everyone can agree on.

SUMMARY

Often it is easier to do an assessment than to analyze the assessment data and develop appropriate expected outcomes and interventions. The patient must participate in the development of desired outcomes and interventions or treatment will fail. The home care nurse must be creative, patient, and flexible in order to help the patient achieve the desired treatment outcomes.

NOTES

1. D. Olsen, "Ethical Cautions in the Use of Outcomes for Resource Allocation in the Managed Care Environment of Mental Health," *Archives of Psychiatric Nursing* 9, no. 4 (1995): 173–178, at 173.

2. L. Mosher and L. Burti, *Community Mental Health: Principles and Practice* (New York: W.W. Norton & Company, 1989), 28.

3. L. Beebe, "Reframe Your Outlook on Recidivism," *Journal of Psychosocial Nursing* 28, no. 9 (1990): 31–33, at 31.

4. Beebe, "Reframe Your Outlook on Recidivism," 32.

5. B. Wittlin, "Practical Psychopharmacology," in *Psychiatric Rehabilitation of Chronic Mental Patients*, ed. R. Liberman (Washington, DC: American Psychiatric Press, Inc., 1988), 117–145, at 132–133.

6. Wittlin, "Practical Psychopharmacology," 139–141.

7. Joint Commission on Accreditation of Healthcare Organizations, *1995 Accreditation Manual for Home Care*, Vol. 1 (Oakbrook Terrace, IL: 1994), 10.

8. Joint Commission on Accreditation of Healthcare Organizations, *1995 Accreditation Manual for Home Care*, Vol. 1, 92.

9. American Nurses Association, *Standards of Home Health Nursing Practice* (Washington, DC: 1986).

10. American Nurses Association, *A Statement on Psychiatric-Mental Health Clinical Nursing Practice and Standards of Psychiatric-Mental Health Clinical Nursing Practice* (Washington, DC: 1994).

11. K. Graybeal, "Clinical Pathway Development: The Overlake Model," *Nursing Management* 24, no. 4 (1993): 42–46, at 42.

12. K. Giuliano and C. Poirier, "Nursing Case Management: Critical Pathways to Desirable Outcomes," *Nursing Management* 22, no. 3 (1991): 52–55, at 53.

13. D. Goodwin, "Critical Pathways in Home Healthcare," *Journal of Nursing Administration* 22, no. 2 (1992): 35–40, at 35.

14. G. Stuart, "Implementing the Nursing Process: Standards of Care," in *Principles and Practice of Psychiatric Nursing*, ed. G. Stuart and S. Sundeen (St. Louis, MO: Mosby–Year Book, 1995), 199–219, at 209.

15. Goodwin, "Critical Pathways in Home Healthcare," 38–39.

16. Giuliano and Poirier, "Nursing Case Management: Critical Pathways to Desirable Outcomes," 53.

17. C. Homan, "Five Hospitals Succeed with Critical Paths for Psychiatric Inpatients," *Hospital Case Management* 2, no. 8 (1994): 135–138, at 135.

18. Graybeal, "Clinical Pathway Development: The Overlake Model," 43.

19. Graybeal, "Clinical Pathway Development: The Overlake Model," 43.

20. J. Kennedy, *Fundamentals of Psychiatric Treatment Planning* (Washington, DC: American Psychiatric Press, Inc., 1992), 5.

21. D. Webster et al., "Introducing Solution-Focused Approaches to Staff in Inpatient Psychiatric Settings," *Archives of Psychiatric Nursing* 8, no. 4 (1994): 254–261, at 255.

22. N. Klebanoff, "Psychosocial Home Care," in *Psychiatric-Mental Health Nursing: Adaptation and Growth*, ed. B. Johnson (Philadelphia: J.B. Lippincott Co., 1993), 758–773, at 764.

23. Klebanoff, "Psychosocial Home Care," 766.

24. Klebanoff, "Psychosocial Home Care," 769–770.

25. R. Liberman, "Social Skills Training," in *Psychiatric Rehabilitation of Chronic Mental Patients*, ed. R. Liberman (Washington, DC: American Psychiatric Press, Inc., 1988), 147–198, at 151.

26. Liberman, "Social Skills Training," 159–163.

27. A. Esser and S. Lacey, *Mental Illness: A Homecare Guide* (New York: John Wiley & Sons, 1989), 168–173.

SUGGESTED READING

Baker, C. 1995. The development of the self-care ability to detect early signs of relapse among individuals who have schizophrenia. *Archives of Psychiatric Nursing* 9, no. 5: 261–268.

Beebe, J. 1990. Reframe your outlook on recidivism. *Journal of Psychosocial Nursing* 28, no. 9: 31–33.

Copeland, M. 1992. *The depression workbook*. Oakland, CA: New Harbinger Publications, Inc.

DeRisi, W., and G. Butz. 1975. *Writing behavioral objectives*. Champaign, IL: Research Press.

Goodwin, D. 1992. Critical pathways in home healthcare. *Journal of Nursing Administration* 22, no. 2: 35–40.

Hamera, C. et al. 1991. Patient self-regulation and functioning in schizophrenia. *Hospital and Community Psychiatry* 42, no. 6: 630–631.

Harris, J. 1990. Self-care actions of chronic schizophrenics associated with meeting solitude and social interaction requisites. *Archives of Psychiatric Nursing* 4, no. 5: 298–307.

Jackson, J., and M. Neighbors. 1990. *Home care client assessment handbook*. Gaithersburg, MD: Aspen Publishers, Inc.

Jernigan, D. 1986. Mental health assessment and intervention: An integral part of nursing service. *Caring* 5, no. 7: 5–10.

Joyce, B. et al. 1990. Staying well: Factors contributing to successful community adaptation. *Journal of Psychosocial Nursing* 28, no. 6: 20–24.

Keating, S., and G. Kelmer. 1988. *Home health care nursing: Concepts and practice*. Philadelphia: J.B. Lippincott Co.

Liberman, R. 1988. *Psychiatric rehabilitation of chronic mental patients*. Washington, DC: American Psychiatric Press, Inc.

Martin, K., and N. Scheet. 1992. *The Omaha system: A pocket guide for community health nursing*. Philadelphia: W.B. Saunders Company.

Munich, R., and E. Lang. 1993. The boundaries of psychiatric rehabilitation. *Hospital and Community Psychiatry* 44, no. 7: 661–665.

Murphy, M., and M. Moller. 1993. Relapse management in neurobiological disorders: The Moller-Murphy symptom management assessment tool. *Archives of Psychiatric Nursing* 7, no. 4: 226–235.

O'Conner, F. 1991. Symptom monitoring for relapse prevention in schizophrenia. *Archives of Psychiatric Nursing* 5, no. 4: 193–201.

Olsen, D. Ethical cautions in the use of outcomes for resource allocation in the managed care environment of mental health. *Archives of Psychiatric Nursing* 9, no. 4: 173–178.

Seifert, P., and C. Beck. 1989. Psychiatric assessment tool. In *Clinical Assessment Tools for Use with Nursing Diagnosis*, ed. C. Guzzeetta et al., 161–171. St. Louis, MO: C.V. Mosby.

❖

Psychopharmacology for the Psychiatric Patient in the Home

CHAPTER

12

The Decade of the Brain
and Psychopharmacology

INTRODUCTION

The 1990s have been called the "Decade of the Brain" due to the explosion of research in the area of psychiatry. This has caused increased stress for psychiatric nursing because it has required change in nursing practice. McKeon stated in 1990 that "the biological view of mental illness integrated into the practice of nursing provides an opportunity for psychiatric mental health nursing to achieve a distinct and valued role in the care of patients who are seriously mentally ill."[1(p.19)] Psychiatric home care might be a place to demonstrate a biopsychosocial synthesis as described by Pothier: "The core of psychiatric nursing will still be the use of ourselves in therapeutic relationships, but the goal of our interpersonal encounters will be to assist patients and families in living and functioning better with chronic disorders, rather than emphasizing psychotherapy in its traditional sense."[2(p.77)]

Home care patients require both excellent medical care and excellent psychiatric nursing care. Many psychiatric illnesses have physiological components, and research will probably discover even more. Medications require monitoring of the patient's physical status and psychological status. Many patients with psychiatric illnesses also have medical illnesses. In addition, the home care nurse cares for patients with medical illnesses who are experiencing psychological responses to their illnesses that require interventions. In the home the patient is a person with all of the biopsychosocial components. It is easier to compartmentalize a patient's needs when he or she is in the hospital on a psychiatric unit, but in the home it is more difficult. The focus of Part IV is biological psychiatry, the biological science that describes the etiology and treatment of mental illness, particularly focusing on psychophysiology, psychobiology, psychoneurology, psychoneuroendocrinology, and psychoneuroimmunology.[3]

257

To emphasize the importance of the recent scientific advances that are changing the understanding of the human brain, mental illness, and biochemical treatments of mental disorders, the American Nurses Association (ANA) created a psychopharmacology task force in 1992. The task force developed psychopharmacology guides for psychiatric mental health nurses that are described in the publication about the project.[4] The information is highly relevant for nurses who work in psychiatric home care, which is a more independent psychiatric nursing role than inpatient psychiatric nursing. The psychiatric home care nurse has less support when providing direct care and must provide the frontline assessment and monitoring of the patient's status, particularly in regard to medications. The ANA guidelines serve as the framework for this discussion of psychopharmacology for the psychiatric home care patient.

GUIDING PRINCIPLES

According to the ANA: "The goal of clinical management of psychopharmacologic interventions is to promote physiological stability that will permit the attainment of psychological, social, and spiritual growth—thus enhancing the quality of the patient's life and health."[5(p.31)] Guiding principles related to psychopharmacology that should be considered as the nurse forms a relationship with the home care patient and the family/significant others (SOs) include ecological advocacy, collaboration, efficacy and progress of treatment, education, and legal and ethical standards.

Ecological Advocacy

The home care nurse and the patient come together to develop a patient-centered treatment plan that, for most patients, will include medication. The principle of ecological advocacy emphasizes that the process and the nurse's philosophical view ensure that medications or the psychopharmacological interventions promote the patient's quality of life.[6] This advocacy requires that the nurse have some understanding of the patient's view of treatment and potential goals. Information must be shared. The nurse gains information from the patient assessment and other sources such as the patient's family/SOs, referring physician, or previous hospital records. The nurse shares information in this interactive relationship with the patient and, as appropriate, with the family/SOs about the psychopharmacological interventions. Questions to consider include the following:

- What does the patient hope to obtain from the use of medications?
- How many side effects is the patient willing to experience?

- How much time will the patient allow for the medication to work?
- What side effects are most troublesome for the patient?
- What are the family's/SOs' expectations about the use of medications?

Responses to these questions may indicate the need to change psychopharmacological interventions. The next principle, collaboration, is directly related to advocacy.

Collaboration

Collaboration requires joint effort on the part of the home care nurse and the patient and family/SOs. On the surface this may appear to be an easy principle to meet, but it is not. It is the rare patient-nurse relationship that immediately agrees on goals and methods for reaching those goals. Most nurses assume, but may not acknowledge, that the patient's goals will eventually be the same as the nurse's goals for treatment. Collaboration eventually requires that choices are made, and the nurse may not always agree with the patient's choice, such as to decrease dosage to prevent a side effect. The nurse must provide the patient with the information needed to make the choice and help the patient develop the necessary decision-making skills; however, ultimately the patient must make the choice. According to the ANA: "The nurse must make a commitment to 'live through the choice with the patient.' This commitment may mean maintaining a supportive and trusting relationship with the patient who chooses a direction that is different from that advocated by the nurse and/or the treatment team."[7(p.32)]

Efficacy and Progress of Treatment

The goal of the principle of efficacy and progress of treatment is to provide an effective psychopharmacologic treatment program with the patient and family/SOs. This requires that goals, outcomes, and interventions are agreed upon and based on both nursing and medical diagnostic reliability.[8] According to the ANA guidelines, the following should be part of the patient-focused health care delivery system:

- Recommendation of medication by health care professionals must be integrated with the patient's perspective of significant life issues.
- Balancing side effects and efficacy is a serious consideration for each patient and each medication.
- Elements that might be agreed upon before treatment begins include the adjustment range within which the patient may alter the dosage pattern, the

methods for dealing with missed doses, and the physiological conditions that require a change in dosage.

- Each medication must be given sufficient time before progress is determined. This monitoring should include an assessment of target symptoms.
- Critical elements of progress include the patient's overall functioning, satisfaction, and self-care activities.
- Adverse effects must be included in monitoring.
- Each patient should be screened for factors that might interfere with medication actions or monitoring (e.g., liver pathology that might interfere with absorption).
- Interactions with food and other drugs are considered throughout treatment.
- Side effects and idiosyncratic responses to medications are identified and treated.
- The nurse must develop practical methods for monitoring side effects, adverse effects, and response to medications (e.g., use of standardized rating measures, patient log of side effects).
- The nurse, in collaboration with the patient and the family/SOs, develops a plan that focuses on potential problems that may arise requiring actions. The plan should be specific to the patient and each medication the patient is taking.

Education

Patient and family/SO education is critical to any success that psychopharmacology might offer the home care patient. According to the ANA psychiatric-mental health standards, "the psychiatric-mental health nurse, through health teaching, assists patients in achieving satisfying, productive, and healthy patterns of living."[9(p.31)] If the patient has been hospitalized and has begun medication, the assumption might be made that the patient received medication education in the hospital. If this education was provided, many factors may affect its effectiveness. With shorter lengths of stay, there is less time to provide comprehensive medication education and assess its effectiveness. Patients are sicker in the hospital, less time is devoted to recovery and more time is devoted to crisis intervention. Thus patients are less able to receive education. With many admissions, sicker patients, and less professional nursing staff, there is less time for education that meets individual needs. Patients may return home before a response to medication is actually observed, or medications may be changed after discharge.

In the long run, the patient and families/SOs must know everything they possibly can about medications as they will ultimately be responsible for its administration and monitoring. A major responsibility for the psychiatric home care nurse is to teach the patient/family/SOs about the medication, its administration, and monitoring its effectiveness. To accomplish this, the nurse must be knowledgeable about psychopharmacology as well as adult education principles and methods. When teaching patients, the nurse must consider the patient's developmental level, reading ability, and cultural and linguistic factors. All education must be documented, including "evidence of what the patient knows, and documentation of how and when the patient's knowledge is changed by symptoms of the disorder.[10(p.33)] According to the Joint Commission on Accreditation of Healthcare Organizations (Joint Commission) standards for home care, this education includes the following:[11]

- name and description of the medication
- dosage, route of administration, duration of drug therapy
- special directions and precautions related to preparation, self-administration, and use of the medication in the home with attention paid to safeguards against microbial contamination and appropriate compounding and administration techniques
- intended use and expected actions of the medication therapy
- significant side effects, interactions, and therapeutic contraindications including avoidance recommendations and action required if side effects occur
- self-monitoring techniques
- storage and expiration dating of medications
- prescription refill information
- action to be taken for a missed dose
- proper disposal of unused or expired medications
- potential drug-food interactions and relevant diet considerations

The ANA standards for home care also emphasize teaching the patient and family/SOs, but these standards are less specific about the education required for self-medication.[12]

Legal and Ethical Standards

As with all areas of nursing, legal and ethical standards must be maintained. These include professional nursing standards, the ANA *Ethical Code,*[13] agency standards, relevant state laws, and rules and regulations related to Medicare. The following are some specific legal issues.

Informed Consent and Medications

Psychopharmacology is not without risks to the patient. As a consequence of this, informed consent is very important. Patients have the right to be told about the recommended medications before they take them and have the right to refuse this treatment. The patient's physician should review the medication and its risks and benefits before the initial dose of medication. Failure to do this may result in charges of negligence or assault and battery. Each state has laws related to these issues, and the home care nurse must be knowledgeable about them and their application in the home care setting.

Noncompliance with Medication

Some patients refuse medications. Each nurse needs to know the appropriate agency policy and procedure about noncompliance. The policy and procedure should be based on state laws. The patient's physician should be notified, and this should be documented in the patient's medical record. Patients should not be deceived about taking medications.

Experimental Drugs

The nurse must follow agency policy and procedure related to experimental drug use. The patient must be informed and give written consent to the physician. Nurses need to be given information about the drug in order to provide appropriate nursing care.

Guidelines Related to Medications and Legal Issues

- The nurse must know about drugs that he or she administers.
- Physician orders must be accurate and transcribed correctly.
- If a nurse has any questions about an order, the physician should be contacted. If the nurse is still not satisfied, the nurse's supervisor should be contacted.
- The patient is identified prior to administering the medication or providing the prescription.
- Allergies are identified during the admission assessment and updated as necessary.
- The nurse monitors side effects and develops appropriate interventions with the patient and family/SOs.
- The patient's rights are maintained at all times.
- The home care staff report medications errors and complete required documentation (such as an incident report).
- Documentation includes side effects, compliance, patient education, effectiveness, identification of target symptoms, and referral of treatment responsibility or consultation.
- Patient consent is obtained prior to release of psychopharmacologic treatment information.

- Delegation of tasks to a paraprofessional requires that the nurse assess the paraprofessional's knowledge, skill, and ability to perform those tasks to ensure that they meet state law requirements.

CLINICAL MANAGEMENT

Psychopharmacological Assessment

Prior to completing a psychopharmacological assessment, the nurse must be knowledgeable about the medications the patient is taking, including the following:[14]

- medication actions
- target effects
- unwanted effects, such as side effects, toxicity, and adverse effects
- medication management, such as dosage, scheduling, lab monitoring, symptom assessment
- precautions/contraindications
- interactive effects, such as with other medications, food, health status, behavior, and the environment

It is difficult to remember all of the information about medications, particularly for medications that are not prescribed frequently; however, reviewing this information is critical. This review will assist during the assessment and during clinical management and patient education.

The psychopharmacological assessment provides baseline data that may later be used to assess patient responses and thus affect clinical decision making. If the nurse knows the patient's medications prior to the initial visit, the first step is to review information about any medication that may be unfamiliar or used infrequently. The agency should have written educational material that the nurse will use at the appropriate time with the patient and family/SO, preferably during the initial visit. The information will be reinforced at each visit. During the admission assessment, the pharmacological assessment is performed focusing on the following specific areas:[15]

- identification of target symptoms and selection of treatment methods
- side-effect profile of selected pharmacologic agents
- response to prior medications
- concomitant drug use
- drug allergies
- patient preference for treatment

- therapeutic response of first-degree (biological) family members to medication for related problems

Asking the patient and family/SOs if they have kept logs or diaries about the patient's medications may reveal important and helpful information. After encountering problems with health care providers about medications, many families/SOs have kept such diaries so that they could use the information. As indicated earlier, the patient's preferences for treatment cannot be ignored, and it is during the assessment that the nurse initially ascertains the patient's view of his or her illness and treatment. As information is collected about the family's medical history, particularly members with similar diagnoses such as depression, it is important to identify medications that were taken and the family member's response to those medications. For example, if a tricyclic antidepressant was taken, did the family member improve? Were adverse reactions experienced? This information may help health care providers determine the proper medication for the patient and avoid interventions that might not be helpful. As with any assessment, identifying allergies is important. Even if the nurse has past medical records from the patient, the nurse should repeat the inquiry about allergies. If the patient experiences any allergies during home care, these must be documented.

The objectives of the psychopharmacological assessment are as follows:[16(p.43)]

- to identify patient-related variables pertinent to the risk/benefit assessment of psychopharmacologic treatment such as demographic (age, gender, ethnicity/race); physical (organ system function, concurrent illnesses); treatment (concurrent treatments); and personal (past history, self-care practices, goals of treatment, ability to pay, and quality of life) characteristics
- to identify drug-related variables important in the risk/benefit assessment of psychopharmacologic agents, such as safety and efficacy, advantages and disadvantages compared to other drugs in the same class, therapeutic range, side-effect profile, toxicities, contraindications, potential interactions with other drugs or diet, polypharmacy considerations, safety in overdose, availability of information on long-term side effects, and cost
- to evaluate the appropriateness and least restrictive nature of psychopharmacologic interventions for each patient
- to assess the ability and willingness of the patient and family/SOs to give informed consent for treatment with psychopharmacologic agents
- to utilize standardized behavioral rating scales to assess and monitor drug effects and changes in target symptoms

Consideration must also be given to the environmental assessment, as this information may influence psychopharmacologic treatment. If there are economic problems, medications may not be obtained easily. Cultural factors may influence the patient's and the family/SO's attitudes toward the use of medications. A chaotic living situation may affect the patient's support that is required for taking medication routinely.

Diagnosis

Diagnostic judgment is used to set treatment priorities and determine psychopharmacological interventions. The nurse does not prescribe the medications; however, an understanding of the patient's medical diagnosis will provide the nurse with background information about the patient's potential symptoms and needs and the reasons for the use of specific medications. Identifying nursing diagnoses will identify patient needs that must be considered as care is planned and implemented. Many of these will relate to medications (e.g., problems with specific side effects such as excessive sleep or constipation; educational needs about diet related to a specific drug such as a monoamine oxidase inhibitor).

Phases of Psychopharmacologic Treatment

ANA recommends a framework in its psychopharmacologic guidelines that is composed of phases of treatment that "facilitate the use of complex and changing information encountered in the treatment of individuals with psychiatric disorders."[17(p.27)] These phases are helpful as interventions are planned with the patient in the home. They help to organize the clinical management of the patient's medication treatment. The four phases are

1. initiation
2. stabilization
3. maintenance
4. medication-free

Initiation

Interventions during the first phase will vary, depending upon the length of time the patient has been taking medications at the time of admission. It is easy to assume that certain interventions have occurred for patients who have taken medications for a long time; later in treatment the nurse may discover that some intervention was not taken, and this is causing problems. For example, the patient may have had inadequate education or informed consent was never obtained. Both of these may lead to patient confusion about medications. The patient may not understand why he or she is experiencing a particular side effect or may feel that he or she was not informed about an adverse side effect prior to making a decision to take a medication. All of this leads to distrust and stress, which can be very detrimental to the patient's progress. The initiation phase focuses on the following:[18]

- *Pharmacokinetics/pharmacodynamics.* The nurse needs to understand how these actions will affect the patient's use of specific medications.
- *Patient education about medication and alternative treatments.* Education begins at the time of admission and continues as long as the patient is in home care. The patient is taught how to self-medicate and monitor his or her medications.
- *Informed consent.* The patient's physician must give the patient information about medications including risks and possible complications prior to prescribing them and as the patient's consent is obtained. Consent to treatment cannot be provided by a minor or someone who is judged incompetent. The criteria for incompetence are difficult at times. According to Laben and McLean: "Unless the individual has been found incompetent to manage his affairs, he is considered able to make decisions for himself."[19(p.13)] Informed consent establishes the requirement of patient participation in treatment and respects the patient's needs to participate and identify concerns. It is also "a continuing educational process rather than a procedure performed merely to comply with the law."[20(pp.182–183)]
- *Identification of target symptoms and rating scales.* With each patient, the nurse must identify those symptoms that are of most concern and monitor the patient's progress related to those symptoms. Rating scales may be used, as well as observation, self-monitoring, and other methods.
- *Early medication effects.* The nurse must be aware of what to expect early in medication treatment and provide this information to the patient. For example, many medications cause sedation early in treatment; however, this decreases later. If the nurse does not know about this effect, he or she might develop elaborate interventions to stimulate the patient when there is no need for this type of intervention. The patient may become discouraged or the family/SOs may complain that the patient is only getting worse on the medication.
- *Alternative treatments.* Along with the physician, the nurse must be aware of alternative treatments such as electroconvulsive therapy (ECT) for depression rather than the use of antidepressants. Some medications may work better on some patients than on others, and changes may need to be made. The physician is responsible for making the change; however, the nurse must understand why the change is made and what other treatment changes could be made. The nurse is the one who has frequent contact with the patient and is most aware of the patient's needs.

- *Development of treatment plans.* The use of medications is part of the treatment plan. Patient education, self-administration, self-monitoring methods, side effects, and compliance are also integral parts of the treatment plan.
- *Implications of information obtained in assessment.* Data collected in the assessment must be analyzed and applied to treatment decisions. If the assessment indicates that a patient has had past problems with compliance or frequently has a specific side effect, then this information must be incorporated into the treatment plan. Assessment data can be overwhelming, as they must be prioritized so that they can be useful.

Stabilization

After the initial phase of medication treatment, the patient gradually stabilizes on the medication or changes are made in treatment. The nurse is concerned with the following:[21]

- *Continued assessment of target symptoms.* Target symptoms are identified in the first phase, and during the stabilization phase they are monitored to assist in evaluating progress or problems.
- *Expected timing of medication effects.* The nurse is aware of specific effects of particular drugs and when they might be expected. This information is used as the patient is monitored (e.g., antidepressants are not effective for at least two to three weeks, so the nurse would not expect a notable change in target symptoms before that time).
- *Recognition and treatment of adverse effects.* The nurse and the patient must be aware of the potential adverse effects. The patient and the family/SOs must have a response plan in the event that adverse effects occur. These are developed with the nurse, the patient, and family/SOs.
- *Therapeutic drug monitoring.* Some medications may be monitored with laboratory tests to determine therapeutic levels or toxicity. The nurse should use these tests when appropriate in consultation with the patient's physician. The patient must be part of this process and communication.
- *When and how to change medication strategies.* The nurse may be the first to recognize that a medication is not effective for the patient. The nurse must inform the patient's physician of observations that may indicate the need to change medication. Medication dose or frequency may need to be adjusted.
- *Ongoing patient education.* Medication education never ends. Questions continue to arise as the patient learns to live with taking medications, and for many patients this may be long term.
- *Transition between treatment settings.* It may be necessary for a psychiatric home care patient to enter another treatment setting. The most common is

when the patient requires hospitalization or partial hospitalization. When this occurs, the nurse assists the patient's transition by providing information about the patient and the patient's medication history to the new treatment setting.

Maintenance

Maintenance carries with it a long-term connotation, and most of the interventions related to it focus on the issues of assisting the patient to continue on medication treatment in the most effective way possible. Interventions relate to the following:[22]

- *Providing education regarding relapse and recognition of stressors.* Each patient has a potential for relapse, and each responds to stressors in different ways. Part of assessment and treatment planning with the patient is to identify specific stressors with the patient that need to be prevented or recognized as important so that interventions can be taken to assist the patient with them when they occur.
- *Monitoring efficacy, side effects, and laboratory values.* Monitoring is ongoing and is part of each visit. The patient must learn how to do this for himself or herself in order to prepare for discharge from home care.
- *Considering potential long-term side effects.* The nurse must know what the long-term side effects are and when to institute interventions that will prevent them.
- *Addressing compliance issues.* Compliance is a difficult issue, but it must be actively considered during the admission assessment. Often the first assumption about patient noncompliance is that it is intentional, and this may not be correct. According to McPherson, "The manner in which home health care patients keep their medications 'straight' and remain compliant should be assessed. Patients may become confused and thereby unintentionally noncompliant, taking too much of one medication and skipping others."[23(pp.72-73)] Self-medication is complex and can cause stress for the patient and the family/SOs. They need help in sorting out the issues around taking medications as well as the mechanics related to self-medication.
- *Determining when and how to discontinue medication treatment.* The patient's physician must order the discontinuation of medication; however, patients themselves sometimes make this decision. The nurse must listen to the patient, provide information, and assist the patient in discussing concerns with the physician.
- *Providing patient education for relapse prevention.* Relapse for psychiatric patients is not unusual. As every treatment plan is developed and as discharge plans from home care are developed, it must be considered. Assess-

ment data may help to identify patients who might relapse. Response to treatment during home care may indicate that the patient may relapse. The choice of treatment after home care may also influence the chance of relapse. This is as complicated an area as compliance and requires some analysis throughout the patient's home care treatment.

Medication-Free

It may be possible for some patients to be medication-free; and it is not unusual for patients to raise this topic. The nurse must consider the duration of treatment for the patient's disorder; tapering methods and schedules; symptom recognition that might indicate the need to restart medication; and relapse prevention.[24] When the patient does stop medication, information must be shared about possible withdrawal, dependence, rebound effects, and return of symptoms of illness. These will vary with the specific medication and patient, but they must be reviewed with all patients. According to the ANA; the nurse should "develop with the patient, family, and significant others a plan for self-care in a post-medication phase that considers assessments of quality of life, predisposing stressors, re-emergence of symptoms, appropriate use of support systems, and contact sources for potential re-evaluation of treatment status."[25(p.45)]

SUMMARY

According to Hayes, "Mental health, even in the presence of mental illness, is advanced by the harmonious functioning of all systems (biological, psychological, and environmental) that make up who we are as human beings."[26(p.221)] The nurse has many responsibilities related to psychopharmacology therapy while working with the patient in the home care setting:

- assessing the patient's mental status on admission and throughout the home care process
- collecting data related to the patient's medication history and, when possible, reviewing the information obtained by other health care providers
- applying information about the patient's medical problems and history to psychopharmacological therapy
- collaborating with the patient to develop a treatment plan that meets the patient's needs
- ensuring that physicians' orders related to medications are complete, appropriate, and followed
- collaborating with the physician when necessary to adjust patient's medication, dose, and frequency
- providing patient/family/SOs education related to patient's medications

- documenting administration of medications and patient education
- evaluating outcomes related to medications

NOTES

1. K. McKeon, "Introduction: A Future Perspective on Psychiatric Mental Health Nursing," *Archives of Psychiatric Nursing* 4, no. 1 (1990): 19–20.
2. P. Pothier, "Toward a Bio/Psycho/Social Synthesis," *Archives of Psychiatric Nursing* 4, no. 2 (1990): 77.
3. A. Hayes, "Psychiatric Nursing: What Does Biology Have To Do With It?" *Archives of Psychiatric Nursing* 9, no. 4 (1995): 216–224, at 216.
4. American Nurses Association, *Psychiatric Mental Health Nursing Psychopharmacology Project* (Washington, DC: American Nurses Publishing, 1994).
5. American Nurses Association, *Psychiatric Mental Health Nursing Psychopharmacology Project*, 31.
6. American Nurses Association, *Psychiatric Mental Health Nursing Psychopharmacology Project*, 31.
7. American Nurses Association, *Psychiatric Mental Health Nursing Psychopharmacology Project*, 32.
8. American Nurses Association, *Psychiatric Mental Health Nursing Psychopharmacology Project*, 32.
9. American Nurses Association, *A Statement on Psychiatric-Mental Health Clinical Nursing Practice and Standards of Psychiatric-Mental Health Clinical Nursing Practice* (Washington, DC: American Nurses Publishing, 1994), 31.
10. American Nurses Association, *Psychiatric Mental Health Nursing Psychopharmacology Project*, 33.
11. Joint Commission on Accreditation of Healthcare Organizations, *1995 Accreditation Manual for Home Care, Vol. 1* (Oakbrook Terrace, IL: 1994), 18–19.
12. American Nurses Association, *Standards of Home Health Nursing Practice* (Washington, DC: 1986), 12.
13. American Nurses Association, *Ethical Code* (Washington, DC: 1985).
14. American Nurses Association, *Psychiatric Mental Health Nursing Psychopharmacology Project*, 27.
15. American Nurses Association, *Psychiatric Mental Health Nursing Psychopharmacology Project*, 29.
16. American Nurses Association, *Psychiatric Mental Health Nursing Psychopharmacology Project*, 43.
17. American Nurses Association, *Psychiatric Mental Health Nursing Psychopharmacology Project*, 27.
18. American Nurses Association, *Psychiatric Mental Health Nursing Psychopharmacology Project*, 27.
19. J. Laben and C. McLean, *Legal Issues and Guidelines for Nurses Who Care for the Mentally Ill* (Thorofare, NJ: SLACK, Inc., 1984), 13.

20. G. Stuart, "Legal Context of Psychiatric Nursing Care," in *Principles and Practice of Psychiatric Nursing*, ed. G. Stuart and S. Sundeen (St. Louis, MO: Mosby–Year Book, 1995), 171–197, at 182–183.

21. American Nurses Association, *Psychiatric Mental Health Nursing Psychopharmacology Project*, 27.

22. American Nurses Association, *Psychiatric Mental Health Nursing Psychopharmacology Project*, 27.

23. M. McPherson, "Drug-Induced Mental Status Changes," *Journal of Home Health Care Practice* 2, no. 3 (1990): 72–73.

24. American Nurses Association, *Psychiatric Mental Health Nursing Psychopharmacology Project*, 27.

25. American Nurses Association, *Psychiatric Mental Health Nursing Psychopharmacology Project*, 45.

26. Hayes, "Psychiatric Nursing: What Does Biology Have To Do With It?" 221.

SUGGESTED READING

Abbondanza, D. et al. 1994. Psychiatric mental health nursing in a biopsychosocial era. *Perspectives in Psychiatric Care* 30, no. 3: 21–25.

Abraham, I. et al. 1992. Integrating the bio into the biopsychosocial: Understanding and treating biological phenomena in psychiatric-mental health nursing. *Archives of Psychiatric Nursing* 6, no. 5: 296–305.

American Nurses Association. 1994. *Psychiatric mental health nursing psychopharmacology project.* Washington, DC: American Nurses Publishing.

Harper-Jaques, S., and M. Reimer. 1992. Aggressive behavior and the brain: A different perspective for the mental health nurse. *Archives of Psychiatric Nursing* 6, no. 5: 312–320.

Hartman, D. 1993. Critical thinking in psychiatric nursing in the decade of the brain. *Holistic Nursing Practice* 7, no. 3: 55–63.

Hayes, A. 1995. Psychiatric nursing: What does biology have to do with it? *Archives of Psychiatric Nursing* 9, no. 4: 216–224.

Kaplan, H., and B. Sadock. 1995. *Comprehensive textbook of psychiatry.* Baltimore, MD: Williams & Wilkins.

Lego, S. 1992. Biological psychiatry and psychiatric nursing in America. *Archives of Psychiatric Nursing* 6, no. 3: 147–150.

McEnany, G. 1992. Psychobiology. In *Psychiatric Nursing*, ed. H. Wilson and C. Kneisl, 99–117. Menlo Park, CA: Addison-Wesley.

McKeon, K. 1990. Introduction: A future perspective on psychiatric mental health nursing. *Archives of Psychiatric Nursing* 4, no. 1: 19–20.

Pothier, P. 1990. Toward a bio/psycho/social synthesis. *Archives of Psychiatric Nursing* 4, no. 2: 77.

Pothier, P. et al. 1990. Dilemmas and directions for psychiatric nursing in the 1990s. *Archives of Psychiatric Nursing* 4, no. 5: 284–291.

Stuart, G., and S. Sundeen. 1995. *Principles and practice of psychiatric nursing.* St. Louis, MO: Mosby–Year Book.

13

Understanding Psychopharmacology and Mental Illness: Neuroscience

INTRODUCTION

The American Nurses Association (ANA) in collaboration with the National Institute of Mental Health funded a special project in 1992, the *Psychiatric Mental Health Nursing Psychopharmacology Project.*[1] At that time there was concern about integrating of scientific advances related to the understanding of the human brain, mental illness, and biochemical treatments of mental disorders into nursing education and clinical practice in all settings, and this continues to be a concern. After gathering information, the ANA developed the guidelines described in Chapter 12 to address issues of nursing education and application of scientific advances into clinical practice. According to the ANA:

> Historically, in non-psychiatric nursing specialty areas, patient care has been well grounded in basic science. Moreover, this knowledge has been viewed as a prerequisite to practice and fundamental to effective treatment. This same emphasis has not traditionally held true for the psychiatric nursing specialty. In psychiatric nursing, historical, philosophical, and political issues converged to create a climate in which psychiatric nurses knew little about neurobiological factors, were not encouraged to obtain this knowledge, and oftentimes viewed neurobiological explanations and treatments as falling outside the domain of nursing practice.[2(p. 22)]

It is important that these guidelines are applied in all settings providing care for psychiatric patients, including home care.

Recent biological research has identified important facts about the nervous system, possible problems related to psychiatric illnesses, and responses to drugs. Further research will undoubtedly lead to many more discoveries and changes in proposed theories. Due to the changing nature of this information, psychiatric home care nurses who work daily with these medications must remain current with the information about these medications and their use with patients in the home setting. To understand and work with medications in the home, the nurse must have a working knowledge of basic brain biology. The ANA guidelines identify those areas that are important, and these are included in Exhibit 13–1. Some aspects of the nervous system will be discussed in this chapter; because this is a very complex area, the nurse should also review other references related to neurology and neuroscience.

Exhibit 13–1 Neuroscience Content for Psychiatric Nurses

I. Neuroanatomy
- cerebrum
- thalamus
- limbic system
- basal ganglia
- cranial nerves
- cerebellum
- hypothalamus reticular system
- corpus callosum
- brainstem
- peripheral nervous system
- extrapyramidal system
- neuronal structure and function
- hemispheres and lobes of the brain

II. Genetic/familial correlates
- genetic structures: RNA, DNA, chromosomes
- principles of genetic investigation
  - familial aggregation studies
  - twin and adoption studies
  - segregation analysis
  - genetic linkage

III. Systems of neuroregulation
- neurotransmitters
  - amino acids
  - monoamines
  - acetylcholine
  - neuropeptides
- enzymes
- cellular neurochemistry/electrophysiology in neurotransmission

continues

Exhibit 13–1 continued

   IV. psychoendocrinology
- hypothalamic-pituitary-thyroid axis (HPT)
- hypothalamic-pituitary-adrenal axis (HPA)
- hypothalamic-pituitary-gonadal axis (HPG)

   V. Psychoimmunology
- basic components of the immune system
  - lymph nodes
  - bone marrow
  - phagocytes
  - leukocytes
- stress response mechanisms
  - differential effects of long-term stress versus short-term stress
  - catecholamines
  - cortisol

   VI. Normal biological rhythms
- sleep-wake
- temperature
- biological rhythm changes

   VII. Psychobiological dysfunctions
- kindling
- sleep disturbances
- biological rhythm changes

   VIII. Biological theories of major psychiatric disorders
- schizophrenia
- anxiety disorders
- seizure disorders
- obsessive-compulsive disorder
- mood disorders
- substance abuse
- Tourette's syndrome
- personality disorders
- delirium/dementias
- trauma/infection

   IX. Brain imaging in diagnosis of mental illness
- computerized tomography (CT)
- magnetic resonance imaging (MRI)
- positron emission tomography (PET)
- single photon emission computerized tomography (SPECT)

   X. Physiological indices of mental illness
- laboratory studies

Source: Reprinted with permission from American Nurses Association, *Psychiatric Mental Health Nursing Psychopharmacology Project,* p. 23, © 1994, American Nurses Association.

CENTRAL NERVOUS SYSTEM: RELATIONSHIP TO MENTAL ILLNESS

Andreasen has stated that "the brain is the source of everything that we are. It is the source of everything that makes us human, humane, and unique. It is the source of our ability to speak, to write, to think, to create, to love, to laugh, to despair, and to hate."[3(p.83)] The focus of psychobiological research is the brain, which is highly complex with many highly specialized parts. Mental and bodily functions cannot take place without the brain. Mapping of brain specialization has been a long-term process, which has assisted in identifying areas of the brain and their functions that are relevant to mental illness. The psychiatric home care nurse is not a neurologist; however, some understanding of the anatomy and physiology of the brain is necessary. Before the nurse can explain the physiological aspects of some mental illnesses to the patient and family/significant others (SOs), the nurse must know the anatomy and physiology of the brain. This information is also important in understanding how psychiatric medications affect the brain.

There is no doubt that this is a difficult area to understand, but some facts can be easily understood and applied in the clinical practice setting. Andreasen suggests a metaphor for the brain: "a very large network of different communication centers that can flash on and off and send messages to one another through electrical impulses. The brain contains many different specialized information centers scattered throughout its three-dimensional space."[4(p.90)] As neuroanatomy and neurophysiology are reviewed, it is important to remember that some areas of the brain perform the same functions. This protects the individual when there is brain damage. This is referred to as the brain's *adaptive capacity* or its *plasticity*. In the brain, messages can be sent through alternate connections.[5] However, brain damage is permanent, even though the individual may be able to regain all or some of a function due to the brain's ability to adapt.

Functional neuroanatomy is important in the understanding of the regulation of neuronal processes. Exhibit 13–2 and Figure 13–1 identify some brain structures relevant to psychiatric disorders.

Basic to all of the parts of the nervous system is the cell. With its critical components, it plays a major role in neuroregulation. This is very important in the areas of psychobiology and psychopharmacology. Nerve cells or neurons are composed of the following parts:

- the cell body containing the nucleus—serve as the metabolic center of the neuron
- the dendrites or processes that arise from the cell body and branch—serve as the recipient areas for information or input from other neurons
- the axon or the single process—serve as the messenger to other neurons

Exhibit 13–2 Structure and Functions of the Brain

Structure	Functions
Sensory strip	Integration of sensory information from various parts of the body
Motor strip	Regulation of voluntary movement
Thalamus	Major relay station for messages from all parts of the body
Hypothalamus	Regulation of metabolism, reasoning, inhibiting
Parietal lobe	Somesthetic and motor discrimination functions
Occipital lobe	Visual discrimination and some aspects of visual memory
Corpus callosum	Communication between the right and left hemispheres
Cerebellum	Fine motor coordination, posture, and balance
Reticular formation	Arousal reactions; information screening
Medulla	Breathing; blood pressure; other vital functions
Frontal lobe	Learning; abstracting; reasoning; inhibiting

- the axon terminals—fine branches that emerge from near the end of the axon forming synapses with dendrites or cell bodies of other neurons releasing neurotransmitters; these serve as a source of interneuronal communication

SYSTEMS OF NEUROREGULATION: EFFECTS ON ILLNESS AND MEDICATION SIDE EFFECTS

Neurons can also be classified according to their neurotransmitters, and it is the neuron and neurotransmitters that are attracting so much research interest. Exhibit 13–3 describes important networks of nuclei implicated in psychiatric disorders.

According to Grebb: "The human body has three great communicative systems—the neural system, the immune system, and the endocrine system. All three systems communicate with each other, and a disease in one can cause dysfunctions in the others."[6(p.3)] These interactions are important in psychiatric disorders. These three systems change regularly with time, neuronal function, immune responses, and the release of hormones.[7]

A neurotransmitter is a chemical messenger between brain cells or neurons. Neurotransmitters may inhibit (act as an antagonist) or activate (act as an agonist) biological responses within the cell. They are synthesized within the cell and released from the axon into the synapse or the space between neurons. A nearby neuron receives the neurotransmitter by means of its dendrite. Laraia uses the following analogy to describe neurotransmitters: "Like a key inserted into a lock,

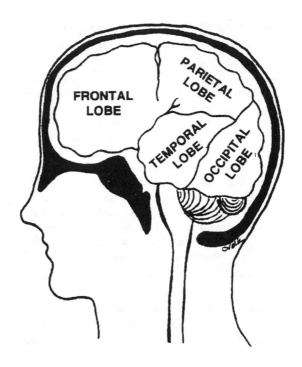

1. **FRONTAL LOBE**
   Center for speech, emotional control, motivation, problem solving, reasoning, insight, movement, and behavior.
2. **TEMPORAL LOBE**
   Center for hearing, memory, organization, and musical awareness.
3. **PARIETAL LOBE**
   Takes in, understands, and uses information from the environment. This includes thinking skills, moving, and positioning the body.
4. **OCCIPITAL LOBE**
   Center for vision and recognition of things seen before (people, objects).

Figure 13–1 Lobes of the Brain. *Source:* Reprinted from St. Joseph Rehabilitation Hospital and Outpatient Center, "Brain Injury," *Patient Education and Discharge Planning Manual,* p. 6, © 1995, Aspen Publishers, Inc.

Exhibit 13-3 Networks of Nuclei Implicated in Psychiatric Disorders

Network	Functions
Cerebral cortex	decision making; higher order thinking such as abstract reasoning
Limbic system	regulates emotional behavior, memory, and learning
Hypothalamus	regulates hormones throughout the body and behaviors such as eating, drinking, and sex
Locus ceruleus	manufactures norepinephrine, which affects the body's stress response
Raphe nuclei	made up of serotonin neurons, which regulate sleep and are involved with behavior and mood
Substantia nigra	dopamine-producing cells which assist in the control of complex movements, thinking, and emotional responses

Source: Reprinted with permission from M. Laraia, "Biological Context of Psychiatric Nursing, in *Principles and Practice of Psychiatric Nursing*, G. Stuart and S. Sundeen, eds., p. 105, © 1995, Mosby–Year Book, Inc.

each of these chemicals fits into specific receptor cells, or proteins, embedded in the membrane of the dendrite, which recognize it."[8(p.104)] The signal given by the neurotransmitter may communicate the message to excite the receiving cell and cause an action, or it may prevent the cell from firing and stop an action. The communication between neurons is both chemical and electric. After this release and response, the neurotransmitter is returned to the axon from which it came. This is called *reuptake*. The neurotransmitter is stored for later use or metabolized and inactivated by enzymes.[9] The three major types of neurotransmitters are the monoamine neurotransmitters, the amino acid neurotransmitters, and the neuropeptide neurotransmitters.

At this time, researchers believe that the *monoamine neurotransmitters* are the most important neurotransmitters; they include the catecholamines (dopamine, norepinephrine, and epinephrine); serotonin; acetylcholine; and histamine neurotransmitters. It is this group of neurotransmitters that is most affected by psychotrophic drugs. These neurotransmitters are either excitatory or inhibitory and have a variety of functions.[10]

- *Norepinephrine* can have an excitatory or inhibitory effect. Its functions include changes in levels of attention, vigilance, and mood regulation. The role of norepinephrine is not fully understood; however, it is thought to play a major role in memory.[11] Its actions are important in affective and anxiety disorders.

- *Dopamine* usually has an excitatory effect. Its functions include control of complex movements, motivation, cognition, and regulation of emotional responses. It is important in movement disorders such as Parkinson's disease and in many deficits found in schizophrenia and other psychoses. Drugs such as cocaine and amphetamines cause dopamine to be released. This has led to the proposal that dopamine plays a role in making experiences pleasurable and that it influences memory.[12]
- *Serotonin's* effect is mostly inhibitory. Its functions include a role in arousal and modulation of general central nervous system activity; an effect on mood and probably the symptoms of delusions, hallucinations, and withdrawal; temperature regulation; and pain control. Its actions are important in affective disorders, anxiety disorders, and schizophrenia.
- *Acetylcholine* has an excitatory or inhibitory effect. Its functions include a role in the sleep-wakefulness cycle and stimulation of muscle activity. In addition, it is thought to play a major role in learning and memory. Its actions are important in Alzheimer's disease and myasthenia gravis.

The second group of neurotransmitters, the *amino acids*, also have a variety of functions but are not as important as the monoamines. These neurotransmitters include the following:[13]

- *Glutamate* has an excitatory effect. It can be toxic to neurons if overexposure is experienced. Its actions are important in strokes and some degenerative diseases such as Huntington's disease. Blocking this neurotransmitter might prevent seizures and neural degeneration from overexcitation.
- *Gamma-aminobutyric acid (GABA)* is a major neurotransmitter for postsynaptic inhibition on the central nervous system. It is important in the treatment of anxiety disorders as well as in treatment to induce sleep.

The third group of neurotransmitters is the *neuropeptides*. Not as much is known about them, and there are many that have not been identified. Even though they are found to be of low concentration, they can exact a strong effect.[14] Future research may indicate that this group is more important in the understanding of psychiatric disorders.

How does neuroregulation relate to psychiatric illnesses and drugs used for treatment? According to Hayes: "The psychobiological mechanism of thoughts, emotions, and behavior are an intricate and not thoroughly understood system. The various neurotransmitter systems do not operate in isolation. There is a hierarchical order depending on need, similar in nature to the functioning of a symphony orchestra. Moreover, it is proposed that the neurotransmitter systems have the capacity to compensate and adapt when there are weaknesses."[15(pp.219–220)] The etiology for many psychiatric illnesses is thought to relate to either an underresponse or overresponse of the neurotransmitter process. Psychotropic drugs can increase or decrease a neurotransmitter's action by

- affecting the receptor site on the postsynaptic cell membrane and thereby enhancing or diminishing the neurotransmitter action
- affecting storage or reuptake of the neurotransmitter and thus the reabsorption of the neurotransmitter by the presynaptic cell when it is no longer needed
- affecting the enzymes involved in the synthesis or breakdown of the neurotransmitter

Most psychopharmacology treatment is an attempt to change or modify the neurotransmission process. This, however, has not been perfected, and drug actions affect not only the areas of the brain thought to be associated with symptoms but also other areas. This can lead to side effects and problems with drug interactions. It is hoped that with additional research over the next few years, these drugs and their actions on the neurotransmitters will become more responsive to the target psychiatric symptom with fewer side effects.

GENETICS AND FAMILY ISSUES

Scientific research in the field of genetics has been highly successful in the past few years. Psychobiological research has also been expanding in this area; however, the results have been less conclusive. The relationship between genetics and mental illness is very complex. According to Hyman and Nestler, "Understanding the mechanisms by which environmental factors—such as life experience, drugs, infections, and injuries—affect the expression of neural genes is critical for an understanding of the pathophysiology of psychiatric disorders."[16(p.136)] It is necessary to conduct more research to arrive at more definitive answers. Factors that make this a difficult area for psychiatry include the following:[17]

- the changeable nature of the psychiatric diagnostic classification system
- the fact that a gene sometimes produces a psychiatric disorder but may not always do so
- the belief that several different genes may be necessary to produce a disorder
- the presence of nongenetic factors that may contribute to the development of a disorder

Genetics is a topic that patients and their families frequently raise. Common questions include: Who gave this to me? Will I pass it on to my children? Although patients and families may not always verbalize these questions, they think about them. The home care nurse should be willing to discuss these concerns openly and share relevant facts about genetics and the patient's specific illness. This requires the nurse to be aware of the facts. Consulting with the patient's physician about this issue is also important so that a coordinated effort can be made to assist the patient and family with their fears.

IMMUNE AND ENDOCRINE SYSTEMS AND MENTAL ILLNESS

The integration and modulation of the central nervous system is maintained by the neural system, the immune system, and the endocrine system. There has been increasing interest in the relationships among these three communicative systems.[18] Immune system research has focused on the relationship between psychosocial stresses and the immune system. Researchers are investigating whether the immune system is depressed by some stressors, thereby making the individual more vulnerable to illness. Illnesses that have been studied are acquired immune deficiency syndrome (AIDS), schizophrenia, Alzheimer's disease, and Parkinson's disease. AIDS research has revealed that glial cells in the brain can be affected by the human immunodeficiency virus and the person will experience symptoms such as dementia, depression, and psychosis.[19] Hormones have been shown to affect behavior in disorders of hormonal dysfunction that can have psychiatric symptoms (e.g., adrenal and thyroid disorders).[20] Research on the immune system and the endocrine system may reveal more information as the research is expanded.

DIAGNOSING MENTAL ILLNESS: BIOLOGICAL METHODS

Psychiatry has lacked the objective diagnostic tools that have been used in many other areas of medicine. This has always been a problem and has made diagnosis more subjective than objective. The recent emphasis on biological research has increased the possibility of developing more diagnostic tools; however, this area is in its infancy. Some of these diagnostic tools are brain imaging and physiological indexes.

Brain Imaging

Brain imaging provides information about brain structure or brain functioning. At this time, brain imaging techniques cannot provide conclusive diagnosis; however, they do provide important information that has been used in research. Structural imaging is provided by computed tomography (CT) and magnetic resonance imaging (MRI). These tests can reveal the changes in brain tissue volume and enlargement of the cerebral ventricles. Functional imaging provides information about the brain's neurochemistry—the metabolism or the activity of the brain. Magnetic resonance spectroscopy (MRS) is noninvasive and does not expose the patient to radiation. The electroencephalogram (EEG) is probably the most common technique used. It should be used to screen any patient who has a history of episodic behavior such as anxiety attacks or dissociative episodes, brain injury, loss of consciousness, other neurological disturbance, and to assess elderly patients to differentiate dementia from depression.[21]

Physiological Indexes

Pharmacokinetics includes the absorption, distribution, metabolism, excretion, and half-life of a drug. These characteristics are important when the physician selects one drug over another for a specific patient. Blood levels can be monitored for some drugs, such as lithium, to determine how much of the medication is in the blood. One aspect of interest is the half-life, or how long it takes for the drug to reach a steady state of concentration. A steady state occurs when the amount of drug excreted equals the amount ingested. Until this state is reached, the drug level changes with each dose; this causes side effects in some patients.[22] According to Laraia, "Until steady state is reached the optimum dose for a particular patient cannot be determined nor is a blood level accurate in determining a proper dose range.[23(p.666)] This factor is very important in assessing the patient's response to a medication. Exhibit 13–4 identifies risk factors for the development of drug interactions, a critical problem requiring understanding and assessment of the patient's medications and educational needs.

SUMMARY

In the past, psychiatric nursing's interest in biological treatment has focused on administration of medications and, for some psychiatric nurses, on assisting with somatic treatments such as electroconvulsive therapy. Abraham et al. state that "In keeping with psychological understandings, the emphasis has been primarily on emotions, and secondarily on behavioral management. Treatment approaches targeting cognitions and their impact on well- and ill-being have been less prevalent."[24(p.299)] Exhibits 13–5 and 13–6 describe psychiatric nursing's past and recent views on the nature and treatment of biological phenomena in psychiatric nursing. Focus areas related to biopsychosocial understanding are described in

Exhibit 13–4 Risk Factors for Development of Drug Interactions

---

Polypharmacy
High dose
Geriatric patients
Debilitated/dehydrated patients
Concurrent illness
Compromised organ system function
Inadequate patient education
History of noncompliance
Failure to include patient in treatment planning

Source: Reprinted with permission from M. Laraia, "Psychopharmacology," in *Principles and Practice of Psychiatric Nursing,* G. Stuart and S. Sundeen, eds., p. 666, © 1995, Mosby–Year Book, Inc.

Exhibit 13–6. With the new developments in research, there is an increased need for patient and family/SO education about illness and somatic treatment including psychopharmacology as well as "pretreatment, peritreatment, and posttreatment psychosocial support; promotion of appropriate and sustained medication behaviors; and assessment of cognitive deficits and development of supportive interventions designed to assist patients to cope with deficits; . . . [and] partial management of emotional, behavioral, cognitive, and social side and interaction effects due to somatic treatments as a follow-up to nursing observation."[25(p.304)]

As indicated in Exhibit 13–7, there are many potential reasons for patient medication noncompliance, a major problem for many psychiatric home care patients. However, thorough understanding of psychopharmacology will provide information for patient education and assessment of the patient's medication needs and responses to medications. This education and assessment will help to decrease the risk of medication noncompliance.

Exhibit 13-5 Past Nursing Understandings and Nursing Treatments of Mental Health and Illness

Focus	Past Nursing Understandings	Past Nursing Treatments
Psychological	Emotion, behavior, and cognition determined by intrapersonal dynamics. Emotion-focused coping.	Individual counseling and therapy, focused primarily on emotion, secondarily on behavior, and tertiarily on cognition.
Social	Emotion, cognition, and behavior determined by dynamics of: family, number of dyadic relationships, friends, small social groups, large social groups, ethnicity, and community.	Counseling and therapy involving significant other, family, and groups. Social integration. Milieu therapy.
Biological	Global, undifferentiated, and system-nonspecific views on biophysical dysfunction, organicity, manifest physical illness, manifest physical impairment.	Administration of pharmacological treatments. Selective involvement in the somatic treatments.
Psychosocial	Intrapersonal determinants of social functioning. Social determinants of intrapersonal functioning. Psychosocial adaptation. Behavior-focused coping. Social support. Relational adequacy. Community integration.	Counseling and therapy aimed at psychosocial functioning and integration.
Psychobiological	Mind and body interaction. Adaptation to physical illness. Intrapersonal impairment due to biophysical impairment.	Observation of emotional improvement and behavioral adaptation due to pharmacological/somatic treatment. Monitoring for side and interaction effects due to pharmacological/social treatment.
Sociobiological	Interpersonal impairment due to biophysical impairment.	Observation of social improvement and adaptation due to pharmacological/somatic treatment. Monitoring for social side effects to pharmacological/somatic treatment.

Source: Reprinted with permission from I. Abraham, J. Fox, and B. Cohen, "Integrating the Bio into the Biopsychosocial: Understanding and Treating Biological Phenomena in Psychiatric-Mental Health Nursing," *Archives of Psychiatric Nursing,* Vol. 6, No. 5, pp. 298 and 300, © 1992, W.B. Saunders Company.

Exhibit 13-6 Biopsychosocial Understandings

Focus	
Psychological	Emotion, cognition, and behavior determined by intrapersonal dynamics. Emotion-focused coping.
Social	Emotion, cognition, and behavior determined by dynamics of family of origin, current family, dyadic relationships, friends, small and large social groups, ethnicity, and community.
Biological	Brain and central nervous system. Other organ systems. Interactions among organ systems. Endocrinology. Genetics. Sensorium. Pharmacodynamics and pharmacokinetics.
Psychosocial	Intrapersonal determinants of social functioning. Social determinants of intrapersonal functioning. Psychosocial adaptation. Social support. Relational adequacy. Community integration.
Psychobiological	Mind and body interaction. Intelligence. Personal cognition. Adaptation to physical and mental illness. Intrapersonal impairment due to biophysical impairment.
Sociobiological	Impact of environmental toxins. Social cognition. Interpersonal impairment due to biophysical impairment.
Biopsychosocial	Schizophrenia sprectrum disorders. Major depressive disorders. Other bipolar disorders. Appetitive disorders. Obsessive-compulsive disorders. Organic syndromes. Anxiety and panic disorders. Dementias. Sexual disorders. Violence.

Source: Reprinted with permission from I. Abraham, J. Fox, and B. Cohen, "Integrating the Bio into the Biopsychosocial: Understanding and Treating Biological Phenomena in Psychiatric-Mental Health Nursing," *Archives of Psychiatric Nursing*, Vol. 6, No. 5, p. 302, © 1992, W.B. Saunders Company.

Exhibit 13-7 Risk Factors for Patient Medication Noncompliance

Failure to form a therapeutic alliance with the patient

Devaluation of pharmacotherapy by treatment staff

Inadequate patient and family education regarding treatment

Poorly controlled side effects

Insensitivity to patient beliefs, wishes, or complaints

Multiple daily dosing schedule

Polypharmacy

History of noncompliance

Social isolation

Expense of drugs

Failure to appreciate patient's role in drug treatment plan

Lack of continuity of care

Increased restrictions on client's lifestyle

Unsupportive significant others

Remission of target symptoms

Increased suicidal ideation

Increased suspiciousness

Unrealistic expectations of drug effects

Concurrent substance use

Failure to target residual symptoms for nonpharmacological therapies

Relapse or exacerbation of clinical syndrome

Failure to alleviate intrafamilial and environmental stressors that precipitate symptoms

Potential for stigmatization

Source: Reprinted with permission from M. Laraia, "Psychopharmacology," in *Principles and Practice of Psychiatric Nursing*, G. Stuart and S. Sundeen, eds., p. 698, © 1995, Mosby–Year Book, Inc.

NOTES

1. American Nurses Association, *Psychiatric Mental Health Nursing Psychopharmacology Project* (Washington, DC: American Nurses Publishing, 1994).

2. American Nurses Association, *Psychiatric Mental Health Nursing Psychopharmacology Project,* 22.

3. N. Andreasen, *The Broken Brain: The Biological Revolution in Psychiatry* (New York: Harper & Row, 1984), 83.

4. Andreasen, *The Broken Brain: The Biological Revolution in Psychiatry,* 90.

5. Andreasen, *The Broken Brain: The Biological Revolution in Psychiatry,* 91.

6. J. Grebb, "Neural Sciences," in *Comprehensive Textbook of Psychiatry,* Vol. 1, ed. H. Kaplan and B. Sadock (Baltimore, MD: Williams & Wilkins, 1995), 1–4, at 3.

7. Grebb, "Neural Sciences," 3.

8. M. Laraia, "Biological Context of Psychiatric Nursing Care," *in Principles and Practice of Psychiatric Nursing,* ed. G. Stuart and S. Sundeen (St. Louis, MO: Mosby–Year Book, 1995), 103–137, at 104.

9. Laraia, "Biological Context of Psychiatric Nursing Care," 105.

10. Laraia, "Biological Context of Psychiatric Nursing Care," 106–107.

11. A. Hayes, "Psychiatric Nursing: What Does Biology Have To Do With It?" *Archives of Psychiatric Nursing* 9, no. 4 (1995): 216–224, 218.

12. Hayes, "Psychiatric Nursing: What Does Biology Have To Do With It?" 217.

13. Laraia, "Biological Context of Psychiatric Nursing Care," 106–107.

14. Laraia, "Biological Context of Psychiatric Nursing Care," 107.

15. Hayes, "Psychiatric Nursing: What Does Biology Have To Do With It?" 219–220.

16. S. Hyman and E. Nestler, "Basic Molecular Neurobiology," in *Comprehensive Textbook of Psychiatry,* ed. H. Kaplan and B. Sadock (Baltimore, MD: Williams & Wilkins, 1995), 136–144, at 136.

17. Laraia, "Biological Context of Psychiatric Nursing Care," 108.

18. Grebb, "Neural Sciences," 3.

19. Grebb, "Neural Sciences," 3.

20. Grebb, "Neural Sciences," 3.

21. R. Coppola and T. Hyde, "Applied Electrophysiology," in *Comprehensive Textbook of Psychiatry,* ed. H. Kaplan and B. Sadock (Baltimore, MD: Williams & Wilkins, 1995), 72–79, at 75.

22. M. Laraia, "Psychopharmacology," in *Principles and Practice of Psychiatric Nursing,* ed. G. Stuart and S. Sundeen (St. Louis, MO: Mosby–Year Book, 1995), 663–701, at 666.

23. Laraia, "Psychopharmacology," 666.

24. I. Abraham et al., "Integrating the Bio into the Biopsychosocial: Understanding and Treating Biological Phenomena in Psychiatric-Mental Health Nursing," *Archives of Psychiatric Nursing* 6, no. 5 (1992): 296–305, at 299.

25. Abraham et al., "Integrating the Bio into the Biopsychosocial," 304.

SUGGESTED READING

Abbondanza, D. et al. 1994. Psychiatric mental health nursing in a biopsychosocial era. *Perspectives in Psychiatric Care* 30, no. 3: 21–25.

Abraham, I. et al. 1992. Integrating the bio into the biopsychosocial: Understanding and treating biological phenomena in psychiatric-mental health nursing. *Archives of Psychiatric Nursing* 6, no. 5: 296–305.

American Nurses Association. 1994. *Psychiatric mental health nursing psychopharmacology project*. Washington, DC.

Davis, J. 1996. Compliance: Key to relapse. *Current Approaches to Psychoses: Diagnosis and Management* 5, no. 1: 6–7.

Harper-Jaques, S., and M. Reimer. 1992. Aggressive behavior and the brain: A different perspective for the mental health nurse. *Archives of Psychiatric Nursing* 6, no. 5: 312–320.

Hayes, A. 1995. Psychiatric nursing: What does biology have to do with it? *Archives of Psychiatric Nursing* 9, no. 4: 216–224.

Kaplan, H., and B. Sadock. 1995. *Comprehensive textbook of psychiatry*. Vol. 1 and 2. Baltimore, MD: Williams & Wilkins.

Lego, S. 1992. Biological psychiatry and psychiatric nursing in America. *Archives of Psychiatric Nursing* 6, no. 3: 147–150.

McEnany, G. 1992. Psychobiology. In *Psychiatric Nursing*, ed. H. Wilson and C. Kneisl, 99–117. Menlo Park, CA: Addison-Wesley.

Pothier, P. 1990. Toward a bio/psycho/social synthesis. *Archives of Psychiatric Nursing* 4, no. 2: 77.

Stuart, G., and S. Sundeen. 1995. *Principles and practice of psychiatric nursing*. St. Louis, MO: Mosby–Year Book.

Townsend, M. 1990. *Drug guide for psychiatric nursing*. Philadelphia: F.A. Davis Company.

Yudofsky, S. et al. 1991. *What you need to know about psychiatric drugs*. Washington, DC: American Psychiatric Press, Inc.

CHAPTER

14

Antianxiety Medications: Home Care Clinical Management

INTRODUCTION

Antianxiety medications are the most widely prescribed of the psychiatric medications. The purpose of these drugs is to prevent or relieve anxiety, and they do not have antipsychotic properties. They are prescribed to patients whose anxiety makes them anxious about many things, including taking medications. These patients need help in understanding the need for medications as well as education related to the use of these medications. Prior to taking antianxiety medications, the patient should have a physical to rule out physical illnesses that may cause anxiety such as hyperthyroidism, hypoglycemia, cardiovascular illness, and severe pulmonary disease. The home care assessment should include questions about the use of some over-the-counter medications, alcohol, and caffeine, because these substances may also cause anxiety symptoms. Anxiety can be a symptom of many psychiatric illnesses; consequently, diagnosis must be done carefully.

THERAPEUTIC EFFECTS

The major therapeutic effect of these medications is to decrease anxiety. These medications are used for generalized anxiety disorder, anxiety associated with phobic disorders, sleep disorders, alcohol and drug withdrawal, anxiety associated with panic attacks, and posttraumatic stress disorder. It is recommended that antianxiety medications be used when the following factors exist:[1]

- Symptoms of anxiety are prolonged.
- There is no reasonable cause for anxiety.
- Anxiety symptoms are so severe that they interfere with daily functioning or keep the patient from enjoying the ordinary pleasures of life.

- The anxiety symptoms do not respond to nondrug treatments, such as psychotherapy, self-help groups, exercise, or decreased use of caffeine and alcohol.

Antianxiety medications should only be prescribed for serious anxiety problems.

MECHANISM OF ACTION

Antianxiety medications enhance the inhibitory neurotransmitter gamma-aminobutyric acid (GABA). This is the major inhibitory neurotransmitter in the brain. In laboratory animals, GABA has a calming effect; however, there is still much to learn about its role.

TARGET SYMPTOMS

Target symptoms are the symptoms monitored to determine the effectiveness of the medication for each patient. The psychological and behavioral target symptoms for anxiety are irritability, uneasiness, insomnia, and a feeling of panic. The physiological symptoms are nausea, diarrhea, muscle tension or aches, increased fatigue, sweating, rapid heartbeat, dizziness, and increased urination. After taking an antianxiety medication, the patient may describe the response as feeling calmer, more relaxed, and less apprehensive.

EXAMPLES OF ANTIANXIETY DRUGS

In the past, barbiturates were the drug of choice for anxiety; however, the use of these medications can lead to serious problems. They are addictive, and patients can develop tolerance. Lethal withdrawal is possible. They also have some dangerous interactions with other drugs. Today, benzodiazepines are more commonly used because these are safer drugs. Examples of benzodiazepines include the following:

- alprazolam (Xanax)
- diazepam (Valium)
- lorazepam (Ativan)
- chlordiazepoxide (Librium)
- flurazepam (Dalmane)
- clorazepate (Tranxene)
- prazepam (Centrax)

A nonbenzodiazepine, buspirone (BuSpar) may also be used to treat anxiety. This medication has no muscle-relaxant, anticonvulsant, or sedative-hypnotic activity, nor does it interact with central nervous system depressants. It may take one to two weeks to be effective. Patients who have been taking benzodiazepines must be withdrawn slowly from them before taking buspirone, and it may be less effective with these patients.

PHARMACOKINETICS

Knowledge about the half-life of these drugs can help determine the best medication for the patient. Fluctuating anxiety will respond better to medications that have a shorter half-life. Steady anxiety responds better to longer half-life medications. Within the benzodiazepine group, there is variation in gastrointestinal absorption. Clorazepate and diazepam have the quickest absorption rate and prazepam and oxazepam the slowest. The use of antacids or a full stomach slow absorption. Absorption is most rapid after oral use. These drugs are primarily metabolized by the liver. Half-life can vary from between 8 and 15 hours, to greater than 18 to 24 hours. Drugs with a longer half-life can be given once a day; those with a shorter half-life must be given more frequently.

UNWANTED EFFECTS

Side Effects

Side effects of benzodiazepines include drowsiness, nausea, hypotension, ataxia and dizziness, impaired coordination, impaired memory and concentration (particularly with lorazepam), and muscular weakness. Buspirone side effects include nervousness, insomnia, dizziness, gastric upset, nausea, diarrhea, and headaches.

Toxicity

Typical toxic symptoms include decreased coordination, slurred speech, decreased concentration, decreased respiration, confusion, and memory problems. Toxicity requires medical assessment and treatment that may include intravenous fluids and careful monitoring of respiratory status. Until fully recovered, the patient should not operate machinery or drive.

Adverse Effects

Sedation can be a major problem, particularly for the elderly patient. There can be a delayed reaction, with sedation occurring when steady-state levels of the medication are reached. Another adverse effect is anterograde amnesia. As a result, the patient may experience decreased memory several hours after taking the medication. Disinhibition with increasing aggression may occur, especially when there is a history of impulse control problems.

Physical dependency on benzodiazepines can develop with long-term use; consequently, the patient should be monitored for withdrawal. Mild withdrawal symptoms include anxiety, vertigo, agitation, blurred vision, dizziness, headaches, tinnitus, anorexia, insomnia, sweating, and tremulousness. Severe symptoms include hypotension, diarrhea, hyperthermia, neuromuscular irritability, seizures, and psychosis. These symptoms can be reduced by tapering off the drug slowly. Symptoms usually occur a few days after tapering begins, increasing for several weeks, and then stopping. There is a greater risk of dependency with alprazolam. Benzodiazepines with long half-lives have less risk for withdrawal and anxiety rebound, particularly chlordiazepoxide, diazepam, and clorazepate. Buspirone does not cause withdrawal or anxiety rebound.

There has been some discussion in the literature about whether depression is a regular or a frequent adverse effect of therapeutic benzodiazepine use. According to Smith and Salzman, "Some evidence indicates that higher doses are associated with increased risk and that lowering the dose may resolve the depression. Besides lowering the dose, discontinuing the drug, switching to a different benzodiazepine, or treating with an antidepressant agent will likely result in resolution of the symptoms."[2(p.1102)]

MEDICATION MANAGEMENT

Medication management in the home includes dosage, scheduling, laboratory monitoring, and symptom assessment as well as nursing interventions that will facilitate the patient's use of the medication. At this time there is no laboratory monitoring of patients who use these medications.

Nursing interventions considered with antianxiety medications include the following:

- Observe the patient for drowsiness when the antianxiety drug is first administered. Safety is a problem, particularly falling. The patient's family/significant other (SOs) may be concerned about the patient's lack of activity. They should be told that drowsiness is a frequent side effect during initial treatment. Eventually the patient will develop tolerance to the sedative effects of benzodiazepines.
- Due to interactions with other drugs, it is important to identify medications that the patient is taking—particularly over-the-counter drugs, caffeine, and alcohol.
- The dose for elderly patients should be the lowest possible dose.

- When the patient stops taking the medication, careful monitoring of withdrawal symptoms is required. Gradual tapering of the medication is best for safe withdrawal.
- When any patient is admitted to home care, regardless of diagnosis, the patient should be assessed for the use of these medications due to the potential of withdrawal symptoms.
- Food in the stomach or the use of antacids slows absorption of the medications.
- Some medical illnesses have inherently high levels of anxiety such as hypoglycemia, hyperthyroidism, and severe pulmonary disease. Patients with these illnesses require careful assessment prior to making a psychiatric diagnosis.
- Due to the side effect of impaired coordination and risk for accidents, the patient should be told not to drive or operate machinery. Sometimes lowering the dose or changing to a different benzodiazepine may decrease this side effect, but it will not eliminate it.
- It is important to monitor the patient for increasing irritability and decreasing ability to control behavior. The home care nurse should plan with the patient and family/SOs how they will seek help if escalating behavior occurs.
- If anterograde amnesia occurs, there is a concern about safety. The patient may forget that medication was taken. It is best to develop a method, such as a log or special medication delivery system, that identifies when medication is taken. Medication should not be left at the bedside, because the patient may take it in the middle of sleep. The amnesia may also affect reading, studying, and remembering what was heard or seen. It affects the transfer of short-term memory to long-term memory. This may frustrate the patient and the family/SOs. There should be open discussion about family/SOs concerns.
- While taking this medication, as with all other medications, the patient should consult with the physician before taking other medications, including over-the-counter medications.
- As a compliance monitor, the nurse should assess how frequently the patient requires a new prescription.
- The patient should be advised not to use alcohol and to decrease or stop the use of caffeine and tobacco. An explanation about why this is important must be provided by the nurse during the discussion.
- If a patient with respiratory disease must take these medications, the patient's respiratory status should be carefully assessed.
- The patient should be told not to share these medications with others.
- If there are children in the home or children visit frequently, medications should have safety caps.

- If a patient with renal impairment must take these medications, the patient's renal status should be carefully assessed (including monitoring of intake and output) to determine if urinary retention is occurring.
- It is best to take these medication with meals, immediately after eating, or with a snack to decrease gastrointestinal symptoms.
- Benzodiazepines can be administered orally, intramuscularly, and intravenously. In the home, the most common method is oral administration. Medication in this form is rapidly absorbed.

PRECAUTIONS AND CONTRAINDICATIONS

Contraindications include compromised respiratory status, narrow-angle glaucoma, pregnancy and lactation, and use with central nervous system depressants. These medications should be used with precaution with patients who are elderly or debilitated, and patients with hepatic and renal dysfunction, a history of drug abuse or addiction, or acquired immune deficiency syndrome (AIDS). This is particularly important when high doses are prescribed.

INTERACTIVE EFFECTS

- *Other medications.* The following drugs interact negatively with these medications:
  1. Alcohol increases all side effects, especially sedation and decreased respiration; increases memory lapses; and decreases blood pressure.
  2. Narcotics increase the sedative effects.
  3. Use with barbiturates and other sedatives increases sedation and decreases respiration.
  4. Drugs that decrease the liver's ability to remove benzodiazepine increase all of the drug's actions and side effects (e.g., cimetidine [Tagamet], propranolol hydrochloride [Inderal], disulfuram [Antabuse], and oral contraceptives).
  5. The use of caffeine and cigarettes will decrease the effects of the medication.
- *Food.* There are no important food concerns with these medications.
- *Health status.* Patients with renal dysfunction, respiratory disease, and AIDS may have problems taking these medications.
- *Age.* Elderly patients do best on shorter-acting drugs such as oxazepam, lorazepam, and buspirone. Patients with Alzheimer's disease are particularly sensitive to antianxiety medications and experience side effects. They require low doses and careful monitoring.
- *Behavior.* If the patient has a history of poor impulse control, these medications may exacerbate problems with impulse control.

- *Environment.* Safety is a concern when children may have access to the medication. Steps may be a problem for the patient due to the side of effects of impaired coordination and drowsiness.

EDUCATION OF PATIENT/FAMILY/SIGNIFICANT OTHERS

Education for the patient and the family/SOs focuses on the following:

- purpose of the medication and target symptoms
- dose and frequency
- action to be taken if dose missed
- method to monitor intake of medication
- side effects
- safety
- precautions and contraindications, particularly the use of alcohol and the use of other medications
- recommendation for decreasing or eliminating caffeine and smoking

SUMMARY

This discussion about antianxiety medications has focused on the general category of drugs. For specific, up-to-date information about individual medications, the home care nurse should consult appropriate reference material and the patient's physician. As with all medications, it is important to know the patient's medication history and to use this information as treatment is planned, implemented, and changed.

NOTES

1. S. Yudosky et al., *What You Need to Know about Psychiatric Drugs* (Washington, DC: American Psychiatric Press, Inc., 1991), 83.
2. B. Smith and C. Salzman, "Do Bezodiazepines Cause Depression?" *Hospital and Community Psychiatry* 42, no. 11 (1991): 1101–1102.

SUGGESTED READING

Arana, G., and S. Hyman. 1991. *Handbook of psychiatric drug therapy.* Boston: Little, Brown and Company.

Glod, C. 1992. Xanax: Pros and cons. *Journal of Psychosocial Nursing* 30, no. 6: 37–37.

Kaplan, H., and B. Sadock. 1995. *Comprehensive textbook of psychiatry.* Vol. 1 and 2. Baltimore, MD: Williams & Wilkins.

Townsend, M. 1990. *Drug guide for psychiatric nursing.* Philadelphia: F.A. Davis.

15

Medications for Obsessive-Compulsive Disorder: Home Care Clinical Management

INTRODUCTION

Obsessive-compulsive disorder (OCD) is responsive to several tricyclic antide-pressants, particularly clomipramine hydrochloride (Anafranil). According to Zetin and Kramer, "Long term treatment with medications appears to be required for most patients with obsessive-compulsive disorder. Response begins over a period of one to two months after treatment is initiated. Relapse is likely when medica-tions are discontinued."[1(p.695)] For patients who are eager for a change, this long wait may be difficult. They require support as their progress on medication is monitored. As successful as some of these medications have been, some patients do not respond to them. If the medication does not alleviate symptoms, the pa-tient is likely to become depressed, and support is critical at this time.

THERAPEUTIC EFFECTS

The therapeutic effect of these medicines is to decrease obsessive thoughts and compulsive behavior that is specific for the patient.

MECHANISM OF ACTION

The tricyclic antidepressants that have been found to be useful in the treatment of OCD block serotonin uptake, which keeps the serotonin in the synapse, allevi-ating OCD symptoms. They also block reuptake of norepinephrine, another neu-rotransmitter that may be important in OCD.

TARGET SYMPTOMS

The target symptoms are obsessive thoughts specific for the patient; compulsive behavior specific for the patient; and anxiety. The obsessive thoughts and compulsive behaviors interfere with the patient's normal daily living.

EXAMPLES OF MEDICATIONS FOR OBSESSIVE-COMPULSIVE DISORDER

The two categories of medications that can be used are antidepressants and anxiolytic medications. Antidepressants are more effective, particularly clomipramine hydrochloride (Anafranil). Cyclic and atypical antidepressants that might be used include the following:

- clomipramine hydrochloride (Anafranil)
- fenfluramine (Pondimin)
- sertraline (Zoloft)
- fluoxetine (Prozac)
- paroxetine (Paxil)

Anxiolytic drugs are used with some patients; however, they alleviate only the anxiety, and do little for the obsessions and compulsive behavior. An example is alprazolam (Xanax).

PHARMACOKINETICS

Generally, tricyclic antidepressant medications that are used for OCD have a long half-life, often 24 hours or longer. As a result of this, they can be taken once a day. After oral use, these drugs are absorbed in the gastrointestinal tract, metabolized by the liver, and excreted in the urine.

UNWANTED EFFECTS

Side Effects

Typical side effects include dry mouth, drowsiness, orthostatic hypotension, gastrointestinal distress, weight gain, blurred vision, constipation, cardiac arrhythmias, and agitation.

Toxicity

Symptoms of toxicity include irritability, agitation, confusion, dilated pupils, delirium, flushing, seizures, hyperpyrexia, hypotension or hypertension, and tachycardia. These can lead to serious complications such as coma, respiratory depression, cardiac arrest, shock, congestive heart failure, and renal failure. The patient will require treatment in the hospital.

Adverse Effects

Some patients may develop agranulocytosis, thrombocytopenia, or leukopenia; however, this is rare. The nurse must be aware of this risk and monitor the patient. The patient should be told about symptoms that require medical treatment. Seizures can be a serious problem, particularly in the home. Overdose with these medications is a major medical concern and requires immediate medical treatment.

MEDICATION MANAGEMENT

Medication management in the home includes dosage, scheduling, laboratory monitoring, and symptom assessment, as well as nursing interventions that will facilitate the patient's use of the medication. Nursing interventions considered with these medications include the following:

- Because it can take 5 to 10 weeks for the medication to be effective, the patient needs education about this delay and support during this period.
- Some patients with OCD do not respond to these medications. They require support and monitoring for depression and increasing anxiety.
- The patient must be assessed to determine if obsessive thoughts and compulsive behaviors have changed and how they have changed.
- The patient should be advised not to use alcohol and to decrease or eliminate smoking.
- During the initial stages of treatment when drowsiness may be excessive, the patient should be advised not to drive or operate machinery.
- It is best to take the medication with food to decrease gastrointestinal disturbances.
- Long-term therapy requires monitoring with complete blood count and liver function tests.

- If the patient is disturbed by dry mouth, try frequent sips of water, sugarless gum, and sucking on hard candy to decrease this side effect.
- If there are children in the home, medications should have safety caps.
- Due to negative interactions with other medications, it is important to identify all medications that the patient is taking.
- If the patient is having problems with orthostatic hypotension, he or she should rise slowly from sitting and lying positions.
- While taking this medication, the patient should consult with the physician before taking any other medications, including over-the-counter medications.
- Patients who have a history of suicidal thoughts or actions must be monitored carefully.

PRECAUTIONS AND CONTRAINDICATIONS

These medications are contraindicated when the patient is recovering from a myocardial infarction, taking a monoamine inhibitor drug, or during pregnancy and lactation.

Precautions are necessary when taking medications for OCD if the patient has a history of seizures, urinary retention, glaucoma, cardiovascular disease, hepatic insufficiency, renal insufficiency, psychosis, or acute intermittent porphyria.

INTERACTIVE EFFECTS

- *Other medications.* The following drugs interact negatively with these medications prescribed for OCD:
  1. cimetidine
  2. amphetamines
  3. central nervous system depressants (e.g., alcohol, barbiturates, benzodiazepines)
  4. oral contraceptives
  5. disulfiram
  6. thyroid medications
  7. monoamine inhibitors

  Cigarettes also interact negatively. Fluoxetine (Prozac) has less interactive problems than these medications.
- *Food.* There are no problems with foods.
- *Health status.* Specific medical problems were discussed as precautions. Any patient who is debilitated requires careful monitoring while taking these

medications. Patients with hyperthyroidism also must be assessed for possible problems.

- *Age.* These drugs should be monitored carefully in the elderly, using the lowest possible dose.
- *Behavior.* Patients who have a history of suicide attempts require monitoring of their use of these medications. Overdoses are very serious. It may be necessary to limit the amount of a prescription medication that the patient receives at one time and to monitor the frequency of refills. This is particularly important if the patient is not responding positively to the treatment and feels hopeless.
- *Environment.* The environment may be very important to the patient due to the specific OCD symptoms; however, there are no particular environmental issues related to the use of medication. As with all medications, safety must be considered if children are in the home.

EDUCATION OF PATIENT/FAMILY/SIGNIFICANT OTHERS

Education for the patient and the family/significant others (SOs) should provide opportunities to discuss realistic views of progress. Many of patients with OCD feel hopeless. They look for the "wonder cure." Education about medications is critical to the patient's and the family/SO's honest appraisal of progress and their active participation in treatment decisions. They need information about the following:

- purpose of the medication and target symptoms
- dose and frequency
- action to be taken if dose is missed
- method for monitoring medication compliance
- side effects
- safety
- precautions and contraindications
- safety

SUMMARY

This discussion of OCD medications has focused on the general category of drugs. The nurse must be knowledgeable about specific, up-to-date information about medications that the patient is taking. In addition, the patient's medication history must be assessed. All of this information must be used as treatment is planned, implemented, and changed.

NOTE

1. M. Zetin and M. Kramer, "Obsessive-Compulsive Disorder," *Hospital and Community Psychiatry* 43, no. 7 (1992): 689–699, at 695.

SUGGESTED READING

Arana, G., and S. Hyman. 1991. *Handbook of psychiatric drug therapy.* Boston: Little, Brown and Company.

Kaplan, H., and B. Sadock. 1995. *Comprehensive textbook of psychiatry.* Vol. 1 and 2. Baltimore, MD: Williams & Wilkins.

Townsend, M. 1990. *Drug guide for psychiatric nursing.* Philadelphia: F.A. Davis.

CHAPTER

16

Antimanic Medications: Home Care Clinical Management

INTRODUCTION

Bipolar disorder is a serious illness that affects the daily life of not only the home care patient but also the family/significant others (SOs). However, treatment for this disorder is successful for many patients. In 1970, treatment improved with the initiation of the use of lithium. However, according to Keltner and Folks, "About 30 percent of patients in the manic phase of bipolar illness either fail to respond to lithium or are intolerant of the side effects."[1(p.36)] Research is focusing on this area. Although the drug of choice continues to be lithium, there are some alternative medications for those patients for whom lithium is not effective.

THERAPEUTIC EFFECTS

The major therapeutic effect of lithium is to decrease mania and to decrease depression for those patients who require it. Antimanic medications are used primarily in acute mania, hypomania, and recurrent bipolar disorder.

MECHANISM OF ACTION

Lithium is a naturally occurring salt whose main affect has not yet been identified. There are several suggested ideas as to its mechanism of action. These include theories that "lithium corrects an ion exchange abnormality; alters sodium transport in nerves and muscle cells; normalizes synaptic neurotransmission of norepinephrine, serotonin, and dopamine; increases the reuptake and metabolism of norepinephrine; and changes receptor sensitivity for serotonin."[2(p.681)]

Valproic acid (Depakene) is a medication that may be used with some patients with bipolar disorder. It is an anticonvulsant that potentiates gamma-aminobutyric acid (GABA), an inhibitory neurotransmitter in the brain. Pope et al. suggested that GABA "may regulate an abnormally long circadian period in manic patients, thus normalizing their basic life rhythms."[3(p.65)]

TARGET SYMPTOMS

Target symptoms of mania usually include irritability, euphoria, manipulation, lability with depression, decreased sleep, difficulty finding time to eat, pressured speech, flight of ideas, hyperactivity, and distractibility. If the patient is depressed, the target symptoms include those typical for depression such as sadness, pessimism, guilt, hopelessness, sleep disturbance, fatigue, constipation, increased or decreased appetite, suicidal ideation, and poor concentration.

EXAMPLES OF ANTIMANIC MEDICATIONS

Lithium is the drug of choice for bipolar disorder, and there are three types of this drug that are used:

1. lithium carbonate (Eskalith, Lithotabs)
2. lithium carbonate sustained release (Eskalith CR, Lithobid)
3. lithium citrate concentrate (Cibalith-S)

Of patients who take lithium, 20 percent to 40 percent do not respond to it.[4] The following factors may indicate a risk that the patient may not respond to lithium.[5]

- rapid cycling, more than two episodes a year
- thought disorder with depression and paranoia
- anxiety
- obsessive features
- onset after age of 40

For patients who are not responsive to lithium, alternative medications are available. Most of these are classified as anticonvulsants. Carbamazepine (Tegretol) is the most commonly used; others include valproic acid (Depakene) and clonazepam (Klonopin).

Lithium and carbamazepine (Tegretol) may have some antidepressant effect for bipolar depression; however, more specific treatment may also be required. Antidepressants, either tricyclics or monoamine oxidase inhibitors (MAOIs), may be used for patients who are depressed. It is important to remember that "virtually all antidepressants possess the capacity to cause a 'switch' into mania, but patients in the depressive phase of bipolar illness may also develop spontaneous manic symptoms regardless of whether they are taking antidepressants."[6] [(p.229)] Careful assessment may assist in identifying those depressed patients who have the potential to develop manic symptoms. Has the patient experienced manic or hypomanic states in the past? Does the patient's family have a history of mania or hypomania or "hyperthymic" temperament? These factors might indicate the need for mood stabilization medication such as lithium with an antidepressant to prevent the swing to depression.[7] The use of antidepressants in unipolar depression and bipolar disorder is different. The most important difference is that the required dose in bipolar disorder is lower, and it is best to make dose changes gradually.

PHARMACOKINETICS

The half-life for lithium is 18 to 36 hours. Because it can reach toxic levels in three hours, the drug cannot be given in one dose. It is safe to use sustained-release capsules during maintenance treatment. During the acute phase of mania it usually takes one to two weeks to observe a change, but it can take as long as four weeks. During this period, the patient may require an antipsychotic medication. Lithium is not metabolized but excreted almost entirely by the kidneys. It is absorbed in the gastrointestinal tract.

Carbamazepine (Tegretol) has a half-life of 25 to 65 hours with the initial dose, and 12 to 17 hours with repeated doses. It takes up to 10 days to be effective. Valproic acid (Depakene) has a half-life of 5 to 20 hours and is effective in several days to one week. Clonazepam (Klonopin) has a half-life of 18 to 39 hours with a similar effective time period. These drugs are absorbed from the gastrointestinal tract, metabolized by the liver, and excreted by the kidneys.

UNWANTED EFFECTS

Side Effects

Side effects for lithium include the following:
- mild nausea
- diarrhea
- polydipsia
- dry mouth
- polyuria
- fatigue and lethargy

- headache
- fine tremor
- enlarged thyroid gland
- excessive weight gain
- edematous swelling of wrists and ankles
- metallic taste in the mouth

Carbamazepine (Tegretol) has some of the same side effects as lithium, as well as the following symptoms:

- increased alertness
- drowsiness
- ataxia
- dizziness
- visual disturbances (e.g., diplopia, blurred vision)
- mucosal ulceration
- low-grade fever
- gastrointestinal disturbances (e.g., nausea, vomiting)

Valproic acid (Depakene) usually causes few problems, and those that do occur diminish over time. Nausea, vomiting, and indigestion are the most common gastrointestinal side effects experienced at the initial stages of treatment with this medication. Enteric-coated pills may prevent or alleviate this problem. Long-term use of this medication may lead to weight gain, especially if there is concurrent use of lithium, antipsychotic drugs, or some antidepressants.[8] Fewer patients may experience rash, tremor, ataxia, headache, sedation, stupor, and transient alopecia.

Toxicity

The initial effects that may be seen in lithium toxicity are ataxia, confusion or stupor, dizziness, anorexia, nausea, vomiting, fasciculation, twitching, drowsiness, hyperactive deep-tendon reflexes, blurred vision, diarrhea, lethargy, coarse hand tremor, and tinnitus.

As toxicity increases symptoms intensify. Lithium intoxication is indicated by decreased urine output, fever, irregular pulse, tachycardia, decreased blood pressure, palpitations, cardiac arrhythmias, seizures, problems with consciousness, and coma. This is a potentially fatal response and requires immediate medical attention. The lithium must be discontinued. Due to the concern for toxicity, patients must have serum blood levels assessed. The therapeutic range for acute mania is 1.0–1.5 mEq/L (milliequivalents per liter), and for maintenance it is 0.6–1.2 mEq/L.[9] Patients who are elderly or medically ill should have a lower level. Levels above 2 mEq/L put the patient at risk for a toxic response.

Adverse Effects

Adverse effects with lithium usually do not indicate that the patient must stop taking the medication. The patient may experience the following:[10]

- thyroid dysfunction that may require hormone replacement
- mild diabetes mellitus that may require diet control or insulin therapy
- nephrogenic diabetes insipidus that may be helped with a decreased dose (Patient should drink fluids, and the use of thiazide diuretics may paradoxically decrease polyuria.)
- small changes to kidney that are not serious

Agranulocytosis and thrombocytopenia are adverse effects for carbamazepine (Tegretol).

MEDICATION MANAGEMENT

Medication management includes dosage, scheduling, laboratory monitoring, and symptom assessment, as well as nursing interventions that will facilitate the patient's use of the medication.

Physical exam and history are very important for patients who are taking lithium. The history should include information about renal disease, thyroid disease, diabetes mellitus, and hypertension in patient and the patient's family. The assessment should also include information about any diuretic use or analgesic abuse. The prelithium workup should include electrocardiogram, fasting blood sugar, and complete blood count, as well as the following tests:[11]

- urinalysis
- blood urea nitrogen (BUN)
- creatinine
- electrolytes
- 24-hour creatinine clearance
- thyroid-stimulating hormone (TSH)
- thyroxine T_4
- resin uptake (T_3RU)
- free thyroxine index (T_4I)

Maintenance assessment is also critical. It may be necessary to remind the patient about ongoing assessment, as it may become less important to the patient after a period of time on the medication. The lithium level must be monitored every three months for the first six months. Reassessment of renal status, lithium level, and TSH should be done every six months. Annually, the patient needs a reassessment of thyroid function and an electrocardiogram.[12]

Due to the fact that there is a two- to threefold difference between therapeutic and toxic concentration, lithium is usually administered in divided doses, avoiding peaks. Doses are often adjusted according to the blood level. The level should be monitored 10 to 12 hours after the last dose. For maintenance, sustained-release capsules may be used. Lithium carbonate is available in capsules and tablets; lithium citrate in liquid form.

Nursing interventions to be considered with patients who are taking lithium include the following:

- Lithium is not effective quickly; often patients require the use of an antipsychotic medication until the lithium takes effect.
- Patients who require low-sodium or fluid-restricted diets will experience serious side effects. If the patient is experiencing fever, diaphoresis, diarrhea, or diuresis, it is very important to assess the patient carefully. According to Townsend: "Lithium and sodium are similar in chemical structure, behaving similarly and competing for various sites in the body. The conditions described deplete the body of its normal sodium, and lithium that would normally be excreted is reabsorbed by the kidneys, increasing its blood level and possibility of toxicity."[13(p.209)]
- It is best to take lithium with meals or after eating crackers to decrease nausea.
- If the patient is concerned about the fine hand tremor that may occur, the nurse and family/SO should provide support.
- Patients must have serum lithium levels monitored regularly. A calendar for these tests and a method to remind the patient and family/SOs about the tests should be established.
- The home care nurse should plan with the patient and family/SOs about how lithium levels will be obtained. This will be particularly important after discharge from home care.
- If a dose is missed, the patient should not take the lithium unless it is within two hours of the scheduled time. The patient should then take the next dose at the next scheduled time.
- Fluid intake should be 2500 to 3000 mL per day.
- Home care staff should assess patient for changes in mood and behavior and assist the patient and family/SOs to monitor mood and behavior. Mild mood swings are still possible after stabilization on the medication.
- Assess for suicidal ideation.
- Laboratory reports should be monitored and discussed with the physician. The home care nurse should explain the results to the patient.

- On each visit, home care staff should monitor vital signs, with special concern for pulse irregularities and changes in blood pressure; intake and output; and weight. Any change in the intake and output ratio, sudden weight increase, or edema should be discussed with the patient's physician.

Nursing interventions for carbamazepine (Tegretol) and valproic acid (Depakene) include the following:

- The patient should be told not to stop the medication without discussing it with the physician, even if the patient is feeling better.
- It is best to take the medication with food.
- If the patient misses a dose, the patient may take this dose if it is within two hours of the missed dose.
- The medication requires weekly blood tests during initial treatment period and then follow-up. Periodic liver function tests are also advised.
- The patient should be assessed for bruising, fatigue, bleeding, mouth ulcers, fever, sore throat, and petechia or purpuric hemorrhage. These symptoms should be reported to the patient's physician.
- During the initial stage of treatment when drowsiness may be a problem, the patient should avoid driving and operating machinery.
- The patient requires assessment of changes in mood and behavior.

PRECAUTIONS AND CONTRAINDICATIONS

Several precautions must be considered with the use of lithium. Patients who have thyroid disorders, diabetes mellitus, urinary retention, or history of seizure disorders need careful monitoring. Contraindications for lithium include severe cardiovascular disease, severe renal disease, severe dehydration, sodium depletion, brain damage, and pregnancy and lactation. Lithium is not metabolized but is almost entirely excreted by the kidneys. Since it has a low therapeutic index, toxic blood levels can be reached rapidly. Sodium and fluid levels in the body are very important to the level of lithium and its action.

Carbamazepine (Tegretol) is contraindicated for use with patients who are hypersensitive to tricyclic antidepressants, have had past bone marrow depression, are lactating, or are using MAOIs. It should be used with precaution in patients who are elderly, debilitated, or pregnant, and in patients with hepatic, cardiac, or renal dysfunction, or increased intraocular pressure. Valproic acid (Depakene) is contraindicated with patients who have hepatic disease, and it should be used with precaution in patients who are elderly or debilitated, during pregnancy and lactation, with patients who have renal or cardiac disease, and with patients who are concomitantly using other anticonvulsants.[14]

INTERACTIVE EFFECTS

- *Other medications.*
  1. Lithium should not be used with aminophylline, mannitol, acetazolamide, sodium bicarbonate, drugs high in sodium content, haloperidol, neuromuscular blocking agents, paroxicam, indomethacin, and other nonsteroidal anti-inflammatory drugs, thiazide diuretics, phenothiazines, phenytoin, carbamazepine, and iodides.[15]
  2. Drug interactions with anticonvulsants used in the treatment of bipolar disorder vary from interactions with lithium. Carbamazepine (Tegretol) interacts poorly with erythromycin, verapamil, isoniazid, propoxyphene, troleandomycin, cimetidine, phensuximide, doxycycline, theophylline, oral anticoagulants, oral contraceptives, phenytoin, ethosuximide, valproic acid, haloperidol, primidone, phenobarbital, and lithium.[16] Valproic acid (Depakene) interacts poorly with diazepam, phenytoin, ethosuximide, carbamazepine epoxide, phenobarbitol, and primidone.[17]
- *Food.* A patient taking lithium must have a diet with adequate sodium. The nurse helps the patient and family/SOs develop menus that meet this requirement.
- *Health status.* Medically ill patients require a lower lithium therapeutic blood level in order to prevent toxicity. Patients with severe cardiovascular disease, severe renal disease, severe dehydration, sodium depletion, and brain damage are at risk while taking lithium.
- *Age.* Elderly patients require a lower lithium therapeutic blood level in order to prevent toxicity.
- *Behavior.* Patients who are very manic may have problems remembering to take their medications due to their hyperactivity. It may be necessary for family/SOs to monitor medications carefully, and they may require assistance in developing methods for medication administration.
- *Environment.* During the summer months or if the home is very hot, the patient must avoid excessive diaphoresis; the patient should maintain a high fluid level and appropriate diet. Because dizziness is a potential side effect with many of the drugs used for bipolar disorder, safety issues (particularly falls) must be considered in the patient's plan of care.

EDUCATION OF PATIENT/FAMILY/SIGNIFICANT OTHERS

Education about medications used for bipolar disorder should include specific information about the medications. It is important to emphasize the need for laboratory testing, diet/fluids, symptoms of toxicity, and the need to take medication as ordered even if the patient feels better. Education should include the following components:

- purpose of the medication and target symptoms
- dose and frequency
- action to be taken if dose missed
- method for monitoring medication compliance
- side effects
- safety
- precautions and contraindications

SUMMARY

This discussion on medications for bipolar disorder has focused on some of the common medications used in treatment, particularly lithium. For specific, up-to-date information about individual medications, the home care nurse should consult appropriate reference material and the patient's physician. As with all medications, it is important to know the patient's medication history and to use this information as treatment is planned, implemented, and changed.

NOTES

1. N. Keltner and D. Folks, "Alternative to Lithium in the Treatment of Bipolar Disorder," *Perspectives in Psychiatric Care* 27, no. 2 (1991): 36–37.
2. M. Laraia, "Psychopharmacology," in *Principles and Practice of Psychiatric Nursing*, ed. G. Stuart and S. Sundeen (St. Louis, MO: Mosby–Year Book, 1995), 663–701, at 681.
3. H. Pope et al., "Valproate in the Treatment of Acute Mania," *Archives of General Psychiatry* 48, no. 1 (1991): 62–68, at 65.
4. *The Medical Letter* 33 (May 17, 1991): 43–50.
5. Laraia, "Psychopharmacology."
6. A. Dantzler and C. Salzman, "Treatment of Bipolar Depression," *Psychiatric Services* 46, no. 3 (1995): 229–230, at 229.
7. Dantzler and Salzman, "Treatment of Bipolar Depression." 230.
8. *The Medical Letter* 36 (August 19, 1994): 74–75.
9. M. Townsend, *Drug Guide for Psychiatric Nursing* (Philadelphia: F.A. Davis), 209.
10. Laraia, "Psychopharmacology," 683.
11. Laraia, "Psychopharmacology," 682.
12. Laraia, "Psychopharmacology," 682.
13. Townsend, *Drug Guide for Psychiatric Nursing*, 209.
14. Townsend, *Drug Guide for Psychiatric Nursing*, 417–418.

15. Townsend, *Drug Guide for Psychiatric Nursing*, 208.

16. Townsend, *Drug Guide for Psychiatric Nursing*, 85.

17. *The Medical Letter* 36 (August 19, 1994): 75.

SUGGESTED READING

American Psychiatric Association. 1995. Practice guideline for the treatment of patients with bipolar disorder. Washington, DC: American Psychiatric Press, Inc.

Arana, G., and S. Hyman. 1991. *Handbook of psychiatric drug therapy*. Boston: Little, Brown and Company.

Ballinger, J. 1988. The use of anticonvulsants in manic depressive illness. *Journal of Clinical Psychiatry* 49, no. 11 (Supplement) 21–24.

Glod, C., and J. Mathieu. 1993. Expanding uses of anticonvulsants in the treatment of bipolar disorder. *Journal of Psychosocial Nursing* 31, no. 5: 37–39.

Kaplan, H., and B. Sadock. 1995. *Comprehensive textbook of psychiatry*. Vol. 1 and 2. Baltimore, MD: Williams & Wilkins.

McEnany, G. 1990. Psychobiological indices of bipolar mood disorder: Future trends in nursing care. *Archives of Psychiatric Nursing* 4, no. 1: 29–38.

Pope, H. et al. 1991. Valproate in the treatment of acute mania. *Archives of General Psychiatry* 48, no. 1: 62–68.

Post, R. 1989. Introduction: Emerging perspectives on valproate in affective disorders. *Journal of Clinical Psychiatry* 50, no. 3 (Supplement) 3–9.

Townsend, M. 1990. *Drug guide for psychiatric nursing*. Philadelphia: F.A. Davis.

CHAPTER

17

Antidepressant Medications: Home Care Clinical Management

INTRODUCTION

Antidepressants have been available since the 1950s, and during this time research has improved these drugs. Today it is generally recognized that biochemical factors influence the etiology of major depressive illness. According to Brasfield: "As time goes on, our understanding of what happens in the depressed brain will improve and better use of current drugs and discovery of antidepressant drugs with more specific activity targeted for specific brain neurotransmitter sites will ensue."[1(p.651)] Despite the information that is known about biochemical factors, antidepressants do not work for 25 to 30 percent of patients who are depressed.[2] Patients and their families/significant others (SOs) think that antidepressants are mood elevators, but they are not. In fact, if someone who is not depressed takes these medications, the person will feel no change in affect or mood. The home care nurse encounters many patients who are taking antidepressants, both those with psychiatric diagnoses and those without.

THERAPEUTIC EFFECTS

The major therapeutic effect of antidepressants is to decrease depression. These medications are primarily prescribed for major depression; however, they are also used for the treatment of other psychiatric disorders, including panic disorder, obsessive-compulsive disorder, and bulimia.

MECHANISM OF ACTION

There are several theories regarding the action of antidepressant drugs and the etiology of depression. The neurotransmitters, norepinephrine and serotonin, are reduced in depression. Antidepressants increase the functional levels of brain norepinephrine. They block the reuptake of these neurotransmitters at the presynaptic neuron. Selective serotonin reuptake inhibitors (SSRIs) block reabsorption of serotonin, normalizing the brain's chemical supply. Monoamine oxidase inhibitors (MAOIs) inhibit the enzyme monoamine oxidase in the brain, which is one of the primary steps in breaking down norepinephrine and serotonin.[3] Antidepressants affect the brain in very specific ways.

TARGET SYMPTOMS

When identifying target symptoms for depression, it is important to identify the week of antidepressant treatment.[4] During the first week, insomnia, appetite disturbances, and anxiety are the focus. During the second week of treatment, the target symptoms are fatigue, poor motivation, somatic complaints, agitation, and retardation. During the third week, the target symptoms are dysphoric mood and subjective depressive feelings (e.g., anhedonia, poor self-esteem, pessimism, hopelessness, self-reproach, guilt, helplessness, sadness, and suicidal thoughts).

EXAMPLES OF ANTIDEPRESSANT MEDICATIONS

In order to discuss examples of antidepressants, it is necessary to identify the three types of antidepressants that are available: tricyclic antidepressants (TCAs), selective serotonin reuptake inhibitors (SSRIs), and monoamine oxidase inhibitors (MAOIs). By grouping specific medications into these three types of drugs, it is easier to discuss and understand their actions and side effects.

The TCAs are the oldest of the antidepressant drugs. They are safe and effective; 70 to 80 percent of people with major depression respond to them.[5] Their limitations are their side effects and their lethality when an overdose is taken. Examples of TCAs include the following:

- amitriptyline hydrochloride (Elavil)
- imipramine pamoate (Tofranil)
- nortriptyline hydrochloride (Pamelor)
- amoxapine (Asendin)
- desipramine hydrochloride (Norpramin)
- clomipramine hydrochloride (Anafranil)

In addition to its use with depression, clomipramine (Anafranil) has become the drug of choice for obsessive-compulsive disorder.

The MAOIs are the second type of antidepressant. This type is as effective as the TCAs. Frequently they are used when a patient is nonresponsive to TCAs. The major limitation of this type of drug is the danger of an adverse reaction—hypertensive crisis. This may occur when the drug is taken with any food, beverage, or other drug that contains tyramine. Examples of MAOIs are phenelzine sulfate (Nardil), tranylcypromine sulfate (Parnate), and isocarboxazid (Marplan).

The third and newest type of drug is the SSRIs. These drugs have proven to be effective and often cause fewer side effects than the other types. Patients with heart disease, dementia, Alzheimer's, and those who have had a stroke tolerate these drugs better than other types of antidepressants.[6] Examples of SSRIs are fluoxetine hydrochloride (Prozac), sertraline (Zoloft), trazodone (Desyrel), and paroxetine hydrochloride (Paxil). Fluoxetine is widely used today. It has been the focus of intense media attention, ranging from speculation that it is the newest wonder drug to speculation that it causes extreme unexpected violence. It has also been effective for obsessive-compulsive disorder.

PHARMACOKINETICS

The half-life of many antidepressants is long, making it easier to give a single daily dose—often at night. Drugs that are particularly good for once-a-day dosing are fluoxetine (Prozac) (which remains in the patient's system the longest, with a half-life of two to four days) and sertraline (Zoloft) (with a half-life of one day). Sertraline (Zoloft) is more powerful than fluoxetine (Prozac). Antidepressants are metabolized in the liver and excreted in the urine. The TCAs have a half-life of 7 to 50 hours, with each medication varying somewhat within this range. One of the major problems with antidepressants is the length of time it takes for a therapeutic effect, which can be from three to six weeks. It may be difficult for the patient to continue to take a medication when no or limited effects are felt. Therapeutic plasma levels can be helpful in determining if there is enough drug in the patient's blood to be effective. Laraia states that "Blood for a plasma level should be drawn 8 to 12 hours after a single (usually bedtime) dose."[7(p.676)]

UNWANTED EFFECTS

Side Effects

Some antidepressants may produce extrapyramidal symptoms (EPS), which are commonly thought to be caused only by antipsychotic medications. Exhibit 17–1 identifies these antidepressants.

The home care nurse must be alert for these side effects to ensure that appropriate interventions are taken. It is easy to assume that EPS is part of the psychiatric illness or to fail to recognize these symptoms. Chapter 19 contains a detailed discussion about EPS.

Exhibit 17–1 Common Antidepressants That May Produce Extrapyramidal Symptoms

---

Tricyclic Agents

amitriptyline (Triavil, Etrafon)
desipramine (Norpramin)
imipramine (Tofranil)
maprotiline (Ludiomil)
amoxapine (Asendin)
doxepin (Sinequan)
nortriptyline (Aventyl, Pamelor)
protriptyline (Vivactil)

Monoamine Oxidase Inhibitors

isocarboxazid (Marplan)
tranylcypromine (Parnate)
phenelzine (Nardil)

Other Agents

fluoxetine (Prozac)
trazodone (Desyrel)

Source: Reprinted with permission from D. Blair and A. Dauner, "Nonneuroleptic Etiologies of Extrapyramidal Symptoms," *Clinical Nurse Specialist*, Vol. 7, No. 4, p. 229, © 1993, Williams & Wilkins.

Side effects for antidepressants can be grouped into the following categories:[8,9]

- Weight gain is a common side effect. Two medications, bupropion (Wellbutrin) and fluoxetine (Prozac) do not cause weight gain and may even lead to weight loss.
- Anticholinergic side effects are categorized by their location. Central nervous system effects include poor concentration, confusion, delirium, memory dysfunction, and temperature dysregulation. Those that occur in the peripheral nervous system include blurred vision, nasal stuffiness, dry mouth, constipation, tachycardia, and urinary hesitancy and/or retention.
- Sedation is a common side effect for which most patients will develop a tolerance. It can be helpful for patients who are experiencing anxiety with their depression; however, for most depressed patients the sedative effect

only adds to their lethargy. Some may require a lowering of dosage, changing to a less sedating medication, or taking the entire dose at bedtime.

- Orthostatic hypotension can lead to dizziness, falling, weakness, and reflex tachycardia. Safety can be a major problem, particularly for the elderly. Patients who are elderly or who have a cardiovascular disorder should be monitored carefully for this side effect.
- Antidepressant medications can lead to cardiac conduction abnormalities due to their quinidine-like properties.
- As antidepressants lower the seizure threshold, seizures can occur. Patients who have a seizure disorder should take a MAOI—desipramine (Norpramin) or trazodone (Desyrel).
- The use of antidepressants may unmask or cause mania in a small number of patients. Agitation and psychosis may be experienced by patients who have disorders that may lead to these symptoms such as schizophrenia or psychotic depression.
- Other side effects that might be experienced are excessive sweating, nausea, and vomiting. In addition the use of SSRIs may lead to diarrhea, insomnia, nervousness, and headache.

Toxicity

Toxicity is difficult to diagnosis due to the similarity of its symptoms to the symptoms of depression. Because toxicity for antidepressant drugs can be lethal, it is very important to recognize it early. Overdose with these medications must always be monitored. Researchers think that risk factors for toxicity, other than overdose, are probably associated with elevated plasma tricyclic levels, age, polypharmacy, and cholinergic defects in susceptible persons.[10] Treatment with antidepressants provides depressed patients who may very well be suicidal with an excellent suicide method. Drugs of particular polypharmacy concern are antihistamines, antispasmodics, some ophthalmic agents, and certain hypnotics.[11] These medications are often taken by patients for associated medical problems without recognition that they put the patients at risk for a toxic reaction. Toxicity usually presents as delirium with the symptoms of decreased concentration, change in psychomotor behavior, change in sleep, confusion, disorientation, decreased memory, hallucinations, and alteration in level of consciousness. The patient requires medical treatment. The antidepressant must be discontinued; however, it takes two to three weeks for its elimination from the body. The patient needs support during this time. If agitated, the patient should not be given an antipsychotic medication, as its anticholinergic action can worsen the toxicity.[12]

SSRIs and some TCAs have been identified with a new potentially fatal reaction, serotonin syndrome (SS) or a toxic hyperserotonergic state.[13] This reaction is similar to neuroleptic malignant syndrome (NMS). The symptoms that these two reactions have in common are hyperthermia, diaphoresis, rhabdomyolysis, coagulation, and acute renal failure.[14] Their differences include more pronounced rigidity, autonomic dysfunction, and pallor in NMS; and more pronounced hyperreflexia, restlessness, unsteady gait, and myoclonus in SS. Making a diagnosis is more difficult in patients who are taking an antidepressant along with an antipsychotic medication. MAOIs also have the potential for this problem if given with SSRIs. When the patient changes from one of these drugs to another, the body must have time to eliminate the first drug. This period can vary from two to five weeks, depending on the specific medications involved.

A hypertensive crisis may develop if MAOIs are taken with food, beverages, or other drugs that contain tyramine. The symptoms are nausea/vomiting, stiff neck, fever, sweating, palpitations, hypertension, visual changes, sensitivity to sunlight, severe headache, facial flushing, and intracranial bleeding. This is a medical emergency that requires medical treatment. Any patient who is placed on an MAOI must comply with the diet restrictions and be willing to alter eating habits. The restrictions apply until two weeks after the medication has been stopped. If the patient is unwilling to do this, an MAOI is not the drug of choice. Exhibit 17–2 provides a list of those items that the patient must avoid while taking an MAOI.

In addition, some other medications should be avoided including cold medications, nasal and sinus decongestants, allergy and hayfever remedies, narcotics (especially meperidine), inhalants for asthma, local anesthetics with epinephrine, weight-reducing pills, pep pills, stimulants, and other MAOIs.[15]

Adverse Effects

Adverse effects from antidepressants include agitation, mania, psychosis, depersonalization, derealization, and cardiac dysrhythmia.

MEDICATION MANAGEMENT

Medication management includes dosage, scheduling, laboratory monitoring, and symptom assessment, as well as nursing interventions that will facilitate the patient's use of the medication.

Nursing interventions considered with these medications include the following:

- Most patients will develop tolerance to the side effects. It frequently helps to increase the dose gradually and, in some cases, to take the full dose at bedtime.

Exhibit 17–2 Restricted Tyramine Diet with Monoamine Oxidase Inhibitors

---

EXCLUDED FOODS

- alcoholic beverages (ale, beer, sherry, red wine, cognac, liquor)
- coffee
- tea
- cola drinks
- cocoa
- cheese
- liver
- canned meats with yeast extract
- buttermilk
- licorice
- broad beans
- Italian green beans (fava beans)
- yeast and products made with yeast
- vanilla
- chocolate
- sour cream
- yogurt
- anchovies
- figs
- chicken liver
- smoked or pickled meat or fish
- chocolate milk
- soup cubes with yeast extract
- soy sauce
- Chinese peas
- spoiled or overripe fruit

- The patient's drowsiness should be monitored when the medication is first begun or if there is a change in dosage. The patient should not drive or operate machinery until he or she has adjusted to this side effect.
- The medication must be taken as ordered to maintain the desired serum level.
- The medication does not work for several weeks. It may be necessary to remind the patient and family/SOs of this because they may become discouraged. As the staff monitor the patient's progress, they can provide more concrete evidence that the medication is slowly becoming effective.
- The patient should consult with his or her physician before taking any other medication (prescription or nonprescription), due to potential drug interactions.

- The patient should be examined regularly for glaucoma.
- Dry mouth can be decreased by using hard candy, gum, or chips of ice. Dry mouth can lead to problems for the patient including tooth decay, gum disease, mouth ulcers, and candidiasis. Regular dental examination is important.
- Vital signs should be monitored early in treatment.
- Tachycardia may occur, and the patient should be reassured that tolerance usually develops.
- If the patient experiences gastrointestinal side effects, taking the medication at mealtimes may prevent these side effects.
- The patient should be monitored for symptoms of liver damage and taught to report jaundice, change in color of stools, and abdominal pain.
- Because agranulocytosis can occur, even though rare, staff must be alert for symptoms of low white blood cell count, infection of the pharynx, fatigue, and malaise. If agranulocytosis occurs, it usually occurs 40 to 70 days after initial treatment.[16]
- Even though rare, the patient may develop symptoms of increased anxiety; mania; depression; insomnia; nightmares; psychotic reactions; or confused states with delusions, hallucinations, and disorientation. If any of these occur, it may be necessary to discontinue the antidepressant medication.[17]
- Patients who are taking SSRIs, particularly fluoxetine (Prozac), may experience nervousness. The patient might use relaxation techniques to alleviate the nervousness. If this is not successful, it may be necessary to try a lower dose or a different type of antidepressant.
- Interventions to prevent or treat constipation include eight glasses of fluids a day, high-fiber and fruit diet, prune juice, and use of stool softeners or laxatives when required.
- To offer support to patients who are discouraged about not feeling better or even feeling worse with the side effects, tell them that the side effects indicate that the medication is working. For most of the side effects, a tolerance will be developed. Most patients do respond positively to these medications; it just takes time.

In addition, for patients who are taking MAOIs the following are important:

- The patient must maintain the diet requirements that exclude tyramine. These restrictions also include any medications that contain tyramine.
- If a hypertensive crisis should occur, the patient must stop the medication and seek medical treatment.
- While taking MAOIs, regular check of blood pressure is required.

PRECAUTIONS AND CONTRAINDICATIONS

The TCAs should be used with caution for patients with cardiac history, glaucoma, or urinary retention. The suicidal patient should be monitored carefully due to the lethality of these drugs if overdosed. These drugs should not be used with MAOIs and a wash-out of several weeks is required before switching from one type of antidepressant to another. All antidepressants should be used with caution during pregnancy and lactation. The SSRI paroxetine (Paxil) is not recommended for patients with kidney or liver dysfunction. In addition, patients with bundle block disease are at risk with these medications. Caution must be taken when these medications are used with patients who have seizure disorders.

INTERACTIVE EFFECTS

- *Other medications.* MAOIs, TCAs, and SSRIs should not be taken together, and a wash-out period is required when changing from one type of medication to another. Other drugs to avoid include alcohol, cocaine, amphetamines, phenytoin, phenylbutazone, aspirin, scopolamine, antipsychotics, oral anticoagulants, cimetidine, methylphenidate, propoxyphene, steroids, oral contraceptives, barbiturates, meprobamate, androgens, clonidine, guanethidine, methyldopa, disulfiram, estrogens, thyroid hormone, and nicotine. These drugs will either decrease the effectiveness of the antidepressant, increase the antidepressant's side effects, interfere with the effectiveness of the other drug, or cause potential serious side effects due to their interaction.[18]
- *Food.* The only food restrictions are for patients who are taking MAOIs (see Exhibit 17–2). All patients on antidepressants should follow a diet high in fiber and fruit and drink eight glasses of fluid daily to prevent constipation.
- *Health status.* Patients should have a physical examination prior to beginning antidepressants. Patients with kidney, liver, or cardiac problems or seizure disorders may not be appropriate for some of these medications.
- *Age.* The use of antidepressants with the elderly needs to be monitored carefully. Low doses and changing dosage slowly is the best approach.
- *Behavior.* Patients who have a history of suicidal behavior or are suicidal must be monitored carefully due to the lethality of tricyclic antidepressants if taken in inappropriate quantities. Patients at risk for suicidal behavior should receive only a few pills at a time.
- *Environment.* Patients who experience side effects of drowsiness and orthostatic hypotension are at risk for falling and accidents, such as falling asleep while smoking. They require education about these risks. The environment requires a safety assessment and, whenever possible, interventions should be taken to prevent falls (e.g., use skid protectors and safety rails for bathtub or

shower area, provide railings with steps and clear steps of obstacles, avoid loose carpets or rugs, wear appropriate shoes, rise slowly from a sitting or lying position).

EDUCATION OF PATIENT/FAMILY/SIGNIFICANT OTHERS

Education for the patient and the family/SOs focuses on the purpose of taking these medications and their dosage, frequency, side effects, precautions, and interventions to take for side effects. Education about tyramine for those who are taking MAOIs is critical. Because antidepressants do not work quickly, the patient and family/SOs must have opportunities to discuss their hopelessness about slow response to the medication and be encouraged about eventual positive response. Education should include the following:

- purpose of the medication and target symptoms
- dose and frequency
- action to be taken if a dose is missed
- method for monitoring compliance
- side effects
- safety
- precautions and contraindications

SUMMARY

If administered correctly and monitored, antidepressants are usually a very effective treatment for depression. This discussion on antidepressant medications has focused on the general category of drugs. For specific, up-to-date information about individual medications, the home care nurse should consult appropriate reference material and the patient's physician. As with all medications, it is important to know the patient's medication history and to use this information as treatment is planned, implemented, and changed.

NOTES

1. K. Brasfield, "Practical Psychopharmacologic Considerations in Depression," *Nursing Clinics of North America* 26, no. 3 (1991): 651–661, at 651.
2. M. Laraia, "Psychopharmacology," in *Principles and Practice of Psychiatric Nursing*, ed. G. Stuart and S. Sundeen (St. Louis, MO: Mosby–Year Book, 1995), 663–701, at 674.
3. K. Brasfield, "Practical Psychopharmacologic Considerations in Depression," 652.
4. Laraia, "Psychopharmacology," 676.

5. S. Yudofsky, *What You Need to Know About Psychiatric Drugs* (Washington, DC: American Psychiatric Press, Inc. 1991), 43.

6. Yudofsky, *What You Need to Know About Psychiatric Drugs*, 47.

7. Laraia, "Psychopharmacology," 676.

8. Brasfield, "Practical Psychopharmacologic Considerations in Depression," 653–656.

9. Laraia, "Psychopharmacology," 677–678.

10. J. Meadow-Woodruff, "Psychiatric Side Effects of Tricyclic Antidepressants," *Hospital and Community Psychiatry* 41, no. 1 (1990): 84–86.

11. Meadow-Woodruff, "Psychiatric Side Effects of Tricyclic Antidepressants," 85.

12. Meadow-Woodruff, "Psychiatric Side Effects of Tricyclic Antidepressants," 85.

13. N. Keltner, "Serotonin Syndrome: A Case of Fatal SSRI/MAOI Interaction," *Perspective in Psychiatric Care* 30, no. 4 (1994): 26–31.

14. Keltner, "Serotonin Syndrome: A Case of Fatal SSRI/MAOI Interaction," 29.

15. Laraia, "Psychopharmacology," 680.

16. Laraia, "Psychopharmacology," 677.

17. Laraia, "Psychopharmacology," 678.

18. Brasfield, "Practical Psychopharmacologic Considerations in Depression," 656.

SUGGESTED READING

Arana, G. 1991. *Handbook of psychiatric drug threrapy.* Boston: Little, Brown and Company.

Berman, I. et al. 1992. Sertraline: A new serotonergic antidepressant. *Hospital and Community Psychiatry* 43, no. 7: 671–672.

Depression Guideline Panel. 1993. *Depression in primary care.* Vol. 2, *Treatment of major depression. Clinical Practice Guidelines,* no. 5. AHCPR publication no. 93-0551. Rockville, MD: U.S. Department of Health and Human Services, Public Health Service, Agency for Health Care Policy and Research.

Glod, C. 1990. Prozac: Pros and cons. *Journal of Psychosocial Nursing* 28, no. 12: 33–34.

Hollister, L. 1994. New psychotherapeutic drugs. *Journal of Clinical Psychopharmacology* 14, no. 10: 50–53.

Kaplan, H., and B. Sadock. 1995. *Comprehensive textbook of psychiatry,* Vol. 1 and 2. Baltimore, MD: Williams & Wilkins.

Townsend, M. 1990. *Drug guide for psychiatric nursing.* Philadelphia: F.A. Davis.

18

Antipsychotic Medications: Home Care Clinical Management

INTRODUCTION

For patients who require the use of antipsychotic medication, this intervention is critical. The need for other interventions depends on the patient's medication compliance. Medications "buffer the patient's vulnerability to relapse."[1(p.118)] Antipsychotic or neuroleptic medications have been available since the early 1950s. These medications do not cure the illness, but rather decrease the symptoms. Because most of these medications have side effects that can be very severe, the search for better medications continues. Until recently, new medications differed only slightly from the original antipsychotics.[2] The newest medications, such as clozapine (Clozaril) and risperidone (Risperdal), have fewer side effects. These discoveries are very important, because side effects play a major role in patients' compliance with treatment. Many patients who require antipsychotic medications need maintenance medication for a long period of time and sometimes for life. For schizophrenia, medications are effective in reducing positive symptoms; the medication "facilitates cognitive functions and improves the patient's ability to learn from his treatment environment. It enables the patient to acquire new skills and use other forms of therapy."[3(p.121)] With any long-term medication use, cost must be considered, and some of the newer drugs are quite expensive. Compliance may be affected by side effects as well as cost. The decision to use an antipsychotic medication is a complex one, based on diagnosis, long-term requirements, side effects, patient compliance, family/significant other (SO) support, cost, and long-term benefits.

THERAPEUTIC EFFECTS

The major therapeutic effects of antipsychotic medications are to decrease hyperactivity, anxiety, withdrawal, hallucinations, and delusions. These medications are primarily used in patients with psychosis, schizophrenia, organic brain disorder with psychosis, and the manic phase of bipolar disorder.

MECHANISM OF ACTION

Patients who benefit from antipsychotics have dopamine overactivity. The primary action of most antipsychotics is to block dopamine receptors in the limbic system of the brain, the emotional part of the brain. However, antipsychotics not only have a therapeutic effect of decreasing psychotic symptoms; they also affect other areas of the brain, which leads to very serious side effects, extrapyramidal symptoms (EPS). There is still much to be learned about how these drugs work and their effect on the brain. The newer drugs are referred to as serotonin-dopamine antagonists (SDAs).[4] The theory is that dopamine and serotonin, natural chemicals that the brain cells use to communicate with one another, are affected by these drugs. This is particularly helpful in patients with refractory schizophrenia who have not responded to typical antipsychotics. Atypical antipsychotics, or SDAs, produce fewer side effects. The critical question is who should receive which type of drugs. According to Huttunen, "At present there are no tests or biologic markers to indicate which patients will respond best to a particular class of drugs, although such tests may be available within a decade."[5(p.3)]

TARGET SYMPTOMS

Target symptoms for antipsychotics are anxiety, agitation, flat affect, poor hygiene and appearance, hyperactivity, hostility, insomnia, poor motivation, poor social functioning, lack of insight, poor judgment, delusions, hallucinations, suspiciousness, and loose associations.[6] With schizophrenia, it is important to distinguish between positive symptoms and negative symptoms. *Positive symptoms* are grossly abnormal behaviors such as hallucinations, delusions, disordered thinking, and conceptual disorganization. Typical antipsychotics affect these positive symptoms, but they do little for the negative symptoms. *Negative symptoms* refers to the absence of certain normal behaviors or emotions such as emotional and social withdrawal, lack of drive, or blunted affect. In the past, health care workers believed these symptoms were the result of long-term hospitalization. Now they are recognized as part of the illness. Atypical antipsychotics affect these symptoms in addition to the positive symptoms. Exhibit 18–1 provides guidelines for instituting antipsychotic drug therapy.

Exhibit 18–1 Guidelines for Instituting Antipsychotic Drug Therapy

- Whenever possible, a period of drug-free evaluation and careful diagnosis should precede treatment.
- Most acute schizophreniform illnesses should be treated with antipsychotics.
- Adequate sedation and control of even acutely agitated patients can be achieved with any antipsychotic medication. All antipsychotic medications are equally effective in equivalent doses.
- In general, high-potency drugs are to be preferred. At adequate antipsychotic doses, their side effects are less problematic than those of low-potency drugs.
- In an acutely psychotic patient, underdosing is a more serious error than excessive dosing. However, the lowest effective medication dose is always the goal.
- Individuals have been shown to vary widely in their drug absorption, distribution, and metabolism patterns. Adequate doses for some patients will therefore be too little or too much for a significant number of other patients.
- An adequate antipsychotic drug trial can be considered to be four to six weeks of a single drug at or near maximal dose range.
- Polypharmacy has not been shown to be more effective than single drug treatment and carries increased risks. The same antipsychotic that the patient receives on a daily basis can be used orally or intramuscularly as needed for agitation.
- Rapidity of dosage increments depends upon the persisting psychotic symptomatology (insomnia, agitation, hallucinations, delusions) and the need for extra doses.
- Single daily bedtime doses are preferred.
- If patients are excessively lethargic or an acute organic brain syndrome develops, decrease or temporarily discontinue medication.
- Reduced doses are required for children and older patients.
- If an adequate trial produces no response to treatment, consider the following:
  - parenteral therapy (rapid metabolizer or covert noncompliance)
  - diagnostic error
  - a different antipsychotic class
  - high-dose therapy (2 to 4 times maximal dose) with consultation and guidance
- Use anti-Parkinson drugs as necessary. Prophylactic use is preferable to potentially unrecognized side effects and lack of drug maintenance.
- Acute extrapyramidal side effects are not necessarily an indication to decrease, discontinue, or change medication. Treatment should be focused on adequate doses to control psychotic symptoms, not side effects.
- Treatment should be continued for six months after a first schizophrenic episode. Two or more episodes probably require maintenance antipsychotic therapy.

Source: Reprinted with permission from B. Wittlin, "Practical Psychopharmacology," in *Psychiatric Rehabilitation of Chronic Mental Patients*, R. Liberman, ed., pp. 131–132, © 1988, American Psychiatric Press, Inc.

Examples of typical antipsychotics include the following:

- chlorpromazine hydrochloride (Thorazine)
- fluphenazine decanoate (Prolixin)
- fluphenazine hydrochloride (Prolixin; the long-acting form)
- perphenazine (Trilafon)
- trifluoperazine (Stelazine)
- chlorprothixene (Taractan)
- thiothixene hydrochloride (Navane)
- haloperidol (Haldol)
- thioridazine (Mellaril)
- molindone hydrochloride (Moban)
- loxapine succinate (Loxitane)
- prochlorperazine (Compazine)

Examples of atypical antipsychotics include the following:

- clozapine (Clozaril)
- risperidone (Risperdal)
- mesoridazine (Serentil)

Another medication that is used in the treatment of schizophrenia is carbamazepine (Tegretol), an anticonvulsant. An advantage to the use of this medication is that it does not produce the side effects that are typical for neuroleptics. It does, however, cause some sedation and mild dysphoria, but these effects are not permanent. According to Norris et al., "When carbamazepine is used along with neuroleptic medications, it appears to potentiate the effect of the neuroleptic. Less neuroleptic is required to produce the same reduction in symptomatology as that observed for individuals receiving only neuroleptic medication. Carbamazepine also has a protective effect against the extrapyramidal side effects of neuroleptics.[7(p.14)]

PHARMACOKINETICS

The half-life for antipsychotic drugs is more than 24 hours. Patients improve slowly over several weeks, and some change occurs over several months. Maintenance therapy is important for most patients. According to Laraia, "Dosage requirements for individual patients vary considerably and must be adjusted as the target symptoms change and side effects are monitored. Initially the patient is dosed several times a day, and the daily dose can be raised every 1 to 4 days until symptoms improve. Some patients respond in 2 to 3 days, some take as long as 2 weeks.[8(p.687)] Most of these medications are metabolized by the liver and excreted primarily by the kidneys.

UNWANTED EFFECTS

Side Effects

The major side effects for antipsychotics or neuroleptics include hypotension, sedation, extrapyramidal symptoms, anticholinergic symptoms, endocrine effects, and tardive dyskinesia.

- Hypotension is more common with high-dose, low-potency drugs such as chlorpromazine hydrochloride (Thorazine). It happens less often with high-potency drugs, because the drug can be used at a low dose. If the patient uses alcohol, sedative or hypnotic drugs, or street drugs, this side effect will be worse. Hypotension can cause fatigue, loss of balance, and potential falls.[9]
- Sedation can be beneficial for some patients, particularly early in treatment, to decrease hyperactivity and provide some rest. However, it can also interfere with cognitive and social functioning. Low doses of high-potency drugs cause less sedation. Tolerance to this side effect is usually developed after a few weeks. If sedation is a major problem for the patient, the best solution is to have the patient take the entire dose or as much as possible at bedtime.[10]
- Extrapyramidal symptoms (EPS) are discussed in Chapter 19. These are serious side effects that are caused by the medication blocking dopamine receptors in the nigrostriatal subcortical part of the brain, the same area that is affected by Parkinson's disease. These symptoms are frightening, interfere with daily functioning, and may affect the patient's compliance with antipsychotic medication.[11]
- Anticholinergic symptoms typically include dry mouth, blurred vision, constipation, nausea, urinary retention or reduced force of urine stream, and memory disturbance. Other symptoms that might occur are skin rashes, photosensitivity, blood dyscrasia, and jaundice. These symptoms usually are found with the use of high doses of low-potency medications. If the patient is taking antiparkinsonian medications for EPS, these medications will increase anticholinergic symptoms.[12]
- Endocrine disturbances may also occur. This may lead to decreased erections, delayed or absent ejaculation, anorgasmia, menstrual irregularities, galactorrhea, weight gain, or an increase in appetite. It is important to discuss these side effects with the patient, because they can be reasons for noncompliance. Usually endocrine disturbances are not permanent and can be corrected by changing the dose or the medication.[13]

- Tardive dyskinesia (TD) is a serious side effect that may occur in patients who have been taking antipsychotics or neuroleptics over a long period of time. There are no effective preventives or antidotes except to reduce the medication or stop it. This will only reduce the severity of TD. Atypical medications such as clozapine (Clozaril) thus far do not appear to cause TD. Chapter 19 discusses TD in more detail.[14]
- Side effects for specific antipsychotic medications may vary.
  - Typical side effects for clozaril (Clozapine) are increased sedation, tachycardia, seizures, constipation, hypersalivation (which for some patients can be excessive), severe hypotensive reactions, and hypothermia.
  - Typical side effects for risperidone (Risperdal) are agitation, anxiety, insomnia, orthostatic hypotension, tachycardia, headache, nausea, constipation, weight gain, fatigue, and dizziness. With higher doses, risperidone can cause extrapyramidal symptoms more easily.
  - Patients who are taking carbamazepine (Tegretol) need to participate in the assessment of their side effects, because dosage is "titrated according to treatment benefit with side effects as a limiting factor."[15] Therapeutic serum level should be monitored carefully, particularly during the first month of treatment when spontaneous decreases in serum concentration may occur.[16]

Toxicity

Symptoms of toxicity may include central nervous system depression, hypotension, confusion, excitement, agitation, restlessness, severe EPS, convulsions, fever, hypothermia, respiratory depression, and cardiac problems.

Adverse Effects

Adverse effects for typical antipsychotics include agranulocytosis, photo-sensitivity, contact dermatitis, electrocardiogram abnormalities, seizures, neuroleptic malignant syndrome, and tardive dyskinesia. Atypical antipsychotics vary in their adverse effects. Risperidone (Risperdal) does not appear to cause agranulocytosis, neuroleptic malignant syndrome, or TD. In fact, it may actually decrease TD.[17] Clozapine (Clozaril) may cause seizure activity that is dose related and agranulocytosis, and the latter requires careful monitoring.[18] Because agranulocytosis is considered to be of serious concern with this medication, patients taking this medication should have regular blood testing including hematology, blood chemistry, and liver function.

Patients who are taking carbamazepine (Tegretol) are at risk for aplastic anemia, hepatotoxicity, or changes in cardiac rhythms. These are rare occurrences;

however, all patients taking this medication require blood testing to assess hepatic and hematopoietic functions.[19] Signs of infection, bruising, and unusual bleeding require follow-up. This medication can also cause problems for patients with narrow-angle glaucoma.

Even though antipsychotic medications are not addictive, abrupt withdrawal from antipsychotics can lead to exacerbation of psychosis. Symptoms that might indicate that this is occurring are anxiety, agitation, restlessness, insomnia, nausea, emesis, anorexia, diarrhea, rhinorrhea, diaphoresis, myalgia, and paresthesia.[20] Patients who stop taking their neuroleptics without informing staff may be putting themselves at risk for these symptoms. When the home care nurse is suspicious that the patient may not be taking medication, the nurse should carefully assess for these symptoms.

MEDICATION MANAGEMENT

Medication management includes dosage, scheduling, laboratory monitoring, and symptom assessment as well as nursing interventions that will facilitate the patient's use of the medication. Antipsychotic medications have a highly variable response rate that is also influenced by the dosage. Every one to four days, the dose can be increased until target symptoms are changed. The patient may begin to respond after two days to two weeks; however, it usually takes up to six weeks to experience the full benefits. Depot injectables are available—such as fluphenazine hydrochloride (Prolixin), which can be given every 7 to 28 days, and haloperidol decanoate (Haldol), which is given every 28 days. This type of administration takes three months to reach steady-state and is used primarily for maintenance therapy. The benefits of depot injectables are that they bypass the liver and gastrointestinal system, providing a higher concentration of the drug to the brain. This may explain why some patients who do not respond well to oral medication respond better to injections. In addition, there is guaranteed delivery. This is helpful with patients who may be noncompliant for a variety of reasons. There are, however, problems with this method of administration. There is increased risk of weight gain, extrapyramidal symptoms, drug-induced depression, and tardive dyskinesia.[21]

Interventions for patients who are taking typical antipsychotics include the following:

- The patient should have a history and physical. The critical focus areas are[22]
  1. history and physical
  2. vital signs
  3. complete blood count

    4. neurologic exam

    5. electrocardiogram

    6. liver and renal tests

    7. prostate exam for men over 40 years of age

    8. ophthalmologic exam

- Blood pressure should be monitored, usually for several days or until stable.
- There is risk for orthostatic hypotension. The patient must be told to rise slowly from a sitting or lying position. If the patient becomes dizzy, safety in the home will be important (e.g., stairways clear and with railings, no loose carpeting and rugs, bathtub and shower with safety devices).
- The patient should be assessed routinely for extrapyramidal symptoms, and this assessment should be documented.
- Bowel movements should be monitored due to increased risk of constipation. The patient's diet should be reviewed for high fiber and adequate fluids. Adequate exercise should also be encouraged to prevent constipation. Some patients may require a stool softener or a laxative.
- If dry mouth occurs, hard candy and gum may make the patient more comfortable. The patient should be told about the importance of good mouth care.
- Due to photosensitivity, exposure to sun should be avoided by using sunscreen and wearing appropriate clothing outdoors.
- Report any symptoms of infection, bruising, or unusual bleeding to the patient's physician.
- Medications used for extrapyramidal symptoms should be taken as prescribed.
- If the liquid form of these medications is used, all those who use it must be warned about the risk for contact dermatitis and how to avoid it.
- When the drug is stopped, the dosage should be tapered. It should never be stopped abruptly. The staff should routinely assess for symptoms of sudden withdrawal from the medication.

In addition to nursing interventions for typical antipsychotics, additional interventions are necessary for clozapine (Clozaril). Many patients and their families/SOs hold this medication up as a "miracle cure." Working with them to recognize the realities of the medication and its response is very important. Most patients begin this medication after they have been taken off of other medications for 7 to 10 days. Patients require intensive nursing care during this time, as symptoms such as hallucinations, regression, and aggression often worsen. The patient who has been hospitalized may have had negative experiences with the wash-out period. This may come up during conversations about medications. The following interventions may be used when the patient is taking clozapine (Clozaril):

- A history and physical are critical before beginning this medication. Exhibit 18–2 provides information about the typical medical workup required before starting this medication.
- Vital signs must be monitored, particularly until blood pressure is stabilized. A baseline orthostatic blood pressure taken one hour before and one hour after the first dose will be helpful information when determining the patient's stabilized blood pressure. If blood pressure changes more than 20 beats per minute or systolic changes greater than 20 mm Hg, the medication should be stopped, and the physician called. The patient should be encouraged to drink fluids. Low pulse rates may indicate medication noncompliance.
- Because there is a risk of seizures, the patient and family/SOs should be told what to do if seizures occur.
- Regular blood work is required while the patient is taking this medication. Plans should be made to obtain laboratory tests and results.
- The patient should take the medication as ordered and should not stop the medication without talking with the home care nurse and the physician.
- Signs of fever, sore throat, bruising, and changes in the patient's white blood cell count must be discussed with the physician. The medication should be stopped until the patient's condition can be thoroughly assessed.
- For some patients sialorrhea or excessive saliva may be a major problem. The nurse can suggest that the patient keep tissues available and cover his or her pillow with absorbent towels. The patient may be very embarrassed by this excessive saliva, and this may cause the patient to be noncompliant.

Exhibit 18–2 Typical Medical Workup for Use of Antipsychotic Medications

- blood pressure and pulse
- eye exam
- neurological exam
- prostate exam for men over 40
- complete blood count
- kidney and liver tests
- electrocardiogram

Source: Reprinted with permission from S. Yudofsky et al., *What You Need to Know about Psychiatric Drugs,* p. 180, © 1991, American Psychiatric Press, Inc.

- Sedation may be excessive; however, the patient and family/SOs need to be told that this symptom usually decreases.
- If the patient experiences nausea, constipation, and/or diarrhea, these may be side effects, but they may also indicate that there is a major problem of hepatic dysfunction. If these symptoms continue, the patient should see a medical physician.

PRECAUTIONS AND CONTRAINDICATIONS

Antipsychotic medications must be used with caution during pregnancy and lactation. There is no tolerance or addiction related to these drugs. The question of addiction may be a concern of the patient and family/SOs. Patients who are taking benzodiazepines may develop respiratory problems.

INTERACTIVE EFFECTS

- *Other medications.* Medications that may have interactive problems with antipsychotics include antacids, lithium, narcotics, antidepressants, monoamine oxidase inhibitors, beta blockers, barbiturates, levodopa, benzodiazepines, guanethidine, clonidine, antihypertensives, vasodilator drugs, antihistamines, and quinidine.[23] Risperidone (Risperdal) should not be given with other antipsychotic medications because they reduce the effectiveness of this medication and increase side effects.[24]
- *Food.* There are no food restrictions with these medications. Due to the potential for constipation, the patient should be encouraged to eat a high-fiber diet; drink adequate fluids; and, if required, use a stool softener or laxative.
- *Health status.* Patients with cardiac disorders, glaucoma, and prostate enlargement may have problems taking antipsychotics and should be assessed carefully.
- *Age.* Patients who are over 60 with preexisting medical illness may find that their medical problems worsen, particularly cardiac disorders, glaucoma, and prostate enlargement. The dosage for elderly patients should always be monitored closely.
- *Behavior.* Noncompliant behavior may be of serious concern. In fact, it is "so common in schizophrenic outpatients that it makes sense to anticipate it."[25(p.1)] Weiden identifies two major reasons for noncompliant behavior— medication side effects and the patient's denial of illness. He comments that patients are not static in their behavior, changing from compliance to noncompliance. Denial is complex and difficult to overcome. Neuropsychologic deficits may interfere with the patient's ability to be aware of his or her ill-

ness. The patient's denial may also be a psychological response to the illness and the sick role, a method for maintaining dignity.[26] Rather than focusing on the patient's denial, it is better to associate taking medications with the patient's specific goals (e.g., taking over more responsibilities at home, attending clinic appointments, taking a course, or getting a part-time job). In assessing the role that side effects play in noncompliant behavior, it is important to identify the side effects that are of most concern and also who is concerned about them (e.g., patient, family/SOs, staff). If family/SOs are concerned about a side effect, they may directly or indirectly influence the patient's noncompliant behavior. At each visit, the patient should be asked about medication compliance. According to Weiden, staff "should not castigate or scold the patient for being truthful, or that will be the last time they will hear about noncompliance from that patient. Instead, phrase the question as though noncompliance were the norm. Ask questions such as 'When was the last time you stopped taking your medication?'"[27(p.6)] Before changing medications staff should make a careful analysis of the reasons for noncompliance. All documentation describing the patient's behavior and mood, target symptoms, and side effects, as well as history of the use of the medication will be very important in this process of assessing noncompliance.

- *Environment.* Sedation and hypotension increase the risk of accidents and falls. It is necessary to conduct a safety assessment of the environment in order to develop interventions that might decrease these risks (e.g., stairways clear and with railings, bathroom shower stalls and tubs with safety devices, discussion with the patient about smoking safety, correction of loose carpeting).

EDUCATION OF PATIENT/FAMILY/SIGNIFICANT OTHERS

Education for the patient and family/SOs focuses on the purpose, dosage and frequency, side effects, and interventions to help alleviate side effects. Compliance is a critical component of this process. Listening to the patient helps staff to identify risk factors for noncompliance and interventions to prevent noncompliance. The patient must learn self-monitoring to identify times when he or she needs more help and to give the patient a sense of control, an important factor in the success of treatment. Particularly important to include in patient education are the following:

- purpose of the medication and target symptoms
- dosage and frequency
- action to be taken if dose is missed

- method for monitoring medication compliance
- side effects
- safety
- precaution and contraindications

SUMMARY

This discussion on antipsychotic medications has focused on the general category of drugs. For specific, up-to-date information about individual medications, the home care nurse should consult appropriate reference material and the patient's physician. As with all medications, the home care nurse must be knowledgeable about individual medications the patient is taking in order to provide quality care. The patient's medication history is very important, and this information is used during treatment planning, implementation, and changing the plan.

NOTES

1. B. Wittlin, "Practical Psychopharmacology," in *Psychiatric Rehabilitation of Chronic Mental Patients*, ed. R. Liberman (Washington, DC: American Psychiatric Press, Inc.), 118–145, at 118.

2. N. Keltner, "Risperidone: The Search for a Better Antipsychotic," *Perspectives in Psychiatric Care* 31, no. 1 (1995): 30–33, at 30.

3. R. Liberman et. al., "Protective Intervention in Schizophrenia: Combined Neuroleptic Drug Therapy and Medication Self-Management Training," in *The Chronically Mentally Ill: Research and Services*, ed. M. Mirabi (New York: Spectrum Publications, 1984), 119–133, at 121.

4. M. Huttunen, "The Expanding Role of Serotonin-Dopamine Antagonists in Psychoses Treatment," interview with M. Huttunen, *Current Approaches to Psychoses: Diagnosis and Management* 4, no. 2 (1995): 2–3.

5. Huttunen, "The Expanding Role of Serotonin-Dopamine Antagonists in Psychoses Treatment," at 3.

6. M. Laraia, "Psychopharmacology," in *Principles and Practice of Psychiatric Nursing*, ed. G. Stuart and S. Sundeen (St. Louis, MO: Mosby–Year Book, 1995), 663–701, at 687.

7. A. Norris et al., "Carbamazepine Treatment of Psychosis," *Journal of Psychosocial Nursing* 28, no. 12 (1990): 13–18, at 14.

8. Laraia, "Psychopharmacology," 687.

9. Wittlin, "Practical Psychopharmacology," 125.

10. Wittlin, "Practical Psychopharmacology," 125–126.

11. Wittlin, "Practical Psychopharmacology," 125.

12. Wittlin, "Practical Psychopharmacology," 126.

13. Wittlin, "Practical Psychopharmacology," 126.

14. Wittlin, "Practical Psychopharmacology," 119, 124.

15. A. Norris, "Carbamazepine Treatment of Psychosis," 17.

16. A. Norris, "Carbamazepine Treatment of Psychosis," 16.

17. Keltner, "Risperidone: The Search for a Better Antipsychotic," 32.

18. N. Jaretz et al., "Clozapine: Nursing Care Considerations," *Perspectives in Psychiatric Care* 28, no. 3 (1992): 19–24.

19. A. Norris, "Carbamazepine Treatment of Psychosis," 15.

20. A. Norris, "Carbamazepine Treatment of Psychosis," 15.

21. P. Driscoll, "Maintenance Medication for Chronic Schizophrenics: Risk/Benefit Assessment," *Perspectives in Psychiatric Care* 22, no. 3 (1985): 104–110, at 108.

22. S. Yudofsky et al., *What You Need to Know about Psychiatric Drugs* (Washington, DC: American Psychiatric Press, Inc., 1991), 180.

23. Yudofsky, et al., *What You Need to Know about Psychiatric Drugs,* 183.

24. W. Land and C. Salzman, "Risperidone: A Novel Antipsychotic Medication," *Hospital and Community Psychiatry* 45, no. 5 (1994): 434–435.

25. P. Weiden, "Antipsychotic Therapy: Patient Preference and Compliance," interview with P. Weiden, *Current Approaches to Psychoses, Diagnosis and Management* 4, no. 2 (1995): 1, 6–7, at 1.

26. Weiden, "Antipsychotic Therapy: Patient Preference and Compliance," 6.

27. Weiden, "Antipsychotic Therapy: Patient Preference and Compliance," 6.

SUGGESTED READING

Arana, G., and S. Hyman. 1991. *Handbook of psychiatric drug therapy.* Boston: Little, Brown and Company.

Awad, A. 1992. Quality of life of schizophrenic patients on medications and implications for new drug trials. *Hospital and Community Psychiatry* 43, no. 3: 262–265.

Barret, N. et al. 1990. Clozapine: A new drug for schizophrenia. *Journal of Psychosocial Nursing* 28, no. 2: 24–28.

Chapman, T. 1991. The nurse's role in neuroleptic medications. *Journal of Psychosocial Nursing* 29, no. 6: 6–8.

Chen, Cheng-Chung. 1991. A follow-up of patients with neuroleptic malignant syndrome. *Hospital and Community Psychiatry* 42, no. 2: 197–198.

Dillon, N. 1992. Screening system for tardive dyskinesia: Development and implementation. *Journal of Psychosocial Nursing* 30, no. 10: 3–7.

Driscoll, P. 1985. Maintenance medication for chronic schizophrenics: Risk/benefit assessment. *Perspectives in Psychiatric Care* 22, no. 3: 104–110.

Feighner, J. 1995. Treatment for schizophrenia patients with depression. Interview with J. Feighner. *Current Approaches to Psychoses: Diagnosis and Management* 4, no. 1: 10–11.

Green, A., and C. Salzman. 1990. Clozapine: Benefits and risks. *Hospital and Community Psychiatry* 41, no. 4: 379–380.

Hamilton, D. 1990. Clozapine: A new antipsychotic drug. *Archives of Psychiatric Nursing* 4, no. 4: 278–281.

Hogart, G. 1994. Using optimal dosing strategies with psychosocial treatment in schizophrenia. Interview with G. Hogart. *Current Approaches to Psychoses: Diagnosis and Management* 3, no. 4: 6–8.

Jaretz, N. et al. 1992. Clozapine: Nursing care considerations. *Perspectives in Psychiatric Care* 28, no. 3: 19–24.

Johnson, D. 1995. Risks of antipsychotic discontinuation. *Current Approaches to Psychoses: Diagnosis and Management* 4, no. 7: 11–12.

Kane, J., and S. Marder. 1996. Update on newer antipsychotic agents. *Current Approaches to Psychoses: Diagnosis and Management* 5, no. 1: 1, 4–5.

Kaplan, H., and B. Sadock. 1995. *Comprehensive textbook of psychiatry*. Vol. 1 and 2. Baltimore, MD: Williams & Wilkins.

Keltner, N. 1995. Risperidone: The search for a better antipsychotic. *Perspectives in Psychiatric Care* 31, no. 1: 30–33.

Land, W., and C. Salzman. 1994. Risperidone: A novel antipsychotic medication. *Hospital and Community Psychiatry* 45, no. 5: 434–435.

Littrell, K., and A. Magill. 1993. The effect of clozapine. *Journal of Psychosocial Nursing* 31, no. 9: 14–18.

Marder, S. 1995. Switching antipsychotic therapies. *Current Approaches to Psychoses: Diagnosis and Management* 4, no. 7: 1, 5–6.

McCarthy, P., and J. Snyder. 1992. Orthostatic hypotension: A potential side effect of psychiatric medications. *Journal of Psychosocial Nursing* 30, no. 8: 3–5.

Norris, A. et al. 1990. Carbamazepine treatment of psychosis. *Journal of Psychosocial Nursing* 28, no. 12: 13–18.

Tesar, G. 1993. The agitated patient, part II: Pharmacologic treatment. *Hospital and Community Psychiatry* 44, no. 7: 627–629.

Townsend, M. 1990. *Drug guide for psychiatric nursing*. Philadelphia: F.A. Davis.

19

Anticholinergic Medications: Home Care Clinical Management

INTRODUCTION

The use of antipsychotic medications or neuroleptics is not without its risks. These medications can lead to serious side effects, commonly referred to as extrapyramidal symptoms (EPS). Some of these side effects may cause the patient to be noncompliant with treatment and stop taking medications, and this can result in hospital readmission. The patient and family/significant others (SOs) may think that these side effects are caused by the illness rather than the treatment. Some of these side effects may lead to serious and even life-threatening medical problems. The home care nurse plays an important role in assessment and prevention of these side effects. Dauner and Blair state that, due to EPS, "it is apparent that treatment may actually become focused on symptoms caused by the very medications used to treat the patient in the first place."[1(p.14)] Anticholinergic drugs are used to prevent or reduce EPS.

This discussion will concentrate on antipsychotic-induced EPS symptoms. Other drugs can cause EPS symptoms, although these are less common. Some of these nonneuroleptic drugs are antidepressants, antiemetics, some anticonvulsant medications, and lithium. When assessing patients who are experiencing EPS, it is necessary to consider these medications, as well. It is common to eliminate the possibility of EPS, based on the fact that the patient is not taking an antipsychotic medication. According to Blair and Dauner, "This can cause patients to be misdiagnosed, treatment to be misdirected or dangerous, and the patient to be forced to become noncompliant, to endure prolonged hospitalization, and to suffer iatrogenic complications."[2(p.226)]

THERAPEUTIC EFFECTS

Treatment for EPS is focused on prevention or treatment of these symptoms. Prevention should always be the first focus.

MECHANISM OF ACTION

Prior to understanding the mechanism of action for anticholinergic drugs, an understanding of why these symptoms occur is essential. Antipsychotic medications have also been called neuroleptics because of the characteristic side effects they produce. The extrapyramidal system includes the nerve pathways from the brain to the skeletal muscles. Its multisynaptic neurons, which are located in the basal ganglia, parts of the reticular formation, and the upper central nervous system, control and integrate motor and some cognitive functions. This system helps to control stability of movement; balance; and coordination in posture, gait, and voluntary movement. For these functions to remain stable, there must be normal levels of two neurotransmitters—dopamine and acetylcholine. Antipsychotic medications antagonize these neurotransmitters, causing a depletion of dopamine; this can lead to extrapyramidal side effects.

Drugs that help prevent or treat EPS vary. The most common are the anticholinergic drugs. The actions of these drugs are to balance dopamine deficiency and acetylcholine excess in the corpus striata. At the same time, the acetylcholine receptor is blocked to diminish cholinergic effect.[3]

TARGET SYMPTOMS

The target symptoms for the anticholinergic drugs are the extrapyramidal symptoms—nonmovement symptoms of dry mouth, blurred vision, and constipation, and the movement symptoms. The movement symptoms are included in the *Diagnostic and Statistical Manual of Mental Disorders,* 4th ed. *(DSM-IV)* as psychiatric diagnoses coded in Axis I.[4]

- neuroleptic-induced parkinsonism
- neuroleptic-induced dyskinesias and dystonias
- neuroleptic-induced akathisia
- neuroleptic-induced tardive dyskinesia
- neuroleptic-induced malignant syndrome

Over time, the body often adapts to some of these symptoms, particularly the nonmovement side effects. The most common movement symptoms are pseudoparkinsonism, representing 40 percent of all EPS, and the dystonias, dyskinesias, and akathisias, representing 50 percent. Laraia reports that "Currently the correlation between plasma blood levels of antipsychotic drugs or serum dopamine receptor binding and clinical response has yet to be determined, but these tests hold promise for refining drug selection and dosing regimens."[5(p.688)] Because the movement disorders cause many problems for patients, they will be discussed in more detail.

Neuroleptic-Induced Parkinsonism[6]

This type of EPS is similar to parkinsonism, but it is drug induced. It usually begins from four days to two weeks after starting treatment with neuroleptics and peaks at two to four weeks. The patient may experience many of the following symptoms:

- Muscular rigidity, often confused with tension or anxiety, is a plastic hypertonicity affecting the head, trunk, and limbs. The patient may complain about muscular tenderness, stiffness, joint discomfort, and body pain.
- There are alterations in posture (e.g., stooping).
- The patient may develop a shuffling gait, described as a *festinating* or *shuffling* gait that may be propulsive.
- Tremors usually begin in one or both upper extremities. As the tremors progress, they include the tongue, jaw, and lower extremities. Tremors are usually first seen a few days after beginning treatment with an antipsychotic, peak at 2 to 6 weeks, and decline at 8 to 16 weeks. Often the tremors can be suppressed when the patient attempts to perform a task.
- A masklike facies may be confused with flat affect; however, the patient with pseudoparkinsonism tries to communicate feelings in other ways. This does not occur with flat affect.
- Drooling may occur due to decreased pharyngeal motor activity.
- Akinesia—slow, stiff movements—may be experienced. Daily activities become difficult to perform.[7] The patient exhibits less spontaneous movements, increased sleeping, and apathy.

It is easy to see how these symptoms might be confused with symptoms of the patient's illness. These pseudoparkinsonian symptoms can be treated with the medications mentioned in this chapter. The *DSM-IV* requirements for a diagnosis of neuroleptic-induced parkinsonism include one or more parkinsonian tremors with coarse, rhythmic resting tremor occurring between three and six cycles per second that affects the limbs, head, mouth, or tongue; parkinsonian muscular rigidity with cogwheel rigidity or continuous "lead-pipe" rigidity; and akinesia.[8]

These symptoms must occur within a few weeks of taking an antipsychotic medication, raising the dosage of an antipsychotic medication, or when an anticholinergic medication has been reduced. There should be no medical reason or use of a medication other than those mentioned that might cause these symptoms. Tolerance of these symptoms does not develop.

Neuroleptic-Induced Dyskinesias and Dystonias[9]

Dyskinesia is described as involuntary, stereotyped, coordinated, rhythmic movements that can occur in the trunk and the limbs. These movements may be confused with seizures or catatonic posturing. These symptoms may occur within several hours of receiving a single dose of an antipsychotic medication. Dystonias are dramatic and frightening uncoordinated, jerking, bizarre movements that can occur in the neck, face, eyes, tongue, arms, legs, and torso. Common movements are

- torticollis or sideways twisting of the neck
- opisthotonos or head and neck extension
- oculogyric crisis or a backward rolling of the eyes in their sockets
- protrusion of the tongue or thickened speech
- spasms of the jaw muscles or grimacing
- impaired swallowing, speaking, or breathing

These side effects are very painful, and they can lead to medical crises such as respiratory distress, difficulty talking, and difficulty swallowing. Treatment with parenteral diphenhydramine (Benadryl) can resolve these problems quickly. These symptoms may occur one hour to five days after the first dose of an antipsychotic medication; however, they may also occur at any time during treatment. The nurse should listen carefully to the patient's complaints about difficulty with chewing or swallowing, or eyes doing "funny things." This will help to prevent a major medical problem for the patient and determine further required treatment. Misdiagnosis may occur with the diagnoses of epilepsy, encephalitis, meningitis, or tetanus. After experiencing these side effects, the patient may be reluctant to take antipsychotic medications again.

Neuroleptic-Induced Akathisia[10]

Akathisia is an agitated restlessness. It is an extremely uncomfortable feeling. The patient may be unable to sit, lie down, or sleep. The patient may be seen shuffling, tapping, rocking, and shifting weight from one foot to the other. The patient may describe it as "nervous inside," "wired," "jumpy," "things crawling or touching the skin," or "wound up like a spring."[11(p.15)] This side effect may occur during the first 2 weeks of treatment; it peaks at 6 to 10 weeks, with decreased chance of occurrence at 12 to 16 weeks of treatment with neuroleptic.

According to Michaels and Mumford, "Akathisia is more easily observed by the nurse and more often reported by the patient than akinesia."[12(p.99)] Akathisia can be misleading and, consequently, patients may be diagnosed as being more psychotic. Aggressive treatment is then taken for the wrong reason. Such treatment might include more neuroleptics and hospitalization. The use of more neuroleptics may actually worsen the symptoms. Milder forms of akathisia can interfere with the patient's daily functioning. These symptoms can also occur after the dosage of the neuroleptic is increased. Use of anticholinergic medications along with the neuroleptic is important for most patients. Another medication that is used to resolve akathisia is amantadine (Symmetrel). If these medications do not help, diazepam (Valium) may be given. It is important that an explanation is given to the patient who may feel that he or she is getting "crazier." The patient will feel more comfortable to know that the symptoms are a side effect to a medication that can be treated and that these side effects are experienced by other patients.

Neuroleptic-Induced Tardive Dyskinesia[13]

Tardive dyskinesia (TD) occurs after a patient has been taking a neuroleptic for a period of time; it rarely occurs within one year of treatment. The only antipsychotic medication that does not appear to cause TD is clozapine (Clozaril). It does not occur suddenly, but rather slowly over time. According to the American Psychiatric Association (APA), "Even with the most judicious and careful use of medications, tardive dyskinesia inevitably develops in some patients, and no proven safe and effective treatment has been found."[14(p.413)] Risk factors include increasing age, women, and occurrence of drug-induced parkinsonian side effects.[15] The syndrome includes a group of involuntary movements that can affect any muscle, but it seems to concentrate on certain ones, such as facial muscles. Symptoms might include the following:

- sucking of the lips
- smacking of the lips
- dartings of the tongue
- lateral jaw movements
- choreiform movements (e.g., rocking movement to-and-fro; movement of the arms; swaying side to side; flexing and extending of the fingers)
- grimacing

- blinking
- frowning

These movements are not spasmodic but rather coordinated and rhythmic. The most common symptoms are the buccolinguomasticatory ones, which include the smacking and sucking lip movements, projection of the tongue, and lateral movements of the jaw. During sleep, these movements stop. When TD first begins, family or staff may notice it before the patient does. As it progresses, TD can interfere with walking, eating, and in extreme cases breathing.

Early assessment of TD is critical. The earliest sign is small, wormlike movements under the tongue's surface. A diagnosis of TD is based on the absence of other neurological disorders, history of treatment with an antipsychotic medication, and the characteristic movements of TD. Various rating scales have been developed to assess TD, such as the Abnormal Involuntary Movement Scale (AIMS). This is the most commonly used rating scale for TD, and it should be part of ongoing assessment for patients taking antipsychotic medications. Using the AIMS encourages the patient to be more involved in treatment. The scale does not require interpretation of the results, but rather asks the nurse to identify the absence or presence of each item using a five-point scale. This scale is found in Exhibit 19–1. Staff should be trained to use rating scales.

These symptoms continue even after the neuroleptic is stopped. Prevention of this syndrome includes using the lowest possible dose of the neuroleptic and stopping neuroleptic treatment as soon as possible. Intermittent treatment with medication-free days might be tried; however, the patient must be monitored and follow a specific schedule for the medication-free days.[16] These interventions are difficult to do with most patients.

Neuroleptic-Induced Malignant Syndrome[17]

Malignant syndrome is a serious reaction to neuroleptics, and its real incidence is unknown. Prompt identification and treatment are critical. It can occur early in treatment with an antipsychotic medication, particularly for patients on high doses of these medications. Symptoms are severe and rapid rigidity, sudden and rapid hyperthermia with diaphoresis and tachycardia, diffuse tremor, dystonic posturing, increased creatine phosphokinase, mental status impairment, and increased white blood cell count.[18] According to Blair, "Respiratory distress is frequent, and mortality is approximately 20 to 25 percent" usually caused by pulmonary embolism, respiratory failure, or renal failure.[19(p.118)] The first step in treatment is to stop medications. This is a medical emergency, and the patient must be taken to the hospital for medical treatment. Most authorities do not believe that there is a problem in restarting antipsychotic medication treatment after neuroleptic-induced

Exhibit 19–1 Abnormal Involuntary Movement Scale: AIMS

Abnormal Involuntary Movement Scale: AIMS

A simple method to determine tardive dyskinesia symptoms: Total score equals the sum of the items

Patient identification: Date:
Rated by: Treatment period:

Either before or after completing the examination procedure, observe the patient unobtrusively at rest.

After the patient is observed, he or she may be rated on a scale of 0 (none), 1 (minimal), 2 (mild), 3 (moderate), and 4 (severe) according to the severity of symptoms at time of interview. Ask whether there is anything in his or her mouth (e.g., gum, candy), and if there is, ask the patient to remove it. Ask the patient about the *current* condition of his or her teeth. Ask if the patient wears dentures. Do the patient's teeth or dentures bother him or her *now*? Ask the patient whether he or she notices any movement in mouth, face, hands, or feet. If yes, ask the patient to describe such movement and to what extent it *currently* bothers him or her or interferes with activities.

0 1 2 3 4   Have the patient sit in a chair with hands on knees, legs slightly apart, and feet flat on the floor. (Look at entire body for movements while in this position.)

0 1 2 3 4   Ask the patient to sit with hands hanging unsupported. If male, between legs; if female and wearing a dress, hanging over knees. (Observe hands and other body areas.)

0 1 2 3 4   Ask the patient to open his mouth. (Observe the tongue at rest within the mouth.) Have the patient do this twice.

0 1 2 3 4   Ask the patient to protrude his tongue. (Observe abnormalities of tongue movement.) Have the patient do this twice.

0 1 2 3 4   Ask the patient to tap his thumb with each finger as rapidly as possible for 10 to 15 seconds separately with right hand then with left hand. (Observe facial and leg movements.)

0 1 2 3 4   Flex and extend the patient's left and right arms (one at a time).

0 1 2 3 4   Ask the patient to stand up. (Observe in profile. Observe all body areas again, hips included.)

0 1 2 3 4   *Ask the patient to extend both arms outstretched in front with palms down. (Observe trunk, legs, and mouth).

0 1 2 3 4   *Have the patient walk a few paces, turn and walk back to the chair. (Observe hands and gait.) Do this twice.

*Indicates activated movements.

Source: Reprinted with permission from W. Guy, *Assessment Manual for Psychopharmacology*, DHEW publication no. 76-338, p. 22, © 1976, U.S. Government Printing Office.

malignant syndrome resolves, but they suggest that the patient wait one to two weeks between recovery and restarting, preferably with a low-potency antipsychotic.[20]

EXAMPLES OF ANTICHOLINERGIC MEDICATIONS

Several different types of drugs may be used to prevent or treat EPS. This chapter focuses on the antiparkinsonian drugs, particularly the following:

- benztropine mesylate (Cogentin): antiparkinsonian and anticholinergic drug
- trihexyphenidyl hydrochloride (Artane): antiparkinsonian and anticholinergic drug
- amantadine (Symmetrel): antiparkinsonian and anticholinergic drug
- biperiden (Akineton): antiparkinsonian and anticholinergic drug
- orphenadrine citrate (Disipol, Norflex): antiparkinsonian and anticholinergic drug
- procyclidine hydrochloride (Kemadrin): antiparkinsonian and anticholinergic drug.

Other drugs are used to prevent and treat EPS, particularly

- diphenhydramine hydrochloride (Benadryl): antihistamine
- propranolol (Inderal): beta blocker
- lorazepam (Ativan): benzodiazepine
- diazepam (Valium): benzodiazepine

Amantadine is effective for a wide range of EPS symptoms, and it is tolerated better than some of the other antiparkinsonian medications. Beta blockers are especially helpful for akathisia and benzodiazepines for dyskinesia.

PHARMACOKINETICS

Antiparkinsonian and anticholinergic drugs are well absorbed. They are metabolized in the liver and excreted in the urine. Their half-life is unknown.

UNWANTED EFFECTS

Side Effects

The most frequent side effects for antiparkinsonian and anticholinergic drugs are dry mouth, constipation, blurred vision, dizziness, and drowsiness. Others that might be experienced are orthostatic hypotension, tachycardia, palpitations, confusion, memory loss, vomiting, and urinary retention, as well as some psychiatric symptoms (e.g., depression, hallucinations, delusions, and paranoia).

Toxicity

Toxicity can occur. Patient assessment would include the symptoms of central nervous system depression preceded or followed by stimulation, increase in psychotic symptoms, anxiety, ataxia, seizures, delusions and paranoia, hyperpyrexia, dry mucous membranes, decreased bowel sounds, tachycardia, urinary retention, difficulty swallowing, cardiac arrhythmia, shock, coma, cardiac arrest, and respiratory depression or arrest.[21]

Adverse Effects

Paralytic ileus may occur while taking antiparkinsonian and anticholinergic drugs. There is also the potential for increased problems with glaucoma. Patients with decreased renal function who take amantadine (Symmetrel) can accumulate the drug.

MEDICATION MANAGEMENT

Medication management includes dosage, scheduling, laboratory monitoring, and symptom assessment, as well as nursing interventions that will facilitate the patient's use of the medication.

- Vital signs should be monitored at every visit.
- Because hypotension is a possibility, the patient should be warned about rising suddenly from a sitting or lying position.
- The patient may experience drowsiness affecting driving or the use of machinery.
- If nausea is a problem, taking the medication after meals may decrease this side effect.
- If dry mouth is a problem, taking the medication before meals and and sucking on hard candies may decrease it. However, according to Yudofsky, "The candy ingredient sorbitol can cause gas, abdominal bloating, cramping, and diarrhea in some people."[22(p.184)] Good oral care is important.

- The patient should be careful in heat due to problems with decreased ability to sweat.
- The patient should be routinely assessed for movement disorders, and this assessment should be documented. Rating scales may assist in this assessment.
- If the patient complains of constipation, abdominal pain, and distention, assessment for paralytic ileus may be required. Absence of bowel signs would indicate that the patient needs to see a physician.
- To prevent problems with constipation, the patient's diet should contain eight glasses of water, fruit, vegetables, and whole-grain products. Metamucil may be required, as well as a stool softener such as docusate sodium (Colace).
- If the patient experiences problems with dizziness and/or drowsiness, safety issues need to be addressed.
- With long-term use of anticholinergic drugs, assessment should include periodic testing of liver function, complete blood count, and intraocular pressure.
- If the patient experiences rapid weight gain or edema, the physician should be notified.
- The patient should be told not to stop the medication abruptly but rather to discuss it with the nurse and the physician. This medication should be taken even if the patient is feeling well.
- Patients taking benztropine mesylate (Cogentin) have a greater risk of decreased ability to perspire. They cannot cool themselves down well and, thus, are at risk for heat stroke. They require education about this possibility.
- The patient should not drink alcohol or take other medications, including over-the-counter medications, without consulting the physician.
- The patient should carry an identification card describing medications he or she is taking whenever the patient leaves the home.

According to Blair: "Since EPS are predictable, not difficult to diagnosis, and in most cases easy to treat, the legal repercussions of neglecting them are substantial. Issues of informed consent, disclosure, negligence, the involuntary medication of patients, and liability are now becoming very important considerations for those who prescribe and administer antipsychotic medications."[23(p.116)] Risk management is very important. Patient-specific risk factors have been identified.[24] Exhibit 19–2 describes important risk factors for the development of EPS. During the initial assessment, these risk factors should be considered for all patients to determine if preventive treatment is required and to monitor the patient's responses to antipsychotic medications.

Exhibit 19–2 Extrapyramidal Symptoms Risk Factors

- age
  - above 55; higher risk
  - 40–55; moderate risk
  - below 40; less risk
- sex
  - female greater risk than males
  - male younger than 30 years equivalent risk as female
- history
  - previous EPS greater risk
  - exposure to ECT; risk present but less
- diagnosis
  - organic brain syndrome greater risk
  - schizoaffective and/or affective disorder; risk present but less
- agent-specific risk factors
  - high-potency medication; highest risk
  - moderate-potency medication; moderate risk
  - exposure of more than 2 years; moderate risk
  - exposure of more than 60 days; lowest risk
  - low-potency medication; lowest risk
  - depot injections; lowest risk
  - two or more antipsychotic agents; lowest risk
- treatment-specific risk factors
  - no prophylaxis and no PRN for anti-EPS medication; highest risk
  - PRN of antipsychotics more than 5 times/week; higher risk
  - ratio of antipsychotic PRNs to anti-EPS PRNs, more than 3:1; higher risk
  - no prophylaxis, but written PRN order for EPS medication; moderate risk
  - PRN of antipsychotics 2–5 times/week; moderate risk
  - prophylaxis and PRN coverage; lowest risk

EPS, extrapyramidal symptoms; PRN, as needed

Source: © *Joint Commission Journal of Quality Improvement.* Oakbrook Terrace, IL: Joint Commission on Accreditation of Healthcare Organizations, 1990, pp. 120–122. Reprinted with permission.

PRECAUTIONS AND CONTRAINDICATIONS

Antiparkinsonian and anticholinergic drugs should be used with precaution in patients with narrow-angle glaucoma; hepatic, renal or cardiac insufficiency; tendency toward urinary retention; hyperthyroidism; hypertension; autonomic neuropathy; and patients who are pregnant, lactating, or debilitated. These medications are contraindicated in angle-closure glaucoma, pyloric or duodenal obstruction, stenosing peptic ulcers, prostatic hypertrophy or bladder neck obstructions, achalasia, myasthenia gravis, ulcerative colitis, and tachycardia secondary to cardiac insufficiency.[25]

INTERACTIVE EFFECTS

- *Other medications.* Anticholinergic drugs should not be used with other drugs that also have these side effects (e.g., phenothiazines, tricyclic antidepressants, antihistamines, amantadine). This would increase the anticholinergic effects and can lead to paralytic ileus. Other medications with interactive problems are levodopa, slow-dissolving digoxin, and central nervous system depressants (e.g., alcohol, barbiturates, narcotics, benzodiazepines), ketoconazole, antacids.[26]
- *Food.* There are no food restrictions with these medications.
- *Health status.* Patients with glaucoma and decreased renal function are at risk while taking anticholinergic medications.
- *Age.* Patients who are above 55 have a greater risk of developing EPS.
- *Behavior.* There are no behavioral issues with these medications, with the exception of those patients who have experienced severe EPS who then refuse to continue to take antipsychotic medication.
- *Environment.* Environments with high temperatures may be a problem. Homes without air conditioning in hot climates may lead to heat stroke for some patients. The home assessment should include information about temperature and availability of air conditioners and fans. It is necessary to make plans during the hot season to protect the patient from excessive heat. If the patient experiences dizziness, the home safety assessment must consider interventions to prevent falling.

EDUCATION OF PATIENT/FAMILY/SIGNIFICANT OTHERS

Education for the patient and family/SOs focuses on the purpose, dosage and frequency, side effects, and interventions that may be used to prevent or cope with side effects. It is important to explain how these medications are used to prevent side effects from antipsychotic medications. The following components should be included in the education:

- purpose and target symptoms
- dosage and frequency

- action to be taken if a dose is missed
- side effects
- safety
- precautions and contraindications

SUMMARY

This discussion on antiparkinsonian and anticholinergic drugs has focused on the general category of drugs. For specific, up-to-date information about individual medications, the home care nurse should consult appropriate reference material and the patient's physician. As with all medications, it is important to know the patient's medication history and to use this information when treatment is planned, implemented, and changed.

NOTES

1. A. Dauner and D. Blair, "Akathisia: When Treatment Creates a Problem," *Journal of Psychosocial Nursing* 28, no. 10 (1990): 13–18, at 14.
2. D. Blair and A. Dauner, "Nonneuroleptic Etiologies of Extrapyramidal Symptoms," *Clinical Nurse Specialist* 7, no. 4 (1993): 225–230, at 226.
3. M. Townsend, *Drug Guide for Psychiatric Nursing* (Philadelphia: F.A. Davis, 1990), 62.
4. American Psychiatric Association, *Diagnostic and Statistical Manual of Mental Disorders*, 4th ed. (Washington, DC: 1994), 679.
5. M. Laraia, "Psychopharmacology," in *Principles and Practice of Psychiatric Nursing*, ed. G. Stuart and S. Sundeen (St. Louis, MO: Mosby–Year Book, 1995), 663–701, at 688.
6. American Psychiatric Association, *Diagnostic and Statistical Manual of Mental Disorders*, 736–737.
7. R. Michaels and K. Mumford, "Identifying Akinesia and Akathisia: The Relationship between Patient's Self-Report and Nurse's Assessment," *Archives of Psychiatric Nursing* 3, no. 2 (1989): 97–101, at 100.
8. American Psychiatric Association, *Diagnostic and Statistical Manual of Mental Disorders*, 739.
9. American Psychiatric Association, *Diagnostic and Statistical Manual of Mental Disorders*, 742–744.
10. American Psychiatric Association, *Diagnostic and Statistical Manual of Mental Disorders*, 744–746.
11. Dauner and Blair, "Akathisia: When Treatment Creates a Problem," 15.
12. Michaels and Mumford, "Identifying Akinesia and Akathisia," 99.
13. American Psychiatric Association, *Diagnostic and Statistical Manual of Mental Disorders*, 747–749.
14. "APA Report Summarizes Recent Developments in Prevention and Treatment of Tardive Dyskinesia," *Hospital and Community Psychiatry* 43, no. 4 (1992): 413–414.

15. "APA Report Summarizes Recent Developments in Prevention and Treatment of Tardive Dyskinesia," 413.

16. "APA Report Summarizes Recent Developments in Prevention and Treatment of Tardive Dyskinesia," 413.

17. American Psychiatric Association, *Diagnostic and Statistical Manual of Mental Disorders*, 739–741.

18. D. Blair, "Risk Management for Extrapyramidal Symptoms," *Quality Review Bulletin* 16, no. 3 (1990): 116–124, at 118.

19. Blair, "Risk Management for Extrapyramidal Symptoms," 118.

20. A. Lazarus, "Neuroleptic Malignant Syndrome," *Hospital and Community Psychiatry* 40, no. 12 (1989): 1229–1230.

21. Townsend, *Drug Guide for Psychiatric Nursing*, 63.

22. S. Yudofsky, *What You Need to Know About Psychiatric Drugs* (Washington, DC: American Psychiatric Press, Inc, 1991), 184.

23. Blair, "Risk Management for Extrapyramidal Symptoms," 116.

24. Blair, "Risk Management for Extrapyramidal Symptoms," 120–122.

25. Townsend, *Drug Guide for Psychiatric Nursing,* 62.

26. Townsend, *Drug Guide for Psychiatric Nursing,* 62.

SUGGESTED READING

Arana, G., and S. Hyman. 1991. *Handbook of psychiatric drug therapy*. Boston: Little, Brown and Company.

Blair, D., and A. Dauner. 1992. Dangerous consequences: Neuroleptic-induced tardive akathisia. *Journal of Psychosocial Nursing* 30, no. 3: 41–43.

Blair, D., and A. Dauner. 1993. Neuroleptic malignant syndrome: Liability in nursing practice. *Journal of Psychosocial Nursing* 31, no. 2: 5–11.

Blair, D., and A. Dauner. 1993. Nonneuroleptic etiologies of extrapyramidal symptoms. *Clinical Nurse Specialist* 7, no. 4: 225–230.

Bostrom, A. 1988. Assessment scales for tardive dyskinesia. *Journal of Psychosocial Nursing* 26, no. 6: 9–12.

Dauner, A., and D. Blair. 1990. Akathisia: When treatment creates a problem. *Journal of Psychosocial Nursing* 28, no. 10: 93–94.

Dillon, N. 1992. Screening system for tardive dyskinesia: Development and implementation. *Journal of Psychosocial Nursing* 30, no. 10: 3–7.

Goldman, M., and D. Luchins. 1984. Intermittent neuroleptic therapy and tardive dyskinesia: A literature review. *Hospital and Community Psychiatry* 35, no. 12: 1215–1219.

Hooper, J. et al. 1989. Neuroleptic malignant syndrome: Recognizing an unrecognized killer. *Journal of Psychosocial Nursing* 27, no. 7: 13–15.

Kaplan, H., and B. Sadock. 1995. *Comprehensive textbook of psychiatry*. Vol. 1 and Vol. 2. Baltimore, MD: Williams & Wilkins.

Littrell, K., and A. Magill. 1993. The effect of clozapine on preexisting tardive dyskinesia. *Journal of Psychosocial Nursing* 31, no. 9: 14–18.

Masters, J., and R. Spitler. 1986. Neuroleptic malignant syndrome. *Journal of Psychosocial Nursing* 24, no. 9: 11–16.

Michaels, R., and K. Mumford. 1989. Identifying akinesia and akathisia: The relationship between patient's self-report and nurse's assessment. *Archives of Psychiatric Nursing* 3, no. 2: 97–101.

Munetz, M., and S. Benjamin. 1990. Who should perform the AIMS examination? *Hospital and Community Psychiatry* 41, no. 8: 912–915.

Townsend, M. 1990. *Drug guide for psychiatric nursing*. Philadelphia: F.A. Davis.

Yudofsky, S. et al. 1991. *What you need to know about psychiatric drugs*. Washington, DC: American Psychiatric Press, Inc.

V

❖

Clinical Problems in the Home

20

Anxiety Disorders: Generalized Anxiety, Panic, Phobic, and Obsessive-Compulsive Disorders

INTRODUCTION

More Americans suffer from anxiety disorders than any other psychiatric disorder, and most never receive psychiatric treatment. Many seek help from family, friends, clergy, and other self-help resources. Identifying the need for help is often difficult. The symptoms of anxiety pervade a number of disorders. Three effects of anxiety on behavior are withdrawal and/or depression, acting out, and somatizing. In addition, it can cause physical illness. Anxiety also has a positive effect, something that is often overlooked. It can be helpful in learning and problem solving.

DEFINING CHARACTERISTICS

Anxiety is a form of tension. It is an emotional reaction to an object or experience that the individual feels is dangerous or a threat. It may be a real or imagined threat. A person with acute anxiety feels too much and thinks too little.[1] Anxiety may be related to some future event, even a happy one such as marriage or childbirth. A person can also feel anxiety when remembering a past event. Anxiety is also associated with guilt. The person may fear punishment, and thus feel anxious about that fear. Anxiety is experienced physiologically, psychologically, and behaviorally. The person experiences feelings of helplessness, isolation, and insecurity. Anxiety itself, however, is not pathological. Usually the person "perceives some future unpleasantness; the dreaded event is about to happen or may happen, but it's not happening now."[2(p.29)] All people experience anxiety at various levels and at different times. All home care patients experience some anxiety, regardless of their diagnosis, medical or psychiatric. According to Stuart, "An individual's level of self-esteem is also an important factor related to anxiety. A person who is easily threatened or has a low level of self-esteem is more susceptible to anxiety."[3(p.331)]

An operational definition of anxiety may help home care staff to understand anxiety and to explain anxiety to patients and families/significant others (SOs). An operational definition is a tool for learning about concepts through the use of a series of steps. In actual practice, these steps are not necessarily discrete, and this is important to explain to patients. The steps for anxiety include the following:[4]

1. The person has expectations for safety and status. These may be conscious or unconscious.
2. These expectations are not met. There are many reasons that this may occur (for example, others will not or are unable to help the person get what is wanted; the person does not have the ability to meet the expectation; the expectation is not communicated or poorly communicated; or others misinterpret the expectation).
3. The person then feels anxiety and powerlessness. This can be felt briefly or over a long period of time.
4. The person then uses automatic behavior to decrease anxiety and sense of powerlessness. This may or may not be successful. The person may be using unhealthy methods for decreasing anxiety such as withdrawal, anger, aggression, somatization, denial, or acting out. Healthy methods might be problem solving, asking a specific helpful person for guidance, relaxation techniques, or exercise.
5. The person feels the need to justify the behavior, particularly behavior that may not be constructive. When working with the patient to understand his or her own anxiety process, it is easy to focus on steps 4 and 5, focusing on the relief behavior and its justification. This will only become a power struggle with the patient. It is more important to discuss the expectations that were not met and feelings about them.

As is true with most major mental illnesses, there is much research being conducted about anxiety; however, no specific etiology has been identified. There are, however, some factors that are becoming clearer. Patients with anxiety tend to be responsive to benzodiazepines (Xanax, Valium, Dalmane, Ativan). The reason for this response is being explored. Specific benzodiazepine binding sites have been found in the brain, particularly in the cerebral cortex, hippocampus, and cerebellar cortex. These may be inherent receptor sites for neurochemical control of anxiety. Another research focus is the relationship between these drugs and the gamma-aminobutyric acid (GABA) system. GABA functions in some areas of the brain as an inhibitory neurotransmitter. Benzodiazepines work by slowing down brain systems that might stimulate arousal and anxiety, such as the norepinephrine system. Consequently, anxiety is decreased.[5] According to Stuart: "It has also been shown that an individual's general health has a great effect on a predisposition to anxiety. Coping mechanisms may also be impaired by toxic influences, dietary deficiencies, reduced blood supply, hormonal changes, and other physical causes."[6(p.333)] Anxiety may accompany some physical disorders, which are discussed in Chapter 26.

Peplau described four stages of anxiety that help health care workers to understand anxiety and to teach patients and families/SOs about anxiety.[7] In stage I, anxiety is mild, and this stage can be helpful. The patient can actually function at a higher level with increased perception and ability to put various aspects together and see a total picture. This is the level of anxiety that is commonly experienced. It might occur before taking an exam, participating in a job interview, making an unpleasant telephone call, or beginning a new job. This level of anxiety helps the person focus, as the body, physically and psychologically, helps the person prepare to take an action.

In stage II, anxiety is moderate. As perception continues to function at a high level, this stage can also be helpful. However, the person begins to focus only on the situation at hand, excluding other matters. The person concentrates on the problem or critical event, often blocking out or altering other tasks. This makes it difficult for the patient to listen to information or suggestions that are not connected to the critical event. For example, during the discharge process from the hospital, the patient may not hear the information about home care due to anxiety felt about the discharge, or the patient may not remember information about the medication dosage discussed during the first home visit.

During stage III, anxiety is severe; this level of anxiety is problematic, with perception inaccuracies and difficulty in viewing the whole. The person cannot solve problems, and it is important for the nurse to recognize this. This is not the time to ask the patient to solve a problem or to try to teach the patient. The priority is to decrease the anxiety to a more tolerable level, eventually increasing the patient's functioning. It is easy to forget this priority during the patient's admission to home care. If a patient or family/SOs are experiencing a high level of anxiety about the patient's return to the home environment, how much information can they really absorb during the admission procedure? The same question can be applied to patient teaching. The patient's level of anxiety is often neglected in the teaching process and not included in the assessment of the patient's readiness to learn.

In stage IV, the patient experiences panic. At this stage, the patient is not able to see the problem or event clearly or to resolve problems. The patient is at risk for acting impulsively and requires immediate intervention. This may mean calling the police, an ambulance, or family or neighbors for additional help.

ASSESSMENT

Guidelines for Assessment

Patients often do not know what is making them anxious while they experience the anxiety. The first step of the assessment is to determine if the cause can be identified. The four common situations that may lead to anxiety are biological factors, self-esteem, an indefinable threat, and the relationship between the physical and the interpersonal environment. The assessment should include data about these areas. Staff tend to judge what should and should not make a patient anxious. There are also times when the staff and the patient are not able to identify a cause for the anxiety. When this is the case, the staff need to focus on helping the patient to alleviate the anxiety rather than becoming bogged down in finding the cause, which will only increase the patient's and staff's anxiety.

During stage I and stage II, mild and moderate anxiety, the patient will notice that something is different as his or her anxiety moves from mild to moderate.[8] The patient may describe somatic complaints such as increases in urinary frequency and urgency, respirations and pulse, and muscle tension. The patient may try to decrease anxiety by pacing or handwringing, and this can be easily identified during the assessment. During this level of anxiety, the patient is able to describe subjective feelings and can respond to open-ended questions. The nurse might ask the patient to rate his or her anxiety on a scale from 0 to 10; with 10 representing the panic level. This might be helpful information to use as a baseline when the patient experiences anxiety in the future. As the patient moves to severe or panic stages of anxiety, he or she may not be able to speak or may be incoherent, and this will affect the assessment. The home care nurse may observe hyperventilation, tachycardia, dilated pupils, or pallor.[9] The patient may report dizziness, confusion, headache, nausea, sleeplessness, or diarrhea. The patient who is experiencing extreme anxiety may have delusions and hallucinations. It is important to remember that the patient may not be able to say how he or she feels.

The first step in any assessment of a patient with anxiety is a thorough history and physical to distinguish medical illness from the symptoms of anxiety. Typical results from diagnostic studies include blood studies with "increased adrenal function, elevated glucose and lactic acid levels, decreased calcium and oxygen levels, and diminished parathyroid function. Urine studies may show increased epinephrine and norepinephrine levels."[10(p.32)]

The nurse depends upon the patient's description of his or her feelings and how these feelings are interfering with daily functioning. There is minimal cognitive impairment with anxiety disorders unless the patient is experiencing severe or panic levels of anxiety. If the patient experiences rambling or circumstantiality (too many associated thoughts coming at one time with an inability to suppress them selectively), staff need to assess the patient for more severe anxiety. It is not likely that the patient with an anxiety disorder will be suicidal, homicidal, or experiencing hallucinations. The latter occurs during extreme anxiety or panic.

Assessment of anxiety requires an assessment of the patient's relief behaviors. These behaviors may include somatization, acting out, psychological responses, and specific actions the patient uses to relieve anxiety. This information will provide the nurse with data about the appropriateness of the patient's relief behaviors and how much the patient needs to learn about anxiety relief behaviors.

There are different approaches to the assessment of anxiety. McFarland and Wasli recommend that the assessment of anxiety include the following focus areas:[11]

- determination of the patient's level of anxiety and related signs and symptoms
- observation of adaptive or maladaptive behavioral responses to anxiety
- observation of stressors or threats to any of the following: value system, ideals, and beliefs; core or essence of personality; self-concept; personal security system; meaningful interpersonal relationships; stability of environment; and role functioning
- assessment of home and interpersonal level of anxiety in the home
- determination of behavioral changes or physiological changes indicating anxiety
- determination of methods the patient has used in the past to decrease anxiety
- identification of the patient's current adaptive and maladaptive strategies for coping with anxiety
- determination of resources and strengths available for the patient to cope with anxiety

Fauman recommends other clinical information that needs to be included in the assessment. These suggestions, which are more specific than those of McFarland and Wasli, include the following:[12(pp.220–221)]

- current and past history of anxiety
- feelings of derealization, depersonalization, or emotional numbing
- fears of losing control or going crazy
- sleep disturbance; bad dreams
- medical illnesses

- physical symptoms
- previous and current psychiatric illnesses
- current medications and abused substances
- current or past traumatic events or stress
- compulsive behavior or rituals
- obsessive, intrusive thoughts
- phobic fears and the context within which they occur

Signs and Symptoms

The signs and symptoms for anxiety can be categorized as physiological, psychological, or behavioral. It may be difficult for the patient to understand that physiological responses may be due to anxiety. A history and physical exam are important components of a complete assessment for any psychiatric home care patient, but it is particularly important for patients with an anxiety disorder or for patients who are experiencing problems with anxiety. It is important to rule out legitimate medical problems before assuming that the patient is experiencing anxiety. Exhibit 20–1 describes typical signs and symptoms of anxiety that might be identified during an assessment.

The patient does not have to experience all of these signs and symptoms to be diagnosed with anxiety. Another categorization of the signs and symptoms of anxiety that is more specific includes the following:[13(p.29)]

- intellectual anxiety
  1. anticipation of unpleasantness
  2. blocking of words
  3. difficulty concentrating
  4. excessive vigilance
  5. feelings of helplessness, confusion, and being restrained
  6. habitual responses
  7. inability to learn or reason
  8. indecisiveness
  9. lack of awareness of surroundings
  10. loss of short-term recall
  11. narrowed sensory perception
  12. overreacting to stimuli
  13. preoccupation with anxious feelings
  14. selective inattention
  15. sense of impending catastrophe
  16. unrealistic thinking

Exhibit 20-1 Signs and Symptoms of Generalized Anxiety Disorder

PHYSIOLOGICAL SIGNS AND SYMPTOMS

- Chest pain/pressure
- Dyspnea
- Tachycardia
- Hyperventilation
- Palpitations
- Elevated blood pressure
- Muscle tension
- Dizziness
- Heartburn
- Nausea
- Sweating
- Muscular aches
- Tremors
- Insomnia
- Paresthesia
- Choking or smothering sensation
- Decrease in appetite

BEHAVIORAL SIGNS AND SYMPTOMS

- Restlessness
- Rapid speech
- Withdrawal
- Pacing

PSYCHOLOGICAL SIGNS AND SYMPTOMS

- Excessive worry
- Feeling on edge
- Mind going blank
- Tenseness
- Irritability
- Fright
- Decreased attention
- Decreased concentration
- Impaired perceptions of others, situations, and events
- Emotionally drained feeling
- Depressed and flat affect
- Judgment errors
- Impaired perceptions of people and/or events

17. worry over outcome of events
- social anxiety
    1. apprehension within groups of people
    2. attention-seeking behavior (e.g., crying)
    3. aversion of gaze
    4. blaming of others for anxiety-producing situations
    5. demanding behavior
    6. desire to be left alone
    7. fear of losing control in social situations
    8. feelings of forlornness, sadness, loneliness, shyness, or uncertainty
    9. frequent touching
    10. irritation or coldness with close friends or family
    11. seeking to communicate with others
    12. stammering or slips of speech
    13. talkativeness or extreme quietness
    14. withdrawal or aggression
- spiritual anxiety
    1. alienation from others
    2. fear of death, failure, or the future
    3. feelings of helplessness, guilt, and despair
    4. inability to cope, love, or find meaning in life
    5. indifference to previously important things
    6. lack of belief in the future
    7. lack of sense of free choice
    8. rejection of long-held beliefs
    9. withdrawal

DIAGNOSIS

Diagnosis of anxiety must consider related diagnoses that may affect interventions selected for the patient. The first consideration is to determine if the patient is experiencing mild or moderate anxiety but does not meet the criteria for an anxiety disorder diagnosis. If the patient does meet the criteria, then a determination is made as to the character of the anxiety. Is it neurosis involving no distortion of reality or is it psychotic or a "breaking into pieces"?[14] Another important differentiation is whether the patient is experiencing anxiety or depression, which frequently overlap. Exhibit 20–2 describes differences between anxiety and depression.

Medical Diagnosis

According to the *Diagnostic and Statistical Manual of Mental Disorders* (*DSM-*

Exhibit 20–2 Differences Between Anxiety and Depression

Anxiety	Depression
• predominantly fearful or apprehensive	• predominantly sad or hopeless with feelings of despair
• difficulty falling asleep (initial insomnia)	• early morning awakening (late insomnia) or hypersomnia
• phobic avoidance behavior	• diural variation (feels worse in the morning)
• rapid pulse and psychomotor hyperactivity	• slowed speech and thought processes
• breathing disturbances	• delayed response time
• tremors and palpitations	• psychomotor retardation or agitation
• sweating and hot or cold spells	• loss of interest in usual activities
• faintness, light-headedness, dizziness	• inability to experience pleasure
• depersonalization (feeling detached from one's body)	• thoughts of death or suicide
• derealization (feeling that one's environment is strange, unreal, or unfamiliar)	• negative appraisals are pervasive, global, exclusive
• negative appraisals (selective and specific and do not include all areas of life)	• sees the future as blank and has given up all hope
• sees some prospects for the future	• regards mistakes as beyond redemption
• does not regard defects or mistakes as irrevocable	• absolute in negative evaluations
• uncertain in negative evaluations	• global view that nothing will turn out right
• predicts that only certain events may go badly	

Source: Reprinted with permission from G. Stuart, "Anxiety Responses and Anxiety Disorders," in *Principles and Practice of Psychiatric Nursing*, eds. G. Stuart and S. Sundeen, eds., p. 343, © 1995, Mosby–Year Book, Inc.

IV), the diagnosis of a generalized anxiety disorder requires that the anxiety must last for at least six months and be associated with at least three of the following symptoms:[15(p.219)]

- restlessness or feeling "keyed up" or on edge
- being easily fatigued
- difficulty concentrating or mind going blank
- irritability
- muscle tension
- sleep disturbance (difficulty falling or staying asleep) or restless, unsatisfying sleep

Fauman suggests that four questions should be considered as the diagnosis is made during assessment.[16(pp.221–222)]

- Could the patient's symptoms be produced by drugs or a nonpsychiatric medical illness?
- Is the onset of the patient's anxiety linked to a specific situational trigger or cue, or is it unexpected?
- If the patient's anxiety is cued, what types of external situational triggers precipitate it?
- Does the patient experience long-term anxiety that is neither unexpected nor situationally triggered?

As the answers to these questions are analyzed, the following *DSM-IV* diagnoses related to anxiety disorders should be considered:[17]

- panic disorder with agoraphobia
- panic disorder without agoraphobia
- agoraphobia without history of panic disorder
- specific phobia
- social phobia
- obsessive-compulsive disorder
- posttraumatic stress disorder
- acute stress disorder
- generalized anxiety disorder
- anxiety due to (identify general medical condition)

Nursing Diagnosis

Nursing diagnosis refers to the diagnoses that can be identified by a registered nurse at any point during treatment. A home care patient may have any number of nursing diagnoses. The North American Nursing Diagnosis Association (NANDA) identifies the following important nursing diagnoses:[18]

- anxiety
- fear

- powerlessness
- ineffective individual coping
- impaired verbal communication
- self-esteem disturbance
- impaired social interaction
- risk for injury
- sleep pattern disturbance
- ineffective breathing pattern
- alteration in nutrition
- alteration in bowel elimination
- alteration in urinary elimination

A patient may not have all of these diagnoses. These nursing diagnoses are helpful in developing the focus for home care interventions.

EXPECTED OUTCOMES

The following are examples of desired outcomes for the patient with an anxiety disorder in the home:

- The patient will experience less anxiety as exhibited by the ability to handle stress, sleep six to eight hours, participate in family activities, and discuss problems without feeling overwhelming anxiety.
- The patient will identify problems/situations that may have contributed to the development of anxiety.
- The patient will apply the steps in the anxiety process to actual situations in his or her own life.
- The patient will use self-monitoring methods to assess anxiety.
- The patient will recognize that mild and moderate anxiety can be useful for learning.
- The patient will participate in his or her treatment planning, assessment of progress, and discharge planning.
- The patient will identify the dangers of alcohol and drug abuse as a method of alleviating anxiety.
- The patient will use constructive coping methods (e.g., relaxation techniques, exercise, imagery).

HOME CARE STAFF: RESPONSES TO THE PATIENT

Anxiety theory can be applied to all staff in their professional and personal lives. Staff anxiety affects care in the home and how staff work together and with the patient's family/SO. Staff need to identify patient or family/SO behaviors that are increasing staff anxiety. If they can be resolved, this must be done. Staff may react to their own anxiety with acting out (for example, excessive anger, silence, hypercritical behavior, apathy, withdrawal, relating to peers competitively rather than in a collaborative relationship, lack of creativity in treatment planning, or miscommunication).

When a patient or family/SO is anxious, communication should be calm with short sentences with a limited number of directions given at one time. If staff think that the patient may be experiencing anxiety, ask the patient what he or she is feeling. Then staff share with the patient what has been observed. This will begin the collaborative process of identifying feelings and related behaviors or responses. When the patient is able to compare with past feelings and behaviors, this will help the patient develop self-assessment skills. Assessing whether the patient or family/SOs have actually heard and understood what has been said is very important. If staff appear to be judgmental or pressured, the environment will not be calm. It is easy to appear pressured when staff are behind schedule, have many visits to make, or are irritated by a patient or family/SOs. Taking a deep breath and going slowly may actually save time and decrease anxiety.

Using a calm voice and moving the patient to a quieter environment may temporarily decrease the patient's anxiety by reducing stimulation. Let the patient know that he or she is safe. If this is successful and when the patient and family/SOs are able to listen, the nurse can discuss the intervention with them. The patient is taught how to remove himself or herself from potentially anxiety-provoking situations. Encouraging the patient to talk by allowing the patient to lead the conversation puts less pressure on the patient to perform in a specific manner. The nurse can then ask relevant questions. The best attitude to convey to the patient is that the situation can be resolved constructively. In some situations, confrontation can be useful, but it must be used with caution as confrontation can increase anxiety. Ultimately, the patient has the responsibility for change, and this includes learning about anxiety and its effect on daily activities and responses to others.

INTERVENTIONS IN THE HOME

Prior to identifying interventions for anxiety that might be used in the home setting, it is important to understand how the patient copes with anxiety. This should be the focus of the interventions that are developed with the patient and the family/SOs. The most common nonconstructive methods for coping with anxiety are inappropriate defense mechanisms and acting out behaviors. A patient can have several different responses to frustrations, losses, and threats. The situation may be considered rationally with the patient trying to work out a solution, admitting to fear and fleeing, or attacking aggressively. If none of these is possible, the patient may use a psychological defense mechanism, which is the means by which a person attempts to decrease anxiety, guilt, or shame. According to Stuart, "Everyone uses defense mechanisms, and they frequently help people cope successfully with mild and moderate levels of anxiety. They protect the person from feelings of inadequacy and worthlessness and prevent awareness of anxiety. They can be used to such an extreme degree, however, that they distort reality, interfere with interpersonal relationships, and limit the ability to work productively."[19(p.331)] Exhibit 20–3 defines some defense mechanisms that may be used by patients in the home or by their families/SOs.

These defenses are triggered automatically by an anxiety signal that is often too brief for the patient to realize consciously. Sometimes a patient uses a defense mechanism consciously. Defense mechanisms can be very helpful in coping with daily living, and all people use them to decrease anxiety. When they fail to decrease anxiety, illness can result. When used excessively, certain defenses are undesirable because of their negative effects on others. It is easy to assume that all behavior is defensive, but it is not. All reasoning is not rationalizing, nor are all criticisms of others' projections. Overinterpreting defenses or misapplying them is not helpful. This is often a clue of staff discomfort. Analysis can be overdone, and psychiatric nursing offers fertile ground for abuse of analysis that is not always constructive. Nondefensive behavior is usually relatively relaxed and is not motivated primarily by anxiety or guilt. The nonanxious patient does not appear to be driven, impatient, overly empathetic, or easily frustrated.

Acting out occurs when a patient shows behaviorally how he or she feels rather than verbalizing feelings, anxiety, fears, etc. Some patients cannot control their acting out, and they do not realize the reasons for their actions. When a person acts out, it is a defense mechanism to avoid anxiety, and it is a type of regression. Examples include refusing to go to bed, refusing to clean up one's bedroom, excessive drinking, refusing to attend family activities, or throwing or destroying objects. Soon the acting out behavior itself becomes the focus, with the patient defiantly expressing himself or herself, and staff or family/SOs trying desperately to stop the patient. If the primary objective is to stop the acting-out behavior, the staff will find a defiant, hostile patient; more acting out; and a power struggle. Families/SOs need to understand this, too. It is easy for them to get trapped into this cycle. Figure 20–1 provides a description of the acting-out cycle.

This diagram can be a useful tool for teaching families/SOs and patients about the acting-out process; however, they must be ready to listen and learn. The process of acting out includes not only the patient but also all who come in contact with the patient during the process. It can be very destructive to the family/SOs and the environment. In some cases, it may eventually lead to the patient requiring more intensive treatment and more structure.

Exhibit 20–3 Defense Mechanisms

- *Repression:* The most basic of the defense mechanisms. It is the exclusion from consciousness of impulses that the person cannot accept as part of himself or herself. It is different from suppression, which is the conscious attempt to put something out of your mind.
- *Regression:* The person returns to an earlier and more comfortable stage of functioning, becoming more independent and less anxious. For a person forced to accept dependency, this mechanism can be used to make the experience more acceptable, such as hospitalization.
- *Denial:* The refusal to acknowledge what one sees, hears, or feels.
- *Projection:* The person perceives and treats unacceptable inner impulses as if they were outside one's self.
- *Intellectualization:* The control of feelings and impulses through thinking them instead of feeling them or acting on them.
- *Displacement:* Redirecting an emotional feeling from the appropriate person or object to a less threatening person or object, allowing for a safe release of feelings.
- *Rationalization:* Offering a socially acceptable or apparently logical explanation to justify or make acceptable otherwise unacceptable impulses, feelings, behaviors, and motives.
- *Splitting:* Viewing people or situations as either all good or all bad.

Source: Adapted from Nurse Review, *Psychiatric Problems*, p. 27, © 1990, Springhouse Corporation; and G. Stuart, "Anxiety Responses and Anxiety Disorders," in *Principles and Practice of Psychiatric Nursing*, G. Stuart and S. Sundeen, eds., p. 337, © 1995, Mosby–Year Book, Inc.

Whenever acting-out behavior is self-destructive or destructive to others, the first intervention objective is to ensure safety. After this has been met or if it is not necessary, the following objectives should be considered as plans for interventions are made:

- to communicate positive expectations to the patient
- to help the patient identify the reason(s) for and meaning of the behavior to the patient
- to explore with the patient possible alternative methods for expressing feelings

It may not be possible to implement these three objectives immediately, depending on the patient's condition. The patient needs to know that the expectation is that the behavior will be terminated. Staff or family/SOs should never promise

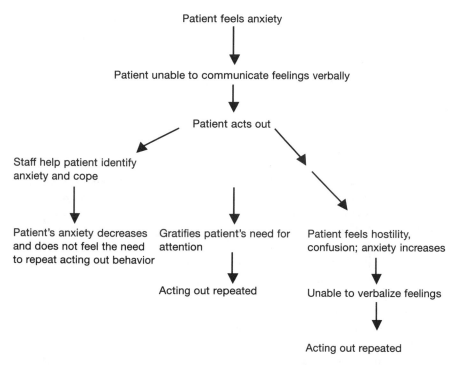

Figure 20–1 Acting Out Behavior. *Source:* Reprinted with permission, Nursecom, Inc.

or threaten anything that they are incapable of carrying out. Trying to discover the reason for the patient's behavior communicates interest in understanding, not judging the patient. At all times the patient is still responsible for his or her behavior. If the patient frequently acts out, staff may be able to identify a pattern. This information can then be used to observe situations in which the patient is beginning to act out and to intervene before the behavior escalates. This process can then be taught to the family/SOs and to the patient. Peplau described interventions for anxiety that can be used to teach the patient and the family/SOs about interventions for anxiety.[20] The five steps are as follows:

1. recognition of anxiety
2. connection of the feeling (anxiety) with the relief behavior
3. identification of the situation immediately preceding the feeling of anxiety and its importance to the person
4. analysis of the information and its relation to past experiences
5. correlation of the causes and effects of the anxiety

Throughout the process, the patient and family/SOs are reminded that the focus is on understanding, not judging. The patient is ultimately responsible for his or her own behavior. Intervention does not imply that the staff or family/SOs are assuming responsibility for the patient's behavior.

Specific interventions that might be used with home care patients who are experiencing anxiety include the following:

- Home care staff recognize that they have anxieties. Patients and their families/SOs can empathize with staff anxiety and vice versa, and this can affect care.
- Staff should assess how the patient has coped with anxiety, both positively and negatively, in the past. During this assessment, staff must listen to the patient and avoid making assumptions. This information is used to help develop a plan to teach the patient better coping skills.
- The nurse should be able to recognize symptoms of anxiety early before panic develops. The nurse observes how much anxiety the patient can handle and helps the patient pull back from situations in order to regain control of feelings and behavior. The patient is taught and asked to use self-monitoring methods such as a diary or log of feelings and responses and to identify specific behaviors that indicate anxiety is increasing or decreasing.
- It is important to remember that anxiety is contagious whenever a patient expresses concern about increasing anxiety or when signs of anxiety are observed. A home situation that has a high level of anxiety can be very detrimental to the patient's progress. If leaving the home is not an option, home care staff must work with the patient and family/SOs to resolve as much of the anxiety as possible. Some patients are more sensitive to others' anxiety, and the family/SOs may not be aware of this sensitivity. Everyone in the home needs to learn about the anxiety process and interventions for self and others in the home. During stressful times, patients should be assessed for increasing anxiety to determine if they require further interventions.
- Because new experiences and situations often increase anxiety, helping the patient relate new experiences to old familiar ways may prevent anxiety or excessive anxiety. Orientation is helpful, as it allows the patient to know in advance what to expect (for example, a home visit, a clinic visit, use of public transportation, attendance at a partial hospitalization program, or a job interview).
- When a patient is experiencing a high level of anxiety, someone should remain with him or her. Leaving the patient alone reinforces the aspect of aloneness and inability to relate to others. Family/SOs need to understand that this is important; however, there may be some family members who are better at providing this type of support than others.
- The patient needs to learn constructive methods for coping with anxiety such as talking with someone, exercising, listening to music, performing a simple

task, using progressive relaxation techniques or guided imagery, thought stopping, and constructive problem solving.

- Staff provide time during home visits for the patient to express feelings and discover the connections between thoughts, actions, and problems.
- Allowing the patient to set his or her own pace will be supportive and help decrease the patient's anxiety.
- All staff must avoid having a judgmental attitude. What makes one person anxious may not make another anxious.
- Correcting false expectations or misconceptions by giving correct information can be reassuring, and the patient needs to have an opportunity to discuss expectations and misconceptions.
- The patient must be respected throughout the treatment process. This can be done by emphasizing mutual respect with the patient; asking about the patient's expectations; asking the patient to participate in evaluation of progress; arriving for home visits on time; calling the patient if a staff member is delayed or needs to cancel; asking the patient where he or she wants to sit during a visit; and asking the patient what would be helpful for him or her.
- The patient may be unaware that he or she is anxious. Providing feedback about what is observed and then asking the patient to talk about this information as well as feelings will help the patient assess his or her own feelings and behavior.
- Safety and security are integral parts of the treatment plan at all times during home care.
- A pattern of late evening anxiety needs to be identified and discussed with the patient. Ask the patient what happens at this time of the day that might be increasing anxiety. Deal with the facts and set up a plan with the patient to limit long discussions about topics that potentially increase anxiety late in the evening or any other reason for this increased anxiety at night. Work with the family/SOs to develop interventions to prevent an increase in anxiety at the end of the day (such as monitoring the viewing of disturbing television programs; timing of the administration of nighttime medication; use of music, hot bath, relaxation techniques, or a warm drink before bedtime; setting a bedtime; and limiting the use of caffeine in the evening). It may be necessary to remind the patient and family/SOs that caffeine is included in many foods and drinks other than coffee and tea such as chocolate and sodas.
- Physical complaints from a patient who is anxious are not unusual. They should be handled with reassurance, appropriate assessment, and interventions. If there is a pattern, it should be discussed with the patient, identifying how feelings are related to the complaints. This, however, should only be done after it is determined that there is no physical basis for the complaint.
- If the patient must have medical testing, the patient will need information about the test and the required preparation. Anyone who accompanies the

patient to the testing should understand the importance of assessing the patient's anxiety during the procedure. Home care staff should speak with medical staff who will be present with the patient and explain the patient's needs. The nurse should develop interventions with the patient that might be used to prevent or decrease the patient's anxiety, such as imagery, relaxation techniques, or thought stopping.

- Staff should encourage the patient to participate in family activities as tolerated. During home visits these activities are discussed, and time is provided for the patient to discuss situations and activities that decrease or increase anxiety.

- Staff work with the patient to identify outlets for anxiety such as exercise, relaxation exercises, music, warm bath, imagery, talking over problems rather than keeping them inside, or using a diary or log. Individual patients resolve or ameliorate symptoms in different ways. Some patients may be comfortable with imagery whereas others may prefer listening to music. Forcing an intervention on the patient will only increase the anxiety. The patient will fail in preventing or decreasing the anxiety, leading to lowered self-esteem, and more anxiety. The patient may then be unwilling to try other interventions.

- The patient should be informed about the dangers of alcohol and drug abuse as methods for alleviating anxiety.

- For most home care patients, too much free time is not helpful. For those with anxiety, it may only increase the anxiety. It might be helpful for staff to remember a time when they had too much free time and were confined (e.g., sick at home, waiting for someone to return home, etc.) and what feelings they experienced. Often these feelings are related to anxiety including frustration, tension, anger, talking to self, or pacing. How does a patient with a serious mental illness feel when he or she is trapped by illness with too much time, with nothing to do? Usually the patient becomes more and more self-absorbed. Working with the patient and the family/SOs to develop a schedule for the patient and to plan activities for the patient is critical. The family/SOs are encouraged to include the patient in daily tasks in the home whenever possible. The patient is encouraged to continue hobbies or develop new ones.

- Home care staff should teach the patient guidelines for coping. Guidelines presented in Exhibit 20–4 and Exhibit 20–5 are helpful.

- Staff can talk with the patient about irrational expectations and beliefs. If the patient feels that he or she must be productive all the time, this is irrational and not helpful. It will be necessary to repeatedly help the patient identify successes and discuss failures from a realistic point of view.

- One exercise the patient might try daily is to think about problems at the end of the day for a specific amount of time. Half of the time the patient should worry about these problems in a totally useless fashion. The other half of the time the patient should use constructive problem solving. This will improve the patient's self-control over the worry.

- The patient should be encouraged to make his or her own living space or bedroom as relaxed as possible by considering colors, lighting, privacy, clutter, and use of music.
- An exercise program can be helpful in decreasing anxiety. Staff should ask the patient if it is followed, and if not, what is interfering. Staff then problem solve with the patient so that the patient will exercise regularly.
- Assisting the patient to correlate cause and effect between stressors and anxiety helps the patient feel more in control. This process will help to decrease anxiety.
- Role playing may be used to teach the patient a coping method for anxiety-provoking situations. If the family/SOs are important to a specific situation, they should be included in the role play.
- Assessment of the patient's use of substances (such as tobacco, alcohol, other drugs, and food) to cope with anxiety is critical with every patient. The treatment plan is then developed to help the patient use different coping methods.
- As preparations are made with the patient for discharge from home care, the patient's activities outside the home are increased. At this time, assessment of anxiety is very important, and the patient needs to participate in the assessment. Activities that are less stressful are important; however, staff, the patient, and family/SOs must recognize that the patient cannot totally avoid stress and anxiety in daily living but can learn to cope better.
- Assessment of the patient's sleep pattern to ensure that the patient is getting adequate sleep is part of the treatment plan. Lack of sleep can affect the anxiety level. Whenever possible, the use of sedatives for sleep should be avoided. Rather than lying in bed worrying about being unable to sleep, the patient might get up but remain inactive or do something boring.
- A diary or log of daily interactions or situations that increase anxiety can be a useful teaching tool and self-assessment monitor. In the diary the patient identifies signs and symptoms, the level of anxiety, responses to the anxiety, and alternative methods for coping. These observations should be discussed at each visit, and staff should provide positive feedback and suggest alternative coping methods.
- The patient may need to be reminded of past successes in order to try something new.

TECHNIQUES TO REDUCE ANXIETY

There are many techniques that can be taught to patients and families/SOs to help them cope with anxiety. The home care agency may want to develop a manual

Exhibit 20–4 Nursing Interventions Related to Anxiety

1. Recognition of anxiety
2. Connection of the feeling (anxiety) with the relief behavior
3. Identification of the situation immediately preceding the feeling of anxiety and its importance to the person
4. Analysis of the information and its relation to past experiences
5. Correlation of the causes and effects of the anxiety

Source: Reprinted from H. Peplau, "Interpersonal Techniques: The Crux of Nursing," *American Journal of Nursing*, Vol. 62, No. 6, pp. 53–54, © 1962. Used with permission of Lippincott-Raven Publishers, Philadelphia, PA.

of these techniques. The staff can then easily review the manual and select techniques that might be helpful for individual patients. This will save staff time and encourage the use of these techniques. The descriptions should be designed so that they can be copied and given to the patient; however, it is very important that staff discuss the technique and practice it with the patient. At subsequent visits the staff should review with the patient the use of the technique and whether it was helpful. Not all techniques work with all patients. Each patient needs to find methods that work best for him or her. Some techniques may work better for different levels of anxiety. The following are descriptions for some of these techniques.

Guided Imagery

Purposeful use of imagination can provide relaxation and a feeling of control. According to Bishai, "Visualization is the conscious programming for change in behavior through positive and creative mental images. It is a natural and automatic mental activity that humans use while daydreaming, thinking of someone, or recalling a past experience. The aim of this technique is to teach the patient how to use and improve his or her already existing power of visualization for better functioning in life."[21(p.120)] The nurse can suggest some possible images, but it must be the patient's image to be successful. Some examples might be walking in a field of flowers, lying on a warm beach, or watching the sunset. Senses should be included in the image. The nurse might ask the patient to try the following procedure: "Find a quiet place and get into a comfortable position. Close your eyes. You may want to use rhythmic breathing and progressive relaxation. Concentrate on an image and picture yourself in it. Slowly experience it with as many senses as possible. Practice going to this place. Develop a specific method for ending the image, such as counting to five. You should not fall asleep."

Exhibit 20–5 What Can You Do To Decrease Anxiety?

- *Talk it out.* Talking things out helps to relieve your strain, helps you to see your worry in a clearer light, and often helps you to see what you can do about it.
- *Escape for a while.* Making yourself "stand there and suffer" is a form of self-punishment, not a way to solve a problem. Escape for a while, but be prepared to come back and deal with your difficulty when you are more composed, and when you and others involved are in better condition to deal with it.
- *Work off your anger.* Do something constructive with your pent-up energy. Working the anger out of your system and cooling off for a day or two will leave you much better prepared to handle your problem.
- *Give in occasionally.* You may find yourself getting into frequent quarrels with others and not willing to give in. You may be right, but sometimes giving in may lessen your anxiety as well as make it easier for others to give in sometimes.
- *Do something for others.* If you feel yourself worrying about yourself all the time, try doing something for somebody else.
- *Take one thing at a time.* For people under tension, an ordinary work load can sometimes seem unbearable. Take on a task at a time.
- *Shun the "superman" urge.* Some people expect too much from themselves and get into a constant state of worry and anxiety because they think they are not achieving as much as they should. Don't take yourself to task if you can't achieve the impossible.
- *Go easy with your criticism.* Some people expect too much from others, and then feel frustrated, let down, disappointed, even "trapped" when another person does not measure up. People who feel let down by the shortcomings (real or imagined) of their relatives, are really let down about themselves. Search for the good points in others.
- *Give the other fellow a break.* When you give the other person a break, you very often make things easier for yourself; if he no longer feels you are a threat to him, he stops being a threat to you.
- *Make yourself "available."* Many people feel that they are being left out, neglected, or rejected. It may be we, not the others, who are depreciating ourselves. Instead of shrinking away and withdrawing, it is much healthier, as well as more practical, to continue to "make yourself available"—to make some of the overtures instead of always waiting to be asked.
- *Schedule your recreation.* Find time to take a time out, a definite schedule for recreation or hobbies.

Source: Reprinted with permission from *How To Deal With Your Tensions*, pp. 4–7, © National Association for Mental Health, 1021 Prince Street, Alexandria, Virginia, 22314, 1-800-969-6642.

Imagery is not suggested for use with patients who are psychotic, as it may only cause or worsen hallucinations or delusions. Prior to recommending the use of imagery, the patient should be assessed to determine the presence of hallucinations or delusions.

Another image that the patient might use is to imagine that what is making the patient anxious is in a balloon. The patient lets go of the balloon and watches it get smaller and smaller as it goes up into the sky.[22]

Quiet-Breathing Technique

Myers suggests the following guidelines for patients who are using breathing techniques:[23(p.173)]

1. Assume a comfortable sitting position.
2. Take a deep, slow breath.
3. As you exhale, envision all your tensions and anxieties flowing outward with each breath.
4. Repeat as needed.

The type of breathing that is important for relaxation is diaphragmatic breathing. The nurse practices with the patient. The patient's stomach should seem to pull in and rise when the patient breathes out. The chest and the shoulders should not move. For some patients lying on the back with knees slightly bent, and hands placed over navel is more conducive to relaxation. The patient can then feel his or her hands rise and fall with breathing.

Progressive Relaxation

Before beginning this technique, the patient should find a quiet place if possible. Some patients do this relaxation exercise sitting and others prefer lying down. Tight clothing should be loosened. Some patients may prefer to remove shoes, glasses, and contact lenses. When muscles are tensed, the patient tries to visualize the tension as well as feel it. The patient tries to visualize relaxation, too. The technique described should be used in a lying position, with a pillow under the knees and arms at the side.

- Concentrate on breathing, using the same type of breathing that is used for quiet breathing. Let your breathing slow down and become more regular.
- Tense by pointing your feet and toes at the same time. You should not feel discomfort but notice the pulling sensation in your calves. Picture the tension, exhale, and then relax. Picture and feel the relaxation.
- Tense by pointing your toes toward your head. Picture the tension, exhale, and then relax. Picture and feel the relaxation.

- Tense the quadriceps muscles on the front part of the legs by straightening out your legs and locking your knees. It will feel like you are pushing your knees into the ground. Picture the tension, exhale, and then relax. Picture and feel the relaxation.
- Tense by digging your heels into the floor or bed. Picture the tension, exhale, and then relax. Picture and feel the relaxation. Relax for 10 seconds feeling the relaxation in your legs, warm and heavy feeling. As you relax, wait 15 more seconds.
- Tense groin and buttocks. Contract the buttocks together as well as the muscles in the genital area between the legs. You may feel this area rising slightly. Picture the tension, exhale, and then relax. Picture and feel the relaxation.
- Tense the stomach muscles. Tighten these muscles to make your stomach hard. Your breathing may be affected. Picture the tension, exhale, and then relax. Picture and feel the relaxation.
- Tense the back by pushing your shoulders against the floor or bed and raising your chest toward your chin. Picture the tension, exhale, and then relax. Picture and feel the relaxation.
- Tense your lower back by pressing it against the floor or bed. Picture the tension, exhale, and then relax. Picture and feel the relaxation. Feel the relaxation in your entire back for 15 seconds.
- Tense your shoulders by squeezing your shoulders downward toward the feet and pressing your arms against your body. Picture the tension, exhale, and then relax. Picture and feel the relaxation.
- Shrug your shoulders and tense, raising the shoulders toward your ears. Picture the tension, exhale, and then relax. Picture and feel the relaxation.
- Tense your forearm by bending your knuckles back toward your elbow pit with fingers bent. Picture the tension, exhale, and then relax. Picture and feel the relaxation.
- Tense your biceps by making fists and pulling your fists up to your shoulders. Picture the tension, exhale, and then relax. Picture and feel the relaxation. Feel your arms relax for 15 seconds.
- Tense your neck by slowly turning to the right and then picture the tension, exhale, and then relax. Picture and feel the relaxation. Then turn slowly to the left and repeat.
- Tense the facial area by making a wide smile, open mouth widely, and tense. Feel it around the cheekbones. Picture the tension, exhale, and then relax. Picture and feel the relaxation. Then frown with corners of mouth down. Picture the tension, exhale, and then relax. Picture and feel the relaxation.
- Tense the jaw muscles by clenching your teeth and pushing your tongue against the upper teeth. Picture the tension, exhale, and then relax. Picture and feel the relaxation.

- Raise your eyebrows high and tense. Picture the tension, exhale, and then relax. Picture and feel the relaxation.
- Imagine warm water flowing all over your body, beginning at the top of your head and down. Use quiet breathing for one minute.

If the patient does not want to go to sleep, it is helpful to count to a specific number to pull out of the relaxation, then stretch and rise slowly.

Problems can occur with progressive relaxation. Patients who have neurologic conditions may find that this technique causes or worsens rigidity.[24] The nurse should consult with the patient's physician before this technique is used.[25] The following pointers will help to prevent problems:

- The patient must assume a comfortable position by sitting or lying down, so that every part of the body is supported. If assuming such a position disrupts relaxation, the effectiveness of the technique must be evaluated.
- To avoid muscle cramps, ask the patient to decrease the tension and apply it more slowly while reducing the period of time.
- Initially, a quiet room is ideal for progressive relaxation. Gradually, the patient needs to learn to relax in a noisier environment.
- Falling asleep decreases the effectiveness of the relaxation, especially when this technique is practiced at bedtime (unless sleep is the desired outcome). Modulating pitch and tone of the voice may correct this problem. Selecting a time for practicing the technique when the patient is not fatigued may also be useful.
- To prevent the patient from experiencing a sense of losing control, ensure that the patient understands the objectives of relaxation and introduce the exercise gradually.
- Identify the annoying or distressing words and phrases that might increase the patient's tension and then ensure that these are avoided.

Thought Stopping[26]

Thought stopping is a technique that can be used to bring thoughts into consciousness and eliminate them. If negative thoughts can be eliminated, their emotions and feelings can also be eliminated.

1. Ask the patient to list self-doubts, fears, or phobias and to identify the ones that are most disturbing. Choose one to work on. To reach a positive result in the beginning, it is best to use a thought that is more logical. When the thought is identified, ask the patient to consider these questions about the thought:
   - Is this thought realistic or unrealistic?
   - Is the thought productive or counterproductive?

- Is this thought easy or hard to control?
- How uncomfortable does this thought make me feel?
- How much does this thought interfere with my life?

2. Ask the patient to think about the thought for several minutes. This can be done after relaxation.
3. The third step is interrupting the thought. Initially, the patient may need to stop the thought using a strong method, such as a timer. When the timer goes off, the patient shouts, "stop." The mind must be emptied of the thought for at least 30 seconds. If it comes back, shout "stop" again. Other methods are wearing a rubber band on the wrist to snap instead of saying "stop," snapping the fingers, raising the hand, etc. Eventually, a normal tone of voice can be used to say "stop." This is used whenever the negative thought occurs.
4. The final step is substituting a positive or assertive thought for the negative one.

Cognitive Therapy

This approach "involves assisting patients to learn how to identify distorted self-statements, the related anxiety reactions, and the accompanying physical reactions (i.e., diaphoresis, racing heart, and shortness of breath)."[27(p.60)] Thinking patterns do affect moods and behaviors. Cognitive therapy requires that the patient and the nurse have a working alliance, a collaborative relationship. The 10 most commonly encountered forms of cognitive distortions are "all or nothing thinking, over-generalization, mental filter, disqualifying the positive, jumping to conclusions, magnification or minimization, emotional reasoning, 'should' statements, labeling and mislabeling, and personalization."[28(p.108)]

PATIENT EDUCATION

Typical patient education goals for patients who are experiencing anxiety might include the following:

- Describe the steps in the anxiety process.
- Identify self-monitoring methods for anxiety.
- Use relaxation exercises at appropriate times.
- Identify the critical elements of stress management and assertiveness for self.
- Identify the potential harmful effects of using alcohol/drugs to decrease anxiety and overusing caffeine.
- Describe the importance of exercise and nutrition in maintaining health.
- Identify name(s) of medications, purpose of taking medication, dosage and frequency, and side effects.

FAMILIES/SIGNIFICANT OTHERS: NEEDS AND STRATEGIES

Families/SOs who must live with a family member who has an anxiety disorder or who is experiencing anxiety due to another illness also experience anxiety themselves. Due to these complex factors, some interactions may increase anxiety for everyone. The home care nurse should assess for the presence of these interactions and then guides the family/SOs to resolve issues with one another. These difficult situations might include the following:

- Excessive questioning of the ill family member may be a problem, even if the intent is to listen supportively.
- Inappropriate advice giving may interfere with the ill family member regaining independence. It is often easier for the family/SOs to tell the patient what to do or how to do it instead of allowing some freedom, even though freedom sometimes means failure. The patient must learn about responsibility. Staff and the family/SOs are there for support and guidance.
- Patronizing or giving insincere praise will be noticed by most patients. It will only lower self-esteem and increase anxiety.
- When an ill family member is complaining and feeling miserable, the family/SO may participate in collusion, agreeing with the ill member rather than offering realistic appraisal of the situation.
- With constructive and reality-based criticism, the patient learns more than from negative feedback, particularly if it is not reality based.
- The home care staff may encounter families/SOs who ridicule, blame, and even attack the ill family member for inadequacies. This can lead to major problems in the home environment and may be one of the reasons the ill family member is experiencing excessive anxiety. This type of family requires intervention or the ill family member will never succeed in the home environment. The nurse should talk with the family/SOs about the behavior that is observed, ask their opinions about what they feel is happening, include the patient in the discussion, and help all learn more positive methods for responding to one another.

EVALUATION

When care for the patient with anxiety is evaluated to determine if outcomes have been met, critical quesions include the following:

- Does the patient appear less anxious?
- Does the patient state that he or she is less anxious?
- Does the patient use adaptive coping mechanisms?
- Did the patient participate in planning and evaluation of progress?
- What is the patient's evaluation of the care and the results?

OTHER ANXIETY DISORDERS

Panic Disorder

The criteria for panic disorder diagnosis are the presence of recurrent, unexpected panic attacks with at least one month of worry that the attack will return. A panic attack is a discrete period of intense fear or discomfort with four or more of the following symptoms that develop abruptly and reach their peak within 10 minutes: palpitations, pounding heart, or accelerated heart rate; sweating; trembling or shaking; sensations of shortness of breath or smothering, choking feeling; chest pain or discomfort; nausea or abdominal distress; feeling dizzy, unsteady, light-headed or faint; derealization or depersonalization; fear of losing control or going crazy; fear of dying; paresthesia; and chills or hot flashes.[29] An estimated one-third of patients with this disorder develop agoraphobia, a fear of places or situations in which they will not be able to get help if they experience a panic attack.[30] Because there is a strong physiological component with this disorder, it is important that the patient receive a complete history and physical to rule out physical problems. If the patient is unable to identify the psychological responses that are experienced, this may lead staff to believe that the patient has a physical problem. "Research indicates that one third of patients with panic disorder develop a secondary major depression, and about one fifth have had a major depressive disorder before developing panic disorder."[31(p.3)] These factors need to be considered during assessment. Because about 70 percent of all people with a panic disorder also have another psychiatric disorder, more than half have an episode of major depression at some time, and a large number have a history of alcohol or drug dependence, assessment in these areas is very important.[32] Treatment may be required for the depression or other illnesses.

With increasing biological research, the etiology for panic disorder is becoming clearer. There does appear to be a genetic component.[33] Biochemically there is thought to be "an overactivity of the noradrenergic system in the brain that mediates the fight-or-flight response, principally the locus ceruleus, which manufactures most of the brain norepinephrine and is thought to control an active response to anxiety-provoking stimuli."[34(pp.118–119)]

Interventions for panic disorder might include the following:

- Staff or family/SOs must stay with the patient during an attack. Family/SOs should understand the need for this support.
- As the patient's perceptual field is decreased during the panic state of anxiety, decreasing the stimuli (such as light, noise, and number of people) will help.
- Prescribed medications may be taken as ordered.
- The patient will need reassurance that the person with him or her, whether staff or family/SOs, will stay with the patient and keep him or her safe. This

needs to be stated. Unless the person knows that the patient will respond positively to touch, it is best not to touch the patient.
- The patient should be encouraged to discuss feelings about what is happening to him or her.
- Simple actions to burn energy, such as pacing, may be encouraged but not forced upon the patient.

Interventions discussed for generalized anxiety disorder also apply to patients with panic disorder.

Phobic Disorders

A phobia is an irrational, persistent fear of situations, objects, or activities. The person avoids these to eliminate the risk of experiencing severe anxiety. Usually phobias begin to interfere with daily living. The patient recognizes that the phobia is unreasonable. If confronted with the phobic stimulus, the person will experience panic, diaphoresis, dyspnea, and/or tachycardia.

In addition to the interventions described for generalized anxiety disorder, the following interventions may be used for patients with phobic disorders:

- The patient may want to withdraw completely. This should be avoided. Home care staff should help the patient and family/SOs to identify small ways that the patient may continue to participate in the family life.
- The patient's phobia should be taken seriously by all as a way that the patient copes with anxiety. This should also be explained to the patient.
- The environment should be supportive and provide a place for the patient to relax.
- If the patient has a phobia about food or fluids, monitoring intake is important. The treatment plan includes a diet that will provide the nutrients the patient requires.
- The patient's phobia may interfere with hygiene. Staff and family/SOs should ensure that hygiene is maintained whenever possible by providing support and not pushing the patient. Moving step by step allows the patient to develop strength to cope with anxiety.
- Desensitization may be used. "The patient is exposed to a series of anxiety-provoking situations beginning with the most provocative."[35(p.40)] Guidance from the patient's physician is very important during this process.

Obsessive-Compulsive Disorder

Obsessive-compulsive disorder (OCD) is another type of anxiety disorder. The patient experiences obsessions and compulsions, either together or alone. These help to prevent extreme anxiety. An obsession is a persistent, unwanted, and uncontrolled idea or impulse that cannot be eliminated by logic or reasoning. The five typical thought content areas related to obsessions are lack of cleanliness, orderliness, aggressive behavior, religious matters, and sexual behavior. According to Brisson, urges and attempts to control obsessions "result in compulsive behavior consisting of repetitive, stereotyped acts or rituals that tend to neutralize the unwanted thought, thus providing temporary and partial relief from anxiety."[36(p.64)] A compulsion is an insistent, repetitive, intrusive, and unwanted urge to perform an act—an obsession in action. If kept from performing the activity, the patient would be overwhelmed with anxiety. Unplanned attempts or interventions to stop obsessive-compulsive behavior may result in the patient experiencing panic.[37]

There is some biological evidence to indicate that OCD is linked to deficiencies in the neurotransmitter serotonin; however, precise information about its role is not yet available. Patients with OCD have also been shown to have abnormalities in the frontal lobes and basal ganglia, but it is not clear what this finding means.[38]

Assessment for OCD includes identification of the following signs and symptoms:

- low self-esteem
- chronic anxiety
- difficulty expressing positive feelings
- depressed mood
- recurrent obsessions and/or compulsions
- interference with everyday functioning
- very judgmental attitude toward self and others
- lack of enjoyment or pleasure
- focus on details
- rigid and perfectionist traits
- tendency to be very productive
- family problems and unsatisfactory relationships
- suicidal thoughts

During the initial assessment, symptoms of depression may be the most obvious symptoms. Rituals can exhaust the patient, particularly if they are complex and center on critical aspects of daily living.[39]

Patient goals for a patient with OCD are as follows:

- to experience less need to use ritualistic behavior
- to experience less anxiety and/or depression as exhibited by ability to cope with stress and to discuss problems without feeling overwhelming anxiety

- to identify and use anxiety-reducing behaviors that are substituted for obsessive-compulsive behavior
- to describe how the obsessive-compulsive behavior and/or thoughts affect his or her life
- to apply problem-solving process to actual problems
- to exhibit appropriate activity level, sleep pattern, eating pattern, and independent self-care within patient's limitations
- to participate in treatment planning, assessment of progress, and discharge planning
- to identify name(s) of medications, purpose of taking, dosage and frequency, and side effects
- to identify coping mechanisms for self that might be used after discharge, such as relaxation techniques, problem solving, or guided imagery
- to attend an OCD support group in the community
- to develop the capacity to express feelings appropriately
- to develop more positive family/SO relationships and social functioning
- to increase self-esteem

Nursing interventions that might be considered for the patient with OCD are varied, and many of them depend upon the patient's specific obsession and compulsive behavior. They include the following:

- The patient's anxiety level and use of obsessive-compulsive behaviors are assessed on admission and throughout home care treatment, particularly noting patterns related to anxiety and behaviors.
- The patient is taught how to cope with anxiety and learns problem-solving skills.
- Interfering with obsessive-compulsive behavior may cause panic. Interventions must be planned carefully with the family/SOs and implemented consistently. The patient requires support. Suicidal risk can be very high at this time.
- If the behavior is causing problems for the family/SOs, this needs to be discussed. The discussion should focus on practical issues and feelings. The goal is to support the patient, but it may be necessary to compromise. The patient needs to participate in the discussion and needs help to recognize the effect his or her behavior has on others.
- The patient's behavior can be very frustrating to the staff. Power struggles can easily start over the ritualistic behavior. Staff assigned to work with the patient should help one another with this frustration before it escalates.
- Nutrition, sleep, activities of daily living, and physical exercise needs must be met. If obsessive-compulsive behavior is interfering and has reached an unhealthy level, active intervention is required.

- The patient is taught relaxation techniques and encouraged to use them.
- Staff should help the patient set reasonable limits on rituals.
- Family/SOs and staff must be careful to avoid reinforcing ritualistic behavior and to reinforce nonritualistic behavior.
- An environment that has structure and predictability will aid in decreasing the patient's anxiety.
- During each visit, home care staff should encourage the patient to discuss thoughts and feelings. Build self-esteem and self-confidence by asking for the patient's assessment of progress and suggestions for the treatment plan.
- Home care staff should work with the patient to plan a daily schedule that includes times for normal activities and time for rituals, gradually decreasing the time for rituals.
- Because OCD patients are compulsive about time and schedules, home care staff should be punctual and consistent.

Interventions for generalized anxiety disorders—such as progressive relaxation, quiet breathing, and thought stopping—can be effective with the patient with OCD if used in conjunction with other interventions. In addition, the following interventions, which require commitment on the part of the nurse and the patient, can be tried:

- *Symptom hierarchy.*[40] The nurse helps the patient learn how to identify the difference between the obsessive thought and the compulsive act. Then each fear and each behavior are clearly described by breaking each item into small manageable steps. Following this, each obsessive thought and compulsive behavior is ranked from the least to most anxiety-provoking, by using a scale of 0 to 100. This process helps the patient begin to separate global fears and anxieties into manageable treatment goals.
- *Cognitive restructuring.*[41] Cognitive restructuring helps the patient discriminate specific distortions of reality and then test them. The first step is to monitor obsessive thoughts and compulsive behaviors. This can be done by having the patient keep a log that details what is thought or done; when; length of time; specific steps; and how the patient feels before, during, and after. The goal is to have the patient connect cognition, affect, and behavior. Evidence for and against distorted thoughts are discussed with the patient. Doubts are discussed in order to develop the patient's reality testing (for example, the patient who worries that he or she will cause a flood in the house every time a faucet is turned on and consequently returns to check each faucet a specific number of times. What is the likelihood that this will really happen? How many times has it really happened?)

Cue cards may be used in conjunction with cognitive restructuring. According to Boyarsky, "These individually tailored, symptom-specific cards formulate reality for the patient, reinforce the concept that he or she is safe in the world and can withstand the anxiety associated with delaying or controlling compulsive rituals, and explain that the compulsions do not really protect him or her from the feared object or circumstance, but rather, cause another set of problems and anxiety."[42(p.302)] Some examples of cue cards follow.[43]

- It's the OCD, not me.
- My worst fear will not happen. I never stop to think about it, but nothing bad has ever happened.
- Relax; I can do it.
- I don't need to doubt myself.
- Trust myself.
- Checking the locks again won't keep me safe. I really am safe in the world.

After the patient has used relaxation techniques, the patient is asked to use imagery to elicit the obsessive thought or to look at the object that he or she uses in the compulsive behavior. Thought stopping is then used to try to stop the thought or behavior. As the patient becomes anxious, he or she reads the cue cards. "This activity prevents, or at least delays, the obsessive thought from spiraling into an uncontrollable anxiety for which he or she must give in to the need to perform a compulsion."[44(p.303)] Homework can be assigned to structure practice sessions for the patient. A contract can be made with the patient to practice a specific amount of times and then to assess anxiety at the conclusion. At each home visit, the nurse discusses the homework with the patient.

Patient education goals for the patient with OCD might include the following:

- Describe the biochemical and psychosocial components of OCD.
- Describe the steps in the anxiety process.
- Identify how OCD behavior is not a healthy coping mechanism and apply to self.
- Identify critical elements of stress management and assertiveness to self.
- Learn relaxation exercises and use as needed.
- Identify the potential harmful effects of using alcohol/drugs to decrease anxiety.
- Identify name(s) of medications, purpose of taking, dosage and frequency, and side effects.
- Identify the importance of exercise and nutrition in maintaining health. (If these are part of the OCD behavior, the patient will need to learn what is appropriate nutrition and exercise.)

SUMMARY

Information about anxiety can be applied to any patient, family/SOs, and home care staff. It is important in all of the care provided in the home, regardless of the patient's medical problems. Anxiety can never be totally avoided. Home care staff who help each patient and the family/SOs learn to cope more effectively with anxiety are providing important care. These coping strategies can be used after the patient is discharged from home care.

NOTES

1. Nurse Review, *Psychiatric Problems* (Springhouse, PA: Springhouse Corporation, 1990), 35.
2. Nurse Review, *Psychiatric Problems*, 29.
3. G. Stuart, "Anxiety Responses and Anxiety Disorders," in *Principles and Practice of Psychiatric Nursing*, ed. G. Stuart and S. Sundeen (St. Louis, MO: Mosby–Year Book, 1995), 327–353, at 331.
4. J. Manaser and A. Werner, *Instruments for Study of Nurse Patient Relationships* (New York: MacMillan, 1964), 103–106.
5. N. Andreasen, *The Broken Brain: The Biological Revolution in Psychiatry* (New York: Harper & Row, 1985), 239–240.
6. Stuart, "Anxiety Responses and Anxiety Disorders," 333.
7. H. Peplau, "A Working Definition of Anxiety," in *Some Clinical Approaches to Psychiatric Nursing*, ed. S. Burd and M. Marshall (New York: MacMillan, 1963), 323–327.
8. J. Kelley and L. Lehman, "Assessment of Anxiety, Depression, and Suspiciousness in the Home Care Setting," *Home Healthcare Nurse* 11, no. 2 (1993): 6–20, at 17.
9. Kelley, "Assessment of Anxiety, Depression, and Suspiciousness in the Home Care Setting," 17.
10. Nurse Review, *Psychiatric Problems*, 32.
11. G. McFarland and E. Wasli, *Nursing Diagnoses and Process in Psychiatric Mental Health Nursing* (Philadelphia: J.B. Lippincott Co., 1986), 52.
12. M. Fauman, *Study Guide to DSM-IV* (Washington, DC: American Psychiatric Press, Inc., 1994), 220–221.
13. Nurse Review, *Psychiatric Problems*, 29.
14. Stuart, "Anxiety Responses and Anxiety Disorders," 339.
15. Fauman, *Study Guide to DSM-IV*, 219.
16. Fauman, *Study Guide to DSM-IV*, 221–222.
17. American Psychiatric Association, *Diagnostic and Statistical Manual of Mental Disorders*, 4th ed. (Washington, DC: 1994), 20–21.
18. North American Nursing Diagnosis Association, *NANDA Nursing Diagnoses: Definitions and Classification 1995–1996* (Philadelphia: 1994), 13, 17, 19, 20, 27, 29, 37, 50, 63, 77, 86, 87.
19. Stuart, "Anxiety Responses and Anxiety Disorders," 331.
20. H. Peplau, "Interpersonal Techniques: The Crux of Nursing," *American Journal of Nursing* 62, no. 6 (1962): 50–54, at 53.

21. M. Bishai, "Visualization and Guided Imagery," in *Decision Making in Psychiatric and Psychosocial Nursing*, ed. A. Baumann et al. (Philadelphia: B.C. Decker, Inc., 1990), 120–121.

22. R. Grainger, "Managing Stress," *American Journal of Nursing* 91, no. 9 (1991): 15–16.

23. D. Myers, *Client Teaching Guides for Home Health Care* (Gaithersburg, MD: Aspen Publishers, Inc., 1989), 173.

24. M. Bishai, "Progressive Relaxation," in *Decision Making in Psychiatric and Psychosocial Nursing*, ed. A. Baumann et al. (Philadelphia: B.C. Decker, Inc., 1990), 118–119.

25. Bishai, "Progressive Relaxation," 118.

26. M. Copeland, *The Depression Workbook* (Oakland, CA: New Harbinger Publications, Inc., 1992), 205–206.

27. D. Antai-Otong, "Generalized Anxiety Disorder," in *Decision Making in Psychiatric and Psychosocial Nursing*, ed. A. Baumann et al. (Philadelphia: B.C. Decker, Inc., 1990), 60–61, at 60.

28. N. Johnston, "Cognitive Therapy," in *Decision Making in Psychiatric and Psychosocial Nursing*, ed. A. Baumann et al. (Philadelphia: B.C. Decker, Inc., 1990), 108–109, at 108.

29. American Psychiatric Association, *Diagnostic and Statisical Manual of Mental Disorders*, 395.

30. "Survey Shows Americans Underestimate Impact of Panic Disorder and Effectiveness of Treatment," *Psychiatric Services* 46, no. 10 (1995): 1089.

31. Nurse Review, *Psychiatric Problems*, 3.

32. "Survey Shows Americans Underestimate Impact of Panic Disorder and Effectiveness of Treatment," 1089.

33. M. Laraia, "Biological Context of Psychiatric Nursing Care," in *Principles and Practice of Psychiatric Nursing*, ed. G. Stuart and S. Sundeen (St. Louis, MO: Mosby–Year Book, 1995), 103–139, at 118.

34. Laraia, "Biological Context of Psychiatric Nursing Care," 118–119.

35. Nurse Review, *Psychiatric Problems*, 40.

36. D. Brisson, "Obsessive-Compulsive Disorders," in *Decision Making in Psychiatric and Psychosocial Nursing,* ed. A. Baumann et al. (Philadelphia: B.C. Decker Inc., 1990), 64–65, at 64.

37. Brisson, "Obsessive-Compulsive Disorders," 64.

38. P. Simoni, "Obsessive-Compulsive Disorder: The Effect of Research on Nursing Care," *Journal of Psychosocial Nursing* 29, no. 4 (1991): 19–23, at 20.

39. Simoni, "Obsessive-Compulsive Disorder: The Effect of Research on Nursing Care," 21.

40. B. Boyarsky et al., "Current Treatment Approaches to Obsessive-Compulsive Disorder," *Archives of Psychiatric Nursing* 5, no. 10 (1991): 299–301, at 301.

41. Boyarsky, "Current Treatment Approaches to Obsessive-Compulsive Disorder," 302.

42. Boyarsky, "Current Treatment Approaches to Obsessive-Compulsive Disorder," 302.

43. Boyarsky, "Current Treatment Approaches to Obsessive-Compulsive Disorder," 302.

44. Boyarsky, "Current Treatment Approaches to Obsessive-Compulsive Disorder," 303.

SUGGESTED READING

American Psychiatric Association. 1995. *Diagnostic and statistical manual of mental disorders.* 4th ed. Washington, DC.

Baloon, D. 1993. Effects on children of having lived with a parent who has an anxiety disorder. *Issues in Mental Health Nursing* 14, no. 2: 187–189.

Beck, A., and G. Emery. 1985. *Anxiety disorders and phobias: A cognitive perspective.* New York: Basic Books.

Boyarsky, B. et al. 1991. Current treatment approaches to obsessive-compulsive disorder. *Archives of Psychiatric Nursing* 5, no. 5: 299–306.

Bulecheck, G., and J. McCloskey. 1985. *Nursing interventions: Treatments for nursing diagnoses.* Philadelphia: W.B. Saunders Company.

Carpenito, L. 1983. *Nursing diagnosis: Application to clinical practice.* Philadelphia: J.B. Lippincott Co.

Cox, H. et al. 1989. *Clinical applications of nursing diagnosis.* Baltimore, MD: Williams & Wilkins.

Doenges, M. et al. 1989. *Psychiatric care plans.* Philadelphia: F.A. Davis.

Elliott, S. 1980. Denial as an effective mechanism to allay anxiety following a stressful event. *Journal of Psychosocial Nursing* 18, no. 10: 11–15.

Fadden, T. et al. 1984. Clinical validation of the diagnosis anxiety. In *Classification of nursing diagnoses: Proceedings of the Fifth National Conference*, ed. M. Kim et al., 183–190. St. Louis, MO: Mosby–Year Book.

Hallam, R. 1992. *Counseling for anxiety problems.* Newbury Park, CA.: Sage Publications.

Hoehn-Saric, R., and D. McLeod. 1993. *Biology of anxiety disorders.* Washington, DC: American Psychiatric Press.

Jenike, M. et al. 1990. *Obsessive compulsive disorders: Theory and management.* 2nd ed. Chicago: Year Book.

Jones, P., and D. Jakob. 1984. Anxiety revisited—From practice perspective. In *Classification of nursing diagnoses: Proceedings of the Fifth National Conference*, ed. M. Kim et al., 285–290. St. Louis: Mosby–Year Book.

Kelley, J., and L. Lehman. 1993. Assessment of anxiety, depression, and suspiciousness in the home care setting. *Home Healthcare Nurse* 11, no. 2: 16–20.

Kolkmeier, L. 1988. Relaxation: Opening the door to change. In *Holistic nursing: A handbook for practice*, ed. B. Dosney et al., 195–222. Gaithersburg, MD: Aspen Publishers, Inc.

Lewis, S. et al. 1989. *Manual of psychosocial nursing interventions.* Philadelphia: W.B. Saunders Company.

Marks, I. 1987. *Fears, phobias, and rituals.* New York: McGraw-Hill.

Mason, J., ed. 1990. *Psychiatric problems: Nurse review.* Philadelphia: Springhouse Corp.

Massion, A. et al. 1993. Quality of life and psychiatric morbidity in panic disorder and generalized anxiety disorder. *American Journal of Psychiatry* 150, no. 4: 600–607.

McFarland, G., and E. Wasli. 1986. *Nursing diagnoses and process in psychiatric mental health nursing.* Philadelphia: J.B. Lippincott Co.

Meares, A. 1963. *The management of the anxious patient.* Philadelphia: W.B. Saunders Company.

Minichiello W. et al. 1988. Behavior therapy for the treatment of obsessive compulsive disorder: Theory and practice. *Comprehensive Psychiatry* 29, no. 2: 123–137.

Rapoport, J. 1989. *The boy who couldn't stop washing.* New York: E.P. Dutton.

Rorden, J. 1987. *Nurses as health teachers.* Philadelphia: W.B. Saunders Company.

Roy-Bryrne, P., and W. Katon. 1987. An update on treatment of the anxiety disorders. *Hospital and Community Psychiatry* 38, no. 8, 1987: 835–843.

Simoni, S. 1991. Obsessive-compulsive disorder: The effect of research on nursing care. *Journal of Psychosocial Nursing* 29, no. 4: 19–23.

Soreff, S. 1985. Indications for home treatment. *Psychiatric Clinics of North America* 8, no. 3: 563–575.

Stuart, G., and S. Sundeen. 1995. *Principles and practice of psychiatric nursing.* St. Louis: Mosby–Year Book.

Suinn, R. 1990. *Anxiety management training.* New York: Plenum Press.

Waddell, K., and A. Demi. 1993. Effectiveness of an intensive partial hospitalization program for treatment of anxiety disorders. *Archives of Psychiatric Nursing* 7, no. 1: 2–10.

Whitley, G. 1989. Anxiety: Defining the diagnosis. *Journal of Psychosocial Nursing* 27, no. 10: 7–12.

Whitley, G. 1991. Ritualistic behavior: Breaking the cycle. *Journal of Psychosocial Nursing* 29, no. 10: 31–35.

Yocum, C. 1984. The differentiation of fear and anxiety. In *Classification of nursing diagnoses: Proceedings of the Fifth National Conference,* ed. M. Kim et al., 352–356. St. Louis: Mosby–Year Book.

Zetin, M., and M. Kramer, 1992. Obsessive-compulsive disorder. *Hospital and Community Psychiatry* 43, no. 7: 689–699.

Depression

INTRODUCTION

The majority of patients admitted to psychiatric units have depression, and it is a common diagnosis encountered in home care. Depression costs this country nearly $44 billion annually, with time lost from work accounting for the largest share.[1] According to Abraham, "The social impact of depression expresses itself also in the ignorance of the lay and, to a significant extent, the professional public. Society does not understand depression as an illness in its many forms and expressions and prefers to shroud it in social taboos. The term 'depression' is unacceptable to many. The elderly, for instance, prefer to use expressions like 'feeling down,' 'feeling blue,' and so forth. Depression is often viewed as a sign of weakness and lack of will power. Depression is something that can be overcome."[2(p.528)]

A depressive disorder is usually responsive to treatment, particularly psychopharmacology; however, most people do not seek treatment. After remission, most people return to healthier functioning, however, a few remain chronically depressed. Despite a typical positive response, depression is poorly recognized and often inappropriately treated in the general health care system. This causes even more problems. "Depression tends to be more debilitating than diabetes, arthritis, gastrointestinal disorders, back problems, and hypertension in terms of physical functioning; interference in work, housework, or schoolwork; and normal social functioning."[3(p.85)] Due to the symptoms of apathy and slow response to medications, the home care patient with depression often engenders frustration, anger, and the feeling of hopelessness in home care staff and the patient's family/significant others (SOs) until improvement is seen.

DEFINING CHARACTERISTICS

Affective disorders, which include depression and bipolar disorder, are disturbances of affect or mood. The patient experiences uncontrolled extremes in his or her affect. The focus in this chapter is on depressive disorders. Howland asserts that "Although depression is associated with significant morbidity and mortality, it is widely believed to have a relatively favorable prognosis compared with other major psychiatric disorders. This belief is due in part to the episodic nature of depression; most patients are expected to return to a completely well state following remission of their acute symptoms."[4(p.633)] Despite this characteristic of depression, for some patients it can be a chronic illness. For these patients the symptoms usually begin early in life and result in significant impairment in psychosocial development.[5] The Agency for Health Care Policy and Research (AHCPR) defines *clinical depression* or a *mood disorder* as "a syndrome (a constellation of signs and symptoms) that is not a normal reaction to life's difficulties."[6(p.9)] It should not be confused with a grief reaction that typically resolves in 2 to 12 months. Exhibit 21–1 identifies early warning signs of depression.

Depressive disorders can begin at any age, but they typically begin in the 20s and 30s. Symptoms develop over several days or weeks. Some patients have a single episode, but 50 percent experience recurrent episodes. The risk factors for depression are[7(pp.6–7)]

- prior episodes of depression
- family history of depressive disorder
- prior suicide attempts
- female gender
- age of onset under 40
- postpartum period
- medical co-morbidity
- lack of social support
- stressful life events
- current substance abuse

Relationships can be very difficult for the depressed patient. Copeland's study of depressed persons indicates that certain patient behaviors tend to make it difficult for the depressed person to develop relationships and maintain them. These include the following:[8(p.116)]

- low self-esteem
- tendency to be very needy and draining
- unreliability
- unpredictability

- difficulty reaching out
- overdependence on one or a few people, wearing them down
- inappropriate behavior, which embarrasses and turns off others
- lack of social skills

Biological research related to affective disorders has advanced rapidly in the last few years. The general consensus is that biochemical factors are part of the cause of major depressive illness. The focus of research has been on neurotransmitters that are located in the brain. Neurotransmitters are the means by which the brain changes and regulates mood, behavior, and all bodily functions. These are chemical messengers that one neuron uses to communicate with another. They are produced by brain neurons and secreted into synaptic clefts, where receptor cells are "turned on" as a result of their selective interaction. They are "turned off" through the reuptake of the neurotransmitter by the neuron that first produced it. Researchers hypothesize that there are impairments in the activity of biogenic amines, particularly the monoamine neurotransmitters, norepinephrine and serotonin, with a depletion that might be related to depression. The site of their actions are the limbic system, the seat of emotion, and the diencephalon (the regulator of sleep, appetite, energy, and psychomotor function). Several hypotheses have been proposed about the etiology of depression.

- *Catecholamine hypothesis.* This hypothesis proposes that there is a deficiency of norepinephrine, which is a neurotransmitter used by the sympathetic nervous system to increase alertness or charge up the body. Both tricyclics and monoamine oxidase inhibitors, medications used to treat depression, increase norepinephrine, but in different ways.
- *Serotonin hypothesis.* Serotonin is a major neurotransmitter that is affected by tricyclics, which increase the amount of serotonin. Some antidepressants affect serotonin and others affect norepinephrine.
- *Neuroendocrine imbalance.* This imbalance has been investigated in relationship to depression with a focus on an abnormality in cortisol secretion.

Because no single hypothesis has been accepted, home care nurses will need to keep abreast of future research results. Up-to-date knowledge will be important for treatment as well as for teaching patients about the illness.

There is significant evidence to support the importance of genetic factors in depression. At this time, however, there is no biologic genetic test to predict depressive disorder. Many families will be concerned about these potential genetic factors, and they will ask questions. The patient may be concerned about his or her children. The nurse must provide information and be honest when questions cannot be answered. Encouraging the patient also to discuss the issue with the physician is important but should not be a way the nurse avoids discussing genetics with the patient or family.

Exhibit 21–1 Typical Early Warning Signs of Depression

• excessive appetite	• difficulty exercising
• lethargy	• low self-confidence
• procrastination	• irritable, impatient
• insecurity	• poor judgment
• obsessive thoughts	• suicidal thoughts
• paranoia	• inactivity
• slow speech	• destructive risk taking
• cry easily	• eat junk food
• physical complaints	• trouble getting dressed
• negative attitude	• feel no one understands
• avoid people	• down on self
• extreme fatigue	• unwillingness to ask for things
• down on future	• negative attitude
• avoid crowds	• hard time getting up
• sleep problems	• repetitive words, actions
• misperceptions	• unable to concentrate
• withdrawal	• unable to experience pleasure
• confused	• inability to show affection
• anxiety	• everything seems disorganized
• low energy level	• increased consumption of alcohol
• fear	

Source: Reprinted with permission from M. Copeland, *The Depression Workbook: A Guide for Living with Depression and Manic Depression*, pp. 52, 107, © 1992, New Harbinger Publications, Inc.

Environmental and social factors influence mood or affect as the patient responds to what is happening in his or her life. Patients who have less ability to cope with negative experience may have a predisposing factor to develop depression. Physical or psychological stressors may be identified for specific patients. In the past, much of the discussion of the etiology and treatment of depression focused on psychodynamic theory, particularly the issue of loss. Today there is less and less emphasis on the psychodynamic causes of depression and more emphasis placed on physiological changes that can be affected by stress and loss. Loss may trigger the predisposing factor, leading to a decreased ability to cope. Depression is often related to loss of a loved person or object that is real or imagined. It may be an attempt by the person to resolve the conflict by turning the negative feelings in toward himself or herself. It is often difficult for staff to see what is a major and minor loss from the patient's perspective, but it is the patient's perspective that is important. Staff cannot be judgmental about what is a good reason to feel depressed. Even if there is a physiological cause of depression, patients continue to need help learning to cope with loss in their lives.

It is important to note that some physical conditions may cause depression (e.g., influenza or other viral infections, childbirth, pancreatitis, pancreatic carcinoma, infectious mononucleosis, hormonal imbalances, hypothyroidism, stroke, brain tumors, Alzheimer's disease, multiple sclerosis, electrolyte disorders, malnutrition).[9] Also, some medications can have the side effect of depression. These include several categories of drugs; antiemetics (large doses and/or over long time), sedatives, tranquilizers, antihypertensives (particularly reserpine), corticosteroids, and oral contraceptives.[10] Alcohol, marijuana, and other abused drugs can also lead to depression, and all patients should be informed about this as well as assessed for their use. Because some physical illnesses and some medications can cause a patient to experience depression, it is important to conduct a complete history and physical including a complete medication history.

As patients are assessed for depression, it is important to remember that a patient can experience a psychotic depression—a mood disturbance with delusions, hallucinations, or both. These patients typically respond poorly to antidepressants and more positively to a combination of an antidepressant and a neuroleptic or electroconvulsive therapy (ECT).[11] Psychiatric depression may be difficult to identify, because it may be concealed, intermittent, or confused with schizophrenia. The common delusions of psychotic depressions are characterized by guilt, sin, and ideas of reference. Of these patients, at least 50 percent will experience more than one type of delusion.[12] Hallucinations may be auditory or visual. Some patients may have tactile and olfactory hallucinations, even though this is more typical for organic brain disease. The typical description of a patient with psychotic depression would be severe and early-onset depression, marked psychomotor retardation or agitation, rumination, gross pseudodementia, frequent hospitalizations, and resistance to antidepressants.[13] Psychotic depression should not be viewed as a part of a continuum of depression. A patient with psychotic depression may have experienced earlier episodes of depression without psychosis; however, after a patient experiences psychotic depression, subsequent episodes are likely to be psychotic depression.[14] There does seem to be a genetic trait and also some relationship to schizophrenia in the family. ECT has been found to be very successful for patients with psychotic depression, who recover more slowly and often require more hospitalizations than nonpsychotic depressed patients. Patients with psychotic depression have a suicide rate that is two to five times higher than nonpsychotic depressed patients.[15] Psychotic depression is a serious illness that needs to be identified so that the patient can receive appropriate treatment.

ASSESSMENT

Guidelines for Assessment

Depression is difficult to assess objectively because the patient's subjective assessment of his or her mood and physical symptoms is very important. Patients may initially deny that they have problems with depression and focus more on somatic complaints such as sleep, appetite, or weight.[16] The assessment includes an interview, observation, history and physical, and may include the use of self-rating scales such as the Beck Depression Inventory or the Zung Self-Rating Depression Scale, as well as rating scales used by the nurse. The major assessment focus areas are the patient's self-concept, stress and coping, perception, mood, communication, and suicidality. Typically the depressed patient exhibits negative verbalizations about himself or herself, others, or life in general.[17] A family history of depression is important to identify as well as the patient's physical health and medication history. A detailed history of previous experiences with depression is very helpful in determining the patient's risk for a major depression and response to treatment. All depressed patients need to be asked about the use of alcohol and other nonprescription drugs that can be abused. Exhibit 21–2 provides sample assessment questions.

As with all medical problems, reassessment is critical and must be ongoing. Is the patient responding to the treatment based on changes in specific symptoms? Has the patient developed other problems? Is the patient experiencing side effects from prescribed medications? Is the patient compliant with treatment? What is the patient's view of his or her progress? What information should be shared with the patient? Is the patient retaining patient information material? How are the family/SOs responding to the patient and the patient's treatment? What needs to be changed in the treatment plan? Assessment data are then used to formulate new interventions and adapt interventions.

Signs and Symptoms

The signs and symptoms of depression can be categorized into three levels: mild, moderate, and severe.[18] It is not necessary for all of these symptoms to be present in each patient with depression. Generally, symptoms are worse in the morning. Depression influences the patient's affect, thought processes, behavior, feelings, communication, and physical status.

Mild Depression

Mild depression is transitory and self-limiting and often related to loss. The patient is usually referred to home care for reasons other than the mild depres-

Exhibit 21–2 Assessment Questions for Depressive Disorders

- How would you describe your mood?
- Have your sleeping habits changed?
- What has changed about your sleeping habits?
- Have your activities changed?
- Would you describe yourself as less active, more active, or about the same?
- Have you been eating less or more?
- How do you cope with stress?
- Is your method for coping with stress helpful?
- Do you feel hopeful about the future?
- What are your most important problems?
- How would you describe yourself?
- What are your strengths?
- Are you feeling any guilt now? About what?
- Is it easy for you to make decisions?
- How is your concentration?
- How is your memory?
- Do you feel you can call on the persons who give you the most support?
- Do you see things improving in your life?

sion; however, the home care nurse identifies it as a problem from assessment data. It affects other psychiatric or physical problems the patient may have at the time. Its symptoms are as follows:

- sadness; crying
- mild anxiety with some irritability
- decreased energy and involvement in interests
- change in sleep, gastrointestinal disturbances, overeating or undereating with possible weight change, somatic complaints
- preoccupation with death, loss, and morbid themes
- lower suicidal risk

Moderate Depression

Patients with moderate depression are more likely to be referred for treatment, such as home care. They exhibit the following symptoms:

- lowered self-esteem
- pessimism
- overt, pervasive anxiety with indirect anxiety
- narrowed thoughts and interests; indecisiveness

- obsessive thoughts
- altered eating patterns with weight change, vegetative signs, increased somatic complaints, altered perceptions of body
- decreased energy
- difficulty with concentration and memory
- feelings of emptiness
- active suicidal risk

Severe Depression

This level of depression is the easiest level to identify, because the patient's affect and behavior are most noticeable. The symptoms for this level include the following:

- intense despair; seems flat or blunted
- anxiety related to delusions
- severe self-deprecation
- hostility directed inwardly
- no interests
- no decision-making ability
- delusions; intense self-persecution probably related to psychotic depression
- poor eating patterns with weight change, severe vegetative signs, self-neglect
- lower suicidal risk due to lack of energy
- slowing of thought processes
- early morning awakening
- extreme guilt
- constipation

DIAGNOSIS

Diagnosis for the patient with depression includes medical diagnoses based on the *Diagnostic and Statistical Manual of Mental Disorders* (*DSM-IV*) and nursing diagnoses. The *DSM-IV* diagnosis will be the admitting diagnosis and the diagnosis that will be used for documentation and reimbursement. The relevant diagnosis is major depression with single episode or recurrent and dysthymic disorder.[19] Selected nursing diagnoses based on the North American Nursing Diagnosis Association (NANDA) are[20]

- anxiety
- ineffective coping
- impaired verbal communication
- disturbance in self-esteem
- impaired social interaction

- potential for injury
- grieving
- self-care deficit
- alteration in sleep
- alteration in nutrition
- potential for violence: self-directed

EXPECTED OUTCOMES

Expected patient outcomes are identified as the initial treatment plan is developed and changed as the patient's condition changes. Desired outcomes that might be identified for a patient with depression include the following:

- The patient will experience a decrease in the symptoms of depression and view problems positively.
- The patient will exhibit the ability to control self-destructive feelings and behavior.
- The patient will identify coping mechanisms for self that might be used after discharge.
- The patient will identify problems/situations that may have contributed to the development of depression.
- The patient will exhibit normal activity level, sleep pattern, eating, and independent self-care within own limitations.
- The patient will identify the name(s) of medications, purpose, dosage and frequency, and side effects.
- The patient will comply with recommended treatment.
- The patient will participate in his or her treatment planning, assessment of progress, and discharge planning.

INTERVENTIONS IN THE HOME

There are three phases of treatment, because depression has three phases.[21] Knowledge of these phases helps the nurse focus the home care on the needs of the patient in each phase.

1. *Acute treatment* lasts from 6 to 12 weeks and focuses on remission of symptoms. A partial response is associated with a poorer prognosis.
2. *Continuation of treatment* lasts from four to nine months and focuses on prevention of relapse. During this phase medication is continued at the full dosage.
3. *Maintenance treatment* focuses on prevention of recurrence in patients who have had prior episodes of depression. Maintenance medication should be considered for patients who have[22]

- first-degree relative with bipolar disorder or recurrent major depression
- history of recurrence within one year after previously effective medication was discontinued
- early onset, before age 20, of the first episode
- two episodes of severe, sudden, or life-threatening depression in the past three years

Interventions must be individualized for each patient, and many interventions should be considered as the treatment plan is developed.

- Medications are a major part of the treatment for depression. Chapter 17 discusses antidepressants and their use in depression. These drugs are not habit forming or addictive and must be taken as prescribed. It is important to understand that it may take as long as six weeks to see the full effect of some antidepresssant medications. This can be frustrating for the patient, family/ SOs, and even the home care staff. The slow response, as well as side effects, may affect the patient's compliance. Compliance should be assessed at each visit. The patient needs to understand that he or she must maintain a serum level of the drug for the medication to be effective. AHCPR reports that "Determinations of antidepressant drug blood levels can establish that patients are receiving a therapeutic dosage, help in the evaluation of adherence, or exclude toxicity. Logically, patients cannot be declared to be nonresponsive to treatment unless the steady-state serum level is within the therapeutic range for at least 2 to 4 weeks."[23(p.62)]
- Home care staff inform the patient when they observe distorted, negative thinking, but this must not be done in a critical or disapproving manner. The patient will need help identifying reality factors. The goal is to clarify perceptions and assist the patient with reality factors. Pacing these discussions will help the patient tolerate them. There will be times when the patient may not be ready to discuss or accept new ideas.
- Acknowledging that depression is painful is important; however, staff should not allow the patient to dwell on this feeling. Staff should never tell the patient that the patient is not sad or depressed or has no reason to be depressed or sad. Value judgments are not helpful. Giving the patient false reassurance or using trite comments, such as "Everything will be alright" will only disturb the patient.
- If the patient is withdrawn, it is best for the patient to have one-to-one interactions rather than interacting with the whole family. When the patient is able to tolerate groups, gradually encourage the patient to increase family/ SO group participation.
- Staff should identify how the patient is making decisions, even if minor, and positively reinforce this behavior. As the patient problem solves, staff can

help identify alternatives. How has the patient coped in the past? Was the patient successful? Has the patient set realistic goals? Is the patient ready to make decisions? The patient may have memory problems and be unable to resolve problems due to the depression. In these circumstances, encouraging the patient to problem solve may only decrease the patient's self-esteem. Has the patient thought about the problem carefully? Is the patient taking an action that might cause problems? Major decisions should not be made while depressed. The nurse needs to be the reality-oriented person and help the patient learn to problem solve, providing feedback during the process. Exhibit 21–3 describes a problematic situation exercise that might be used with patients.

- Admission assessment and assessment throughout home care should include physical status, such as constipation, weight gain or loss, and lack of personal hygiene that may lead to physical problems. Patients with depression can have medical problems, medical problems may be causing the depression, and medications that are taken for medical problems may lead to depression. These factors must be routinely assessed.

- Doing too much for the patient can decrease the patient's self esteem. The patient may feel that staff and/or family/SOs do not think that the patient can care for self. Often there is a fine line between independence and dependence. There needs to be a doing "with" the patient and, as function increases, a letting go. Staff approach and attitude is very important. It is critical to allow the patient to do as much as he or she can and to take initiative. Reassessment of personal hygiene and activities of daily living (ADLs) is required, recognizing when the patient can be more independent. Care needs to be taken when assisting the patient to improve personal appearance, such as changing hair, makeup, etc. The patient may think it proves that "I don't look good." If the patient is interested in working on personal hygiene, family/SOs may be helpful in this area.

- Staff and family/SOs should be careful about being overly cheerful with the patient. This often is the natural response when people feel uncomfortable around a depressed person. This response, however, may only irritate the patient, and the patient may withdraw. If the patient withdraws, staff and the family/SOs should discuss this with the patient. This does not mean that they need to appear sad and depressed themselves. If the patient has particular problems with the family/SOs, staff should encourage the patient and the family/SOs to talk with each other. This may be done during a staff visit, in which case the nurse should follow up on the results of the discussion. Staff need to help the patient deal with the here and now and not run away from problems and relationships. Do not tell the patient what he or she is feeling, but rather allow opportunities for the patient to discuss feelings.

Exhibit 21–3 Problematic Situation Exercise

Problematic situation:

Effect of this situation on your life and the way you feel:

Strategies that might help:

Plans for implementing these strategies:

How these strategies have worked:

Source: Reprinted with permission from M. Copeland, *The Depression Workbook: A Guide for Living with Depression and Manic Depression*, p. 160, © 1992, New Harbinger Publications, Inc.

- False reassurance or use of trite comments such as, "Everything will be alright," is not a productive intervention. This only negates the patient's pain. Staff should help the patient focus on the meaning of loss, somatic symptoms, behavior, and feelings. Patients need honest answers and information about their illness, medical tests, etc.
- Nutrition is an area in which a depressed patient may have problems. Some may overeat, and others may not eat enough. The patient may have problems just getting to the dining room or kitchen due to a lack of energy or desire; however, the patient should be encouraged to attend meals. If there is minimal tension at mealtimes, this can be a positive time for the family/SOs to be together. Constantly badgering the patient to eat will not help the patient eat and may drive the patient away from the table. Providing the food that the patient likes might increase his or her appetite. Small, frequent feedings may be needed until the patient's appetite improves. Force feeding is an extreme intervention and should be avoided unless the patient's physical status is critical. This intervention requires more intensive care and, if the patient is not cooperative, it cannot be done in the home. Fluids are also important, and monitoring of intake and output may be required; however, as the patient is independent, this can be difficult for some patients to do in the home. Keep-

ing track is very difficult, particularly if the patient is uncooperative or confused. Cooperation of the family/SOs is very important.

- The admission assessment includes a description of the patient's sleep pattern prior to depression and during depression. The nurse may ask the patient or family/SOs to maintain a sleep log to assess sleep and changes in the sleep pattern, particularly noting the time of day the patient is sleeping, if the patient wakes up early or at intervals, and the number of hours of sleep. It is helpful to have this information when the patient says, "I didn't sleep," but the sleep log indicates the patient did sleep. Staff should identify problems and then intervene. During the assessment the patient is asked about his or her usual nighttime routine. How can the home environment accommodate the patient's needs without interfering with others who live in the home? What are the patient's activities before sleep? The patient should avoid in-depth discussions prior to sleep. Some activities may increase the patient's anxiety and should be avoided prior to sleep. It may be necessary for the nurse to consider the timing of medications and their dosage. Antidepressants given at bedtime may be more conducive to sleep, particularly if the patient experiences the side effect of drowsiness. The patient may use relaxation tapes or radio to assist with sleep. The patient should not eat or drink anything with caffeine after a certain time and may need to decrease intake during the day. Staff and the family/SOs should emphasize the need to be out of bed by a particular time and to be prepared for the day. To ensure that the patient's day has structure, a daily schedule should be developed with the patient. Staff then should discuss with the patient and the family/SOs how the schedule is maintained, adjusting the schedule as needed.
- If the patient is spending a lot of time alone, it may be necessary to develop a room plan or treatment contract to encourage the patient's interactions with the family/SOs. Use this information to plan with the patient. The patient should not be allowed to eat in his or her room or to stay isolated in his or her room. Staff should identify with the patient at least one activity that the patient will do or participate in during the day. Activities are gradually increased. If television is used to avoid people and consume time, it may be necessary to limit viewing time. The patient requires some time alone but with moderation. Staff and family/SOs should avoid becoming rigid policemen, as this will make everyone feel uncomfortable. As the patient gradually improves, flexibility becomes important. Frequent, short interactions with family/SOs may be more productive than long interactions. Sitting quietly with someone is less isolating than sitting alone in a room. It is also easy to ignore a family member who is depressed and isolated, and this is not helpful. The nurse can ask the family/SOs about the quality and quantity of their interactions with the patient.

- During the initial stages of home care when depression may be extreme, some dependency is expected. Gradually, when the patient is more able to tolerate it, independence should be encouraged.
- The patient needs time to discuss feelings and concerns about depression reoccurring. At this time, the patient will be more responsive to learning coping techniques for stress that can be used after discharge (such as stress management, relaxation, and use of recreation and time for self). Exhibit 21–4 provides an example of a daily checklist that may be used to identify early warning signs of depression. The patient must actively participate by first identifying his or her own early warning signs and then monitoring them.
- It is very important to assess suicidality routinely and intervene as needed. This is discussed in more detail in Chapter 29.
- As the patient prepares for discharge from home care, support groups may help the patient make the transition to independence and put the patient more in control of his or her illness and health. Exhibit 21–5 provides examples of organizations that sponsor support groups. The experience of a support group helps the patient feel that he or she is not alone, that others can understand, and that there is hope as others are seen getting better. Typically, support group meetings do the following:[24]
  1. provide people opportunity to share their problems and experiences, mutual counseling, advice, and support
  2. provide opportunity for people to share their pertinent educational speakers and programs
  3. offer referral to appropriate services and resources
  4. share activities, such as crafts, games, field trips, cooking, and watching videos
  5. lobby for services to benefit people with mood disorders
  After the patient attends a support group meeting, the home care staff should follow up and discuss the experience with the patient. Questions that might be asked include the following:[25]
  1. What did you hope to get out of going to the meeting?
  2. Did it meet your expectations?
  3. How did you feel at the meeting?
- The patient should pace himself or herself and avoid setting unrealistic expectations. Home care staff and family/SOs may help with setting realistic schedules. It took time for the depression to develop, and it will take time for it to go away.
- Compliance is usually a problem when the patient has a personality disorder or concurrent substance abuse in addition to depression, has a lack of acceptance of the diagnosis or treatment plan, and/or experiences problems with

Exhibit 21–4 Daily Checklist: Early Warning Signs of Depression

Early Warning Signs of Depression	Mon.	Tues.	Wed.	Thurs.	Fri.	Sat.	Sun.
Strategies To Cope with Depression	Mon.	Tues.	Wed.	Thurs.	Fri.	Sat.	Sun.

Source: Reprinted with permission from M. Copeland, *The Depression Workbook: A Guide for Living with Depression and Manic Depression*, pp. 107–108, © 1992, New Harbinger Publications, Inc.

Exhibit 21–5 Resources for Patient and Family/Significant Others

National Alliance for the Mentally Ill (NAMI)
   2101 Wilson Blvd., Suite 302
   Arlington, VA 22201
   Toll free: 800-950-6264
National Depressive and Manic Depressive Association (NDMDA)
   730 N. Franklin St., Suite 501
   Chicago, IL 60610
   Toll free: 800-826-3632
National Foundation for Depressive Illness (NFDI)
   P.O. Box 2257
   New York, NY 10116-2257
   Toll free: 800-248-4344
National Mental Health Association (NMHA)
   National Mental Health Information Center
   1021 Prince Street
   Alexandria, VA 23314-2971
   Toll free: 800-969-6642

medication side effects. Assessment data should note if the patient has a previous history of noncompliance, negative attitude toward treatment, significant lack of information or understanding about depression, or a potential need for maintenance therapy.[26]

- Cognitive therapy has helped many patients with depression. This is a goal-oriented approach, focusing on the here-and-now. According to AHCPR, the therapy "aims at symptom removal by identification and correction of the patient's distorted, negatively biased, moment-to-moment thinking and theoretically aims at prevention of relapse/recurrence by identifying and correcting silent assumptions."[27(p.75)] It is based on the theory that someone with depression views situations and people in a negative way. Cognitive distortions usually lead to negative emotions and inaccurate perception.[28] The patient must participate actively in solving current problems and be willing to learn more adaptive responses. Methods that are used in cognitive restructuring include the following:[29]

  1. *Monitoring thoughts and feelings.* The patient needs to become more self-aware and monitor thinking and feeling. Keeping a diary or log of dysfunctional thoughts will provide data to help the patient distinguish between thoughts and feelings and identify adaptive responses that would be alternatives. This will also help the patient recognize the connection between thoughts and maladaptive emotions and behaviors.

  2. *Questioning evidence.* The patient may need assistance in examining the evidence that supports a specific belief as well as the source of the belief. Distorted thinking tends to make the patient give equal weight to all sources or only accept data that support the distorted thinking.

  3. *Examining alternatives.* A depressed patient may feel that there are no options. The nurse can help to identify options with the patient.

  4. *Decatastrophizing.* This is the "what if" technique. The patient may be overestimating a situation, and it becomes a catastrophe. Suggested questions include these examples:
     −What is the worst thing that can happen?
     −Would it be so terrible if that really took place?
     −How would other people cope with such an event?

  5. *Reframing.* Reframing is a strategy that helps the patient view a situation or behavior from both positive and negative perspectives.

  6. *Thought stopping.* Thought stopping is a helpful strategy for the patient to use when negative thoughts occur.

- When a patient is depressed, tasks may seem overwhelming. Home care staff can help the patient break a task down into smaller parts. It may be easier to tackle a small task and then gradually to increase to complete the entire task. The patient can then receive positive feedback for accomplishing something, even if only part of a larger task.

- The nurse asks the patient to describe or list how depression has contributed to lowering his or her self-esteem. The examples should be specific and clear in order to facilitate a discussion about the relationship of feelings to behavior. Following this discussion, the patient is then asked to identify actions that could be taken to increase self-esteem. The patient should try these actions and evaluate them with assistance from the home care nurse.

THE HOME CARE PATIENT AND ELECTROCONVULSIVE THERAPY

The home care nurse may be assigned a patient who is receiving electroconvulsive therapy (ECT) as an outpatient. Patients who receive ECT usually meet one or more of the following criteria:[30]

- severe major depression that has not responded to adequate trial(s) of antidepressant medications
- psychotic depression
- antidepressant or neuroleptic medications pose a medical risk
- severe psychomotor retardation, suicidal behavior, or any clinical situation that requires a rapid response
- previous good response to ECT
- mixed manic episodes
- schizoaffective disorder responding only partially to medication
- catatonia

There are risks with the use of ECT. The patient and family/SOs may ask about these and should be informed of them by the physician prior to signing the consent for the treatments. The home care nurse may be asked about the risks during visits. Risks include the following:[31]

- has specific and significant side effects (e.g., short-term retrograde and anterograde amnesia)
- poses risks of general anesthesia
- is costly when hospitalization required
- is associated with substantial social stigma
- is contraindicated for some medical conditions or is considered high risk (e.g., space-occupying brain lesions and other causes of increased intracranial pressure, recent myocardial infarction, recent intracerebral hemorrhage, bleeding or otherwise unstable aneurysms or vascular malformations, and other conditions associated with increased anesthetic risk)[32]
- usually requires prophylaxis with antidepressant medication, even if a complete, acute-phase response to ECT is attained

To support and teach the patient and the family/SOs about the ECT procedure, the nurse must be knowledgeable about the procedure and its side effects. If the home care nurse is caring for an ECT patient and the nurse has limited experience with ECT, observing a treatment would be helpful. The patient may or may not have previously received ECT in an inpatient setting and may be frightened about the procedure and about coming home after it. Prior to beginning a series of treatments, the patient needs to have a history and physical within three months of the treatments; to undergo pre-ECT laboratory tests; and, after a discussion about the procedure with the physician, to sign the consent for ECT.

The patient should be informed about the procedure, preparation, anesthesia, recovery, and side effects. The night before each treatment, the patient is asked to avoid taking anything by mouth after midnight. The patient needs transportation to return home from the treatment due to the effects of general anesthesia. It is best if the patient wears comfortable clothing and no jewelry. Immediately prior to the treatment, atropine is given or other medications as ordered. The patient is asked to void and to remove dentures, contacts, and/or eyeglasses. Vital signs are taken and recorded. The patient should be told that experienced staff will administer the treatment and that the room will look like a treatment room in the hospital with medical equipment. The patient is given anesthesia and should not feel pain during the procedure. As the patient awakens from the procedure, nursing staff monitor vital signs, ensure that the patient is in good condition, and help orient the patient. As the patient becomes more alert, staff help the patient with ambulation. When able to eat, the patient is given food. The patient will experience some memory loss, but this is temporary. Staff should discuss the memory loss with family/SOs, because they will be coping with the loss daily in the home. When the patient returns home, staff and family/SOs assess the patient's mood and behavior as treatments continue. Home care staff document all relevant changes.

PATIENT EDUCATION

Copeland stated after completing a study of 120 people who had experienced a depressive disorder that "those people who personally take responsibility for their own wellness achieve the highest levels of stability, the highest levels of wellness, control over their own lives, and happiness. Learn all you can about mood disorders."[33(p.41)] Home care staff play a critical role in patient education and help the patient meet education goals. Examples of these goals include the following:

- The patient will identify cause, symptoms, and natural history of depression.
- The patient will describe treatment options, including indications, mechanisms of action, costs, risks, and benefits.
- The patient will identify when he or she needs support and help.
- The patient will identify name(s) of medications, purpose of taking, dosage and frequency, and side effects.

- The patient will identify potential difficulties with compliance and methods for resolving them.
- The patient will, if appropriate, describe the loss process and how it applies to self.
- The patient will identify early warning signs of relapse or recurrence.
- The patient will identify critical elements of stress management and assertiveness related to self.
- The patient will identify the importance of exercise and nutrition in maintaining health.
- The patient will identify the potential harmful effects of using alcohol/drugs to decrease depression.
- The patient will identify the importance of support groups and use them as appropriate.
- The patient will return to psychosocial and occupational functioning.

The AHCPR guidelines for treatment of depression in primary care suggest that the following content is included in patient education:[34(p.10)]

- Depression is a medical illness, not a character defect or weakness.
- Recovery is the rule, not the exception.
- Treatments are effective, and there are many options for treatment. An effective treatment can be found for nearly all patients.
- The aim of treatment is complete symptoms remission—not just getting better, but getting and staying well.
- The risk of recurrence is significant: 50 percent after one episode, 70 percent after two episodes, 90 percent after three episodes.
- Patient and family/SOs should be alert to early signs and symptoms of recurrence, and if depression returns, seek treatment early.

SEASONAL AFFECTIVE DISORDER

The major research on seasonal affective disorders (SAD) began in 1981. SAD is a syndrome of recurrent depressions occurring annually at the same time each year. Researchers believe that it is a reaction to changes in environmental factors such as climate, latitude, or light. These patients usually do not require hospitalization unless the depression is severe. The treatment can be provided on an outpatient basis. It is unlikely that a patient with this diagnosis would be referred for home care unless the depression is severe. However, the home care nurse may be caring for a patient who is referred for another reason, either psychiatric or nonpsychiatric, and encounter patient or family/SOs with this form of depression.

The biological origin of SAD has been identified. Light may affect physiology, causing a biochemically based depression in some people. The two factors that are thought to be related to this response are people who live farther from the equator and people who are unusually sensitive to light. The neurotransmitters melatonin and serotonin are thought to be involved.[35(p.231)]

During depressed periods, these patients experience symptoms that are found in most depressions as well as some that are specific to SAD. These include the following:

- anxiety
- sadness, crying
- decreased energy
- decreased ability to complete tasks or work
- irritability
- changes in appetite; overeating; craving carbohydrates
- weight gain
- decreased sexual interest
- sleep disturbances; hypersomnia

It is important to obtain a complete history and assessment to determine the nature of the symptoms, the recurrence, and time frame. This type of depression usually lasts about four months, beginning between October and December and ending in March. The course of the depression is variable, with some patients experiencing relatively little interference with functioning, and others experiencing great difficulties during this period.

Phototherapy is the most common treatment. This is done with a high-intensity light of 2500 lux or more. The patient uses it early in the morning and late in the evening to induce a summer-type environment and response. Patients can use this in their home. It takes time, but many patients find it helpful. Education about SAD is important. Patients are concerned about the depression returning and its effect on their personal lives. They need to discuss this openly. Teaching the patient about the use of phototherapy is critical, as they will be the ones providing the treatment.

Antidepressant medication may be used if phototherapy is not used or is unsuccessful.

FAMILY/SIGNIFICANT OTHERS: NEEDS AND STRATEGIES

Depression has been shown to result in negative interactions between the depressed family member and his or her family/SOs. Copeland identifies feelings and behaviors that patients with depression have identified, such as the following:[36]

- was or became a dysfunctional family
- they think it's all in my head

- disruption
- tension, stress
- estrangement
- anxiety
- denial
- lack of trust
- financially draining
- emotionally draining
- embarrassment
- confusion
- loss of hope
- patronizing attitudes
- lack of understanding
- everyone is affected by the stigma
- turmoil
- exclusion
- loss
- fear
- anger
- overprotection
- physically draining
- unpleasantness
- worry
- grief
- they're tired of me
- divorce
- they feel helpless
- I'm devalued by family members
- caused depression in other family members
- family members refuse to learn about my illness or take part in my treatment

In addition, Copeland found that patients identified supportive family members as family members who provide the following:[37]

- communication
- encouragement
- concern
- availability
- family members educated themselves about the problem
- monitoring
- financial support
- calling, writing, visiting

- understanding
- listening
- love
- tolerance
- attention
- education, advice, and counsel
- protection
- living space
- activities

This information is useful in helping home care staff understand the family dynamics during the experience of depression in a family member.

Badger identified other aspects of the family/SO and patient relationship during the time of depression,[38] including five protective strategies ("holding our ground"):

1. affirming affection to reassure the member with depression
2. suggesting alternatives to increase pleasurable activities
3. reducing conflict to decrease potential disagreements and tension
4. seeking social support to mobilize social networks
5. maintaining vigilance to protect physical and psychological safety

These strategies are used to prevent the family structure and its relationships from deteriorating further and to protect the ill member.

Families/SOs may also use coercive or "moving forward" strategies to force progress and recovery. These strategies include the following:

- excluding their ill member to eliminate or avoid communication or contact
- demanding change to force improvement, treatment involvement, or role resumption
- expressing emotions about ill member either verbally or physically
- threatening to leave the relationship
- managing resources to control all aspects of care

In addition to protective and coercive strategies, family/SOs may also use strategies to work the system. They can advocate with the physician and other health care professionals for appropriate diagnosis and treatment. Mobilizing resources to cope with access, quality, and cost issues will become very important to the family/SOs. Badger describes the strategies used by families/SOs with a depressed family member as similar to those used with families/SOs experiencing Alzheimer's, heart transplant, and other chronic illnesses; however, there are two differences.[39] First, stigma is a critical component with depression. Second, in comparison to other illnesses, depression has a different course; it usually can be treated, and death is not the usual result. Both of these factors are important to recognize as home care staff provide care in the home.

As the home care nurse discusses the illness and treatment with the patient and the family/SOs, the content must be relevant to the patient and family/SOs. Examples of typical topics that might be discussed are[40]

- understanding the illness
- medical intervention
- medications
- family dynamics
- relationships
- general mental health
- feelings and behavior
- protection methods
- mutual concerns
- getting outside help
- acceptance
- building trust
- doing more things together
- housing
- childhood issues
- ways to get along better
- communication
- support
- stigmatization
- forgiveness
- monitoring
- suicide
- financial issues

The patient's family may be very concerned about the genetic aspects of affective disorders and they may feel guilty about who caused the illness. The home care nurse "can teach that the illness is not an individual's fault but is rather for most a biologically inherited vulnerability."[41(p.69)] Patient and family/SO education is very important and supportive to the family/SOs working together without guilt.

SUMMARY

The depressed patient is a common referral to psychiatric home care, requiring patience and careful planning. The range of severity can be great, but usually treatment is successful. Treatment includes biological interventions—particularly medications, ECT, and exposure to light; patient education; and use of more effective coping skills.

NOTES

1. "News and Notes," *Hospital and Community Psychiatry* 45, no. 1 (1994): 85–86.

2. I. Abraham, "Depression: Nursing Implications of a Clinical and Social Problem," *Nursing Clinics of North America* 26, no. 3 (1991): 527–544, at 528.

3. "News and Notes," 85.

4. R. Howland, "Chronic Depression," *Hospital and Community Psychiatry* 44, no. 7 (1993): 633–639, at 633.

5. Howland, "Chronic Depression," 636.

6. Agency for Health Care Policy and Research, *Depression in Primary Care,* Vol. 1, *Detection and Diagnosis* (Rockville, MD: U.S. Department of Health and Human Services, 1993), 9.

7. Agency for Health Care Policy and Research, *Depression in Primary Care,* Vol. 1, *Detection and Diagnosis*, 6–7.

8. M. Copeland, *The Depression Workbook: A Guide for Living with Depression and Manic Depression* (Oakland, CA: New Harbinger Publications, Inc., 1992), 116.

9. W. Field, "Physical Causes of Depression," *Journal of Psychosocial Nursing* 23, no. 10 (1985): 7–11, at 9–10.

10. Field, "Physical Causes of Depression," 8–9.

11. S. Dubovsky and M. Thomas, "Psychotic Depression: Advances in Conceptualization and Treatment," *Hospital and Community Psychiatry* 43, no. 12 (1992): 1189–1198, at 1189.

12. Dubovsky and Thomas, "Psychotic Depression: Advances in Conceptualization and Treatment," 1190.

13. Dubovsky and Thomas, "Psychotic Depression: Advances in Conceptualization and Treatment," 1190.

14. Dubovsky and Thomas, "Psychotic Depression: Advances in Conceptualization and Treatment," 1190.

15. Dubovsky and Thomas, "Psychotic Depression: Advances in Conceptualization and Treatment," 1194.

16. Agency for Health Care Policy and Research, *Depression in Primary Care,* Vol. 1, *Detection and Diagnosis*, 75.

17. J. Kelley and L. Lehman, "Assessment of Anxiety, Depression, and Suspiciousness in the Home Care Setting," *Home Healthcare Nurse* 11, no. 2 (1993): 17–18.

18. Kelley and Lehman, "Assessment of Anxiety, Depression, and Suspiciousness in the Home Care Setting," 17–18.

19. American Psychiatric Association, *Diagnostic and Statistical Manual of Mental Disorders,* 4th ed. (Washington, DC: 1994), 20.

20. North American Nursing Diagnosis Association, *Nursing Diagnoses: Definitions and Classification,* 1995–1996 (Philadelphia: 1994), 13–14, 29, 37, 38, 50, 63, 65–69, 73, 81–82, 86.

21. Agency for Health Care Policy and Research, *Depression in Primary Care: Detection, Diagnosis, and Treatment,* Quick Reference Guide for Clinicians, no. 5 (Rockville, MD: U.S. Department of Health and Human Services, 1993), 9.

22. Agency for Health Care Policy and Research, *Depression in Primary Care: Detection, Diagnosis, and Treatment,* 18.

23. Agency for Health Care Policy and Research, *Depression in Primary Care,* Vol. 2, *Treatment of Major Depression* (Rockville, MD: U.S. Department of Health and Human Services, 1993), 62.

24. Copeland, *The Depression Workbook: A Guide for Living with Depression and Manic Depression*, 132.

25. Copeland, *The Depression Workbook: A Guide for Living with Depression and Manic Depression*, 132.

26. Agency for Health Care Policy and Research, *Depression in Primary Care*, Vol. 2, *Treatment of Major Depression*, 30.

27. Agency for Health Care Policy and Research, *Depression in Primary Care*, Vol. 2, *Treatment of Major Depression*, 75.

28. Copeland, *The Depression Workbook: A Guide for Living with Depression and Manic Depression*, 18.

29. G. Stuart, "Cognitive Behavioral Therapy," in *Principles and Practice of Psychiatric Nursing*, ed. G. Stuart and S. Sundeen (St. Louis, MO: Mosby–Year Book, 1995), 747–765, at 757–758.

30. Agency for Health Care Policy and Research, *Depression in Primary Care*, Vol. 2, *Treatment of Major Depression*, 95.

31. Agency for Health Care Policy and Research, *Depression in Primary Care*, Vol. 2, *Treatment of Major Depression*, 26–27.

32. Task Force Report of the American Psychiatric Association, *The Practice of Electroconvulsive Therapy: Recommendations for Treatment, Training, and Privileging* (Washington, DC: American Psychiatric Association, 1990), 58.

33. Copeland, *The Depression Workbook: A Guide for Living with Depression and Manic Depression*, 41.

34. Agency for Health Care Policy and Research, *Depression in Primary Care: Detection, Diagnosis, and Treatment*, 10.

35. M. Hensley and S. Rogers, "Shedding Light on 'SAD'ness," *Archives of Psychiatric Nursing* 1, no. 4 (1987): 230–231.

36. Copeland, *The Depression Workbook: A Guide for Living with Depression and Manic Depression*, 145–146.

37. Copeland, *The Depression Workbook: A Guide for Living with Depression and Manic Depression*, 147–148.

38. T. Badger, "Living with Depression: Family Members' Experiences and Treatment Needs," *Journal of Psychosocial Nursing* 34, no. 1 (1996): 21–29, at 23.

39. Badger, "Living with Depression: Family Members' Experiences and Treatment Needs," 28.

40. Copeland, *The Depression Workbook: A Guide for Living with Depression and Manic Depression*, 150.

41. S. Simmons-Alling, "Genetic Implications for Major Affective Disorders," *Archives of Psychiatric Nursing* 4, no. 1 (1990): 67–71, at 69.

SUGGESTED READING

Abraham, I. et al. 1991. Depression: Nursing implications of a clinical and social problem. *Nursing Clinics of North America* 26, no. 3: 527–543.

American Psychiatric Association. 1990. *The practice of electroconvulsive therapy: Recommendations for treatment, training, and privileging.* Washington, DC.

American Psychiatric Association. 1993. *Practice guideline for major depressive disorder in adults.* Washington, DC.

American Psychiatric Association. 1994. *Diagnostic and statistical manual of mental disorders.* 4th ed. Washington, DC.

Badger, T. et al. 1990. Assessment and management of depression. *Archives of Psychiatric Nursing* 4, no. 4: 235–240.

Beeber, L., ed. 1989. *Depression: Old problems, new perspectives in nursing care.* Thorofare, NJ: SLACK, Inc.

Berman, I. et al. 1992. Sertraline: A new serotonergic antidepressant. *Hospital and Community Psychiatry* 43, no. 7: 71–72.

Bushnell, F., and V. DeForge. 1994. Seasonal affective disorder. *Perspectives in Psychiatric Care,* 30, no. 4: 21–25.

Coffey, C., and R. Weiner. 1990. Electronconvulsive therapy: An update. *Hospital and Community Psychiatry* 41, no. 5: 515–521.

Depaulo, J., and K. Ablow. 1989. *How to cope with depression.* New York: McGraw-Hill.

Doenges, M. et al. 1989. *Psychiatric care plans.* Philadelphia: F.A. Davis.

Dubovsky, S., and M. Thomas. 1992. Psychotic depression: Advances in conceptualization and treatment. *Hospital and Community Psychiatry* 43, no. 12: 1189–1198.

Field, W. 1985. Physical causes of depression. *Journal of Psychosocial Nursing* 23, no. 10: 7–11.

Hagerty, B. 1995. Advances in understanding major depressive disorder. *Journal of Psychosocial Nursing* 33, no. 11: 27–33.

Hensley, M., and S. Rogers. 1987. Shedding light on 'SAD'ness, *Archives of Psychiatric Nursing* 1, no. 9: 230–235.

Howland, R. 1993. Chronic depression. *Hospital and Community Psychiatry* 44, no. 7: 633–639.

Kelley, J., and L. Lehman. 1993. Assessment of anxiety, depression, and suspiciousness in the home care setting. *Home Healthcare Nurse* 11, no. 2: 6–20.

Klein, D., and P. Wender. 1988. *Do you have a depressive illness?* New York: New American Library.

McFarland, G., and E. Wasli. 1986. *Nursing diagnoses and process in psychiatric mental health nursing.* Philadelphia: J.B. Lippincott Co.

Meador-Woodruff, J. 1990. Psychiatric side effects of tricyclic antidepressants. *Hospital and Community Psychiatry* 41, no. 1: 84–86.

Rorden, J. 1987. *Nurses as health teachers.* Philadelphia: W.B. Saunders Company.

Ryan, L. et al. 1987. Impact of circadian rhythm research on approaches to affective illness. *Archives of Psychiatric Nursing* 1, no. 9: 236–240.

Simmons-Alling, S. 1987. New approaches to managing affective disorders. *Archives of Psychiatric Nursing* 1, no. 4: 219–224.

Simmons-Alling, S. 1990. Genetic implications for major affective disorders. *Archives of Psychiatric Nursing* 4, no. 1: 67–71.

Stuart, G., and S. Sundeen. 1995. *Principles and practice of psychiatric nursing.* St. Louis, MO: C.V. Mosby.

Tirrell, C., and D. DeForest. 1987. Neuroendocrine factors in affective disorders. *Archives of Psychiatric Nursing* 1, no. 4: 225–229.

Townsend, M. 1988. *Nursing diagnoses in psychiatric nursing.* Philadelphia: F.A. Davis.

Wehr, T. et al. 1986. Phototherapy of seasonal affective disorder. *Archives of General Psychiatry* 43, no. 9: 870–875.

22

Bipolar Disorder

INTRODUCTION

Almost 2 million Americans have bipolar disorder or manic-depressive illness. It is an illness that can cause extreme suffering for the patient and the family/ significant others (SOs). However, it can usually be treated effectively with medications. The illness typically begins in adolescence or early adulthood and continues throughout life. It is not always easy to diagnose. Patients with this illness can continue their usual functioning with periods of relapse, but relapse is less likely if medication is continued.

DEFINING CHARACTERISTICS

Biological research related to bipolar disorder has focused on two areas: genetic and neurochemical. Bipolar disorder has a genetic component. Family studies have shown that the genetic risk factor for bipolar disorder is higher than that for major depressive disorder. The evidence indicates the following:[1(p.421)]

- one parent with bipolar disorder: 25 percent occurrence in a child
- two parents with bipolar disorder: 50–75 percent occurrence in a child
- one monozygotic twin bipolar: 40–70 percent occurrence in other twin
- one dizygotic twin bipolar: about 20 percent occurrence in other twin
- one parent with depressive disorder: 10–13 percent occurrence in a child

The development of the disorder may be related to nutrition, infection, and psychological factors. Genetic factors only make the person more vulnerable. People under 50 have a higher risk of a first attack.[2] Being female is a risk factor. Bipolar disorder has high morbidity and mortality associated with suicide; 10 to

15 percent of untreated patients commit suicide. This suicide rate is 15 to 20 times higher than that found in the general population.[3]

Two neurotransmitters, serotonin and norepinephrine, are important in bipolar disorder. These neurochemicals are responsible for the functions of mood, sleep, appetite, and sexual activity. These functions are disturbed in bipolar disorder, as well as in depression. In depression, norepinephrine levels are lowered. In bipolar disorder they are elevated, and it is thought that this elevation causes elation and euphoria.[4] In addition, certain changes in biological rhythms and related physiology occur in mood disorders, such as body temperature and hormones reach their peak earlier.[5] The absence of sunlight may negatively affect a depressed patient.

In the early stages of the illness, the patient may experience hypomania. During this time the patient experiences a high level of energy, excessive moodiness, and impulsive behavior. This may feel good to the patient, and the patient may then deny that there is a problem. However, the patient may experience problems in school or work performance. The illness can also be covered over with alcohol or drug abuse.

Both the manic and depressive phases focus on alterations in mood. Each phase includes problems with self-esteem and aggression and operate in a cyclic manner. There are variations among individuals, and thus it is important to identify each person's pattern or cycle. During the manic phase, the patient may experience extremes in mood with excitability, elation, impulsivity, inability to sleep, excessive or decreased appetite, and increased physical activity. Some patients appear to be the "life of the party" at this time; however, suddenly they can become very irritable and difficult to control. During the depressive phase, the patient may experience symptoms of depression. If the patient moves quickly from manic to depressive phase, there is increased risk of suicidal feelings.

Even though it is generally accepted that there is treatment for bipolar disorder, a 1991 study indicated that the news is not as positive as once thought.[6] This study was a seven-and-a-half-year follow-up of formerly hospitalized patients with bipolar disorder. About 40 percent of the patients who received lithium, sometimes combined with other treatments, continued to experience marked emotional highs and lows, as well as serious problems at work and home. Overall functioning consistently improved among one in three lithium-treated patients. Several other studies have also reported poor outcomes. Factors that might account for these poor outcomes are

- failure to take lithium
- failure to follow prescription instructions
- occurrence of "mixed states" when symptoms of mania exist with symptoms of depression
- rapid alterations between periods of mania and depression

ASSESSMENT

Guidelines for Assessment

Assessment can be difficult because the patient often does not recognize that there is a problem. If the patient does admit that there is a problem, the patient may identify the cause of the problem as something other than mental illness. The patient may be uncooperative during assessment due to this denial or due to manic behavior that makes it difficult for the patient to focus on the assessment. "When encountering a patient experiencing a manic episode, you'll notice first his elevated energy level, increased enthusiasm, and euphoric outlook. The feelings of deep depression that underlie this surface elation may occasionally surface in bouts of sadness and withdrawal or outbursts of irritability and anger. Most of the time, however, the patient has little control over his incessant animation."[7(p.83)]

Mania can be secondary to some prescription medications and some medical illnesses. Medications of particular concern are steroids, levodopa, amphetamines, methylphenidate, cocaine, monoamine oxidase inhibitors, tricyclic antidepressants, and thyroid hormones.[8] Illnesses that can cause mania are influenza, St. Louis encephalitis, Q fever, general paresis (tertiary syphilis), possibly hyperthyroidism, systemic lupus erythematosus, rheumatic chorea, multiple sclerosis, and diencephalic and third ventricular tumors.[9] A complete history and physical including a medication history is required to rule out these possible causes for the patient's mania. Toxicology screens are also useful to determine if the patient has been using alcohol or other drugs.

Signs and Symptoms

The signs and symptoms for bipolar disorder are categorized by the two phases, the manic phase and the depressive phase.

Manic Phase

The signs and symptoms of the manic phase include the following:

- increased activity; restlessness; inability to complete a project or task
- denial of problems
- inability to recognize fatigue
- high self-esteem; grandiose ideas; unrealistic beliefs in one's abilities and powers
- decreased ability to sleep to the extreme of no sleep
- increased or decreased appetite; no time to eat
- decreased ability to concentrate

- increased irritability with sudden changes
- racing thoughts
- loose associations
- increased talking with pressure of speech
- increased sexual urges
- impulsive acts (e.g., spending excessive amounts of money)
- change in dress to extreme of bright colors and excessive makeup
- limited time for personal hygiene
- increased voice volume
- doing activities in excess
- lack of confidence in solving problems
- delusions
- hallucinations
- attention-seeking behavior
- insulting or hypercritical comments about others
- extreme independence; dislike for directions from others
- poor judgment
- testing limits
- denial of responsibility for self
- sarcasm
- demanding attitude

Important physiological signs and symptoms are dehydration, inadequate nutrition, weight loss, and a lowered sleep requirement. These symptoms are caused by the excessive behavior; if the patient does not receive treatment, these symptoms can lead to serious problems.

Depressive Phase

Signs and symptoms of the depressive phase include the following:

- fatigue, often without cause
- decreased ability to enjoy people or activities
- decreased sleep; sleeping mostly during the day; sleep disturbances
- decreased appetite
- decreased sexual urges
- sad for no specific reason
- suicidal thoughts or attempts, particularly if patient feels guilty, hopeless, worthless
- difficulty in making decisions and following through
- hallucinations
- delusions

- decreased activity
- difficulty concentrating or remembering
- chronic pain or other persistent bodily symptoms that are not caused by physical disease

DIAGNOSIS

Diagnosis for bipolar disorder can be complicated, because consideration must be given to both depressive and manic features as well as recurrence. According to the American Psychiatric Association (APA): "Recurrence is indicated by either a shift in the polarity of the episode or an interval between episodes of at least 2 months without manic symptoms. A shift in polarity is defined as a clinical course in which a major depressive episode evolves into a manic episode or a mixed episode or in which a manic episode or a mixed episode evolves into a major depressive episode."[10(p.351)]

The medical diagnoses are categorized into bipolar I disorder, bipolar II disorder, and cyclothymic disorder.[11]

- *Bipolar I disorder* is defined as a "current or past experience of a manic episode, lasting at least 1 week, when one's mood was abnormally and persistently elevated, expansive, or irritable. The episode is sufficiently severe to cause extreme impairment in social or occupational functioning."[12(p.434)] The patient's illness is classified according to the presence of mania with only manic episodes, depressed with a history of manic episodes and a current depressive episode, or a mixed illness having both manic and depressive episodes.
- *Bipolar II disorder* includes one or more major depressive episodes and at least one hypomanic episode with no manic episodes. Hypomania is similar to mania but not as severe.
- *Cyclothymic disorder* includes a "history of 2 years of hypomania in which the person experienced numerous periods with abnormally elevated, expansive, or irritable moods."[13(p.434)]

Nursing diagnoses are based on the North American Nursing Diagnosis Association (NANDA) diagnoses, particularly the following:[14]

- anxiety
- individual coping ineffective
- impaired verbal communication
- disturbance in self-esteem
- risk for injury
- alteration in thought processes
- alteration in sensory perceptions

- grieving
- self-care deficit
- sleep pattern disturbance
- alteration in nutrition
- sexual dysfunction
- risk for violence: self-directed

EXPECTED OUTCOMES

Establishing expected outcomes is important but difficult with the patient who has a bipolar disorder. This patient may deny the illness or be unrealistic. The home care nurse should guide the patient carefully as outcomes are developed. Examples of desired outcomes include the following:

- The patient exhibits behavior that is appropriate (neither manic or depressed).
- The patient exhibits appropriate sleep pattern, eating, and independent self-care within own limitations.
- The patient participates in treatment planning, assessment of progress, and discharge plan.
- The patient identifies and uses coping mechanisms for hyperactivity as well as for depression.
- The patient identifies name(s) of medications, purpose of taking, laboratory tests required, dosage and frequency, and side effects.
- The patient maintains compliance with medication and lithium serum level laboratory testing.
- The patient makes realistic statements about self.
- The patient performs activities of daily living.
- The patient maintains interpersonal relationships.

INTERVENTIONS IN THE HOME

- Home care staff assess changes in mood and behavior during each home visit. Increased irritability, increased physical activity, or symptoms of depression are of particular importance. If there is a pattern of changes in behavior and mood, this is identified.
- Suicidality and escalating behavior are always assessed. The patient has poor judgment, and safety is always an issue.
- The patient needs to know that the home care staff and family/SOs expect the patient to behave appropriately. This should not be communicated in a threatening manner, but in a manner that communicates a calm and caring attitude.
- Setting limits on inappropriate behavior is a frequent intervention during the manic phase. The patient should not be allowed to embarrass himself or her-

self or hurt others. Family/SOs must understand the importance of setting limits.

- A calm environment helps to decrease manic behavior. Increased stimulation is not helpful. Use of time-outs in the patient's room; treatment contracts; removing the patient from areas of loud music, television, and group activities in the home may be interventions to decrease excessive behavior. Whenever group activities are used, the patient must be observed carefully because too many people may not be helpful.

- Contact with reality may be distorted; however, the patient still perceives the environment and what is occurring, even if at a faster pace. All efforts must be made to reinforce and focus on reality.

- Arguing or trying to reason with the patient (particularly about grandiose ideas and delusions) will only increase the patient's anxiety and escalation.

- The family/SOs should suggest that the patient leave situations in which the patient has become the "life of the party" as this often leads to more escalation.

- Communication should be with a quiet, firm voice; use simple, short sentences. Due to the patient's distractibility and rapid thoughts and speech, the patient's concentration is poor. Detailed explanations are not appropriate or useful when the patient is manic.

- Outlets for physical activity such as exercise or physical work projects may be helpful, but the patient may not be able to do the same activity for long periods of time.

- Home care staff and family/SOs should not participate in the patient's "high" behavior. Staff as well as family/SOs may be the focus of irritability, jokes, etc., and this can increase the patient's anxiety. Staff and family/SOs need appropriate outlets for their own anxiety.

- Staff and family/SOs must be alert for the patient's involvement in "schemes" such as spending excessive amounts of money, shopping sprees, excessive use of telephone, overuse of alcohol, making unrealistic plans, and promiscuity. The patient may try to get others involved in these excessive activities.

- It is easy to miss a problem related to nutrition and fluid with a patient who looks very active, so these areas need frequent assessment. If the patient cannot sit down to eat, "on-the-run" foods (foods the patient can eat standing or moving) may be helpful. High-protein, high-calorie foods, and, in some cases, supplemental feedings may help prevent nutritional problems. The patient's weight should be checked periodically.

- The patient may not recognize when he or she is tired. Monitoring rest and sleep is critical, and if there is a problem, interventions to induce sleep may be required. A sleep log to assess sleep deprivation may be useful. During manic symptoms when the patient may be getting less sleep at night, a rest period may be suggested during the day. Dimming room light and reducing noise stimuli may help the patient rest. The patient may require adjustment in medication. If medication begins to sedate the patient, staff should recognize that this is a temporary problem as the patient adjusts to the medication.

- The patient may not be able to identify physical problems or side effects from medications, so staff and family/SOs must play an important role in assessing the need for interventions.
- Lithium does not decrease symptoms quickly. The patient may require antipsychotic medication until lithium begins to decrease symptoms.
- Some patients require assistance in maintaining personal hygiene. If the patient is dressed inappropriately, staff and family/SOs set limits and assist the patient to dress more appropriately.
- When there is inappropriate sexual behavior, limits on this behavior must be set immediately.
- As the patient learns about the illness, it is critical for the patient to understand that the illness cannot be cured and that continued treatment is very important.
- Food and beverages with caffeine (such as coffee, tea, chocolate, and cola) need to be avoided. These increase anxiety and hyperactivity.
- Activities that are competitive and require a long attention span or fine motor skills are usually unsuccessful and stressful for the patient.
- During a manic episode, it is difficult for the patient to stay focused when experiencing so many thoughts and so much energy. According to Copeland, "The goal is to stay grounded and focused enough to get something done, rather than being very scattered and initiating lots of projects that remain unfinished. A daily plan or schedule can help meet this goal."[15(p.83)]
- When a task is overwhelming or the patient is unable to complete a task due to decreased concentration, breaking the task down into smaller parts is helpful. When the patient's energy level is constantly changing, a smaller part of a task may be easier for the patient to focus on and complete.
- It is not uncommon for a patient to feel embarrassed and guilty after a manic episode when the patient may have acted in a bizarre manner. The patient will need support from family/SOs and the home care staff to accept this behavior as part of the illness.
- The patient may experience an increase in the intensity of mania toward the end of the day. The nurse should work with the patient to identify strategies that might be used during these times (e.g., adjusting medication, writing in a journal or diary, doing relaxation exercises, talking with someone, reading a book, listening to music, or decreasing stimuli).
- Some patients experience a seasonal pattern to their mania. Copeland found that patients experienced mania more in the spring than summer or fall, and patients experienced mania least in the winter.[16] If a patient experiences a seasonal pattern, the patient can be alert to symptoms during these periods

and try to prevent the mania from increasing by maintaining medication, consulting with the physician, relaxing as much as possible, monitoring sleep and nutrition carefully, and using more support from others.

- Medication compliance should be monitored. The effectiveness of lithium requires that the serum level is maintained. Lithium serum levels must be monitored with blood testing to determine compliance and to assess toxicity levels. The patient will need to have blood drawn, and arrangements should be made for this procedure. The home care nurse should be aware of the results and discuss them with the patient's physician and with the patient.
- The patient may fear reporting symptoms that may indicate the need for more intensive treatment such as hospitalization. Manic behavior is obvious to all around the patient; however, the subtle cues or triggers that may indicate that the patient is going into the manic phase may be difficult for others to identify. Self-monitoring is important, but the patient must also feel comfortable enough to ask others for help. Exhibit 22–1 provides a list of typical warning signs of mania identified by patients. Exhibit 22–2 is a tool that may be used to monitor warning signs for an individual patient. Encouraging self-monitoring is important.
- Thought stopping may be useful for this patient.
- To encourage active patient participation in treatment planning and assessment of outcomes, home care staff should ask the patient to participate in identifying strategies to alleviate or eliminate mania. A tool that can be used for this is found in Exhibit 22–3.

Interventions for the depressive phase are found in Chapter 21 on depressive disorders.

RELAPSE

Relapse is a critical issue in bipolar disorder. According to Pollack, "Relapse reduction programs need to be based upon an awareness that relapse is most likely to occur when barriers are encountered, and that people with the disorder perceive barriers to be everywhere. Efforts are needed to teach patients problem-solving skills and how to deal with and overcome barriers."[17(p.128)] Those factors that have been considered important in preventing relapse are treatment organization; laboratory and clinical monitoring; the choice of drug, dosage, and treatment regimen; patient and family education; and psychotherapeutic and social support.[18]

Pollack addressed the issue of relapse and stability in bipolar disorder in her study that included 33 patients who were hospitalized with bipolar disorder.[19] Even though her study focused on hospitalized patients, the ideas presented have

Exhibit 22–1 Typical Early Warning Signs of Mania

- insomnia
- surges of energy
- flight of ideas
- writing pressure
- sleeping much less
- spending too much money
- unnecessary phone calls
- wanting to keep moving
- increased appetite
- euphoria
- feeling superior
- increased superiority
- overambition
- taking on too much responsibility
- nervous and wound up
- anxious
- overly self-involved
- negativism
- feeling unreal
- more sensitive than usual
- out of touch with reality
- inappropriate behavior
- poor judgment
- oblivious
- increased alcohol consumption
- dangerous driving
- increased community involvement
- tingly feeling
- friends notice behavior change

- others seem slow
- speech pressure
- making lots of plans
- irritability
- inappropriate anger
- money loses its value
- difficulty staying still
- restlessness
- compulsive eating
- feeling great
- feeling very important
- obsessions
- unusual bursts of enthusiasm
- very productive
- doing several things at once
- inability to concentrate
- outbursts of temper
- disorganization
- ability to foresee things happening
- noises louder than usual
- bizarre ideas, thoughts
- laugh to self uncontrollably
- thrill seeking
- more sexually active
- danger to self and others
- spotless, energetic housekeeping
- itching
- flushed and hot
- increased sociability

Source: Reprinted with permission from M. Copeland, *The Depression Workbook: A Guide for Living with Depression and Manic Depression*, pp. 77–78, © 1992, New Harbinger Publications, Inc.

relevance to patients with bipolar disorder in the home. Seeking information and self-management are important in all settings but particularly in the home setting. Patients with this illness will encounter barriers on a long-term basis. The most important barrier is denial, which can occur at any stage of the illness. The results of Pollack's study suggest that a person with bipolar disorder will go through various phases; however, these phases may not always be experienced in an or-

Exhibit 22–2 Daily Checklist: Early Warning Signs of Mania

Early Warning Signs of Mania	Mon.	Tues.	Wed.	Thurs.	Fri.	Sat.	Sun.
Strategies To Cope with Mania	Mon.	Tues.	Wed.	Thurs.	Fri.	Sat.	Sun.

Source: Reprinted with permission from M. Copeland, *The Depression Workbook: A Guide for Living with Depression and Manic Depression,* p. 109, © 1992, New Harbinger Publications, Inc.

derly manner. The first phase is realization of need, which must be present to motivate the patient to seek information to help manage the illness. There are times when the patient may not want to give up the positive aspects of a manic mood, because the patient feels very good. In order for the patient to accept the illness and be motivated to learn, the patient needs to feel positive about himself or herself. The second phase is information seeking. Some of the important influences affecting information seeking are a desire for normalcy, the severity of the illness, the pain it inflicts, and concerns for family/SOs.[20] The patient should know about appropriate information and support resources. The third phase is the critical point in the self-management process. At this time, the patient must evaluate the information obtained. The ability to analyze is important, and the patient must feel that it is applicable specifically to himself or herself. In order to use self-management, the patient must have energy, be stabilized on medication, have the will to succeed in managing the illness, and have access to resources. Barriers to self-management include fear of success; fear of failure; and suicidal, depressed, and hopeless feelings.[21] The fourth and last phase is self-management, which is an advanced activity. It can fail due to a lack of information on self-management activities, poor living arrangements, insufficient tolerance and giving up too soon, medication noncompliance, inability to communicate to others that one is not feeling well or suicidal, not trying to do one's best, denial, or stubbornness.[22]

Exhibit 22–3 Strategies for Alleviating or Eliminating Mania

Activities	Have Tried Successfully	Should Use More Often	Would Like To Try
Exercise			
Long walks			
Yoga			
Reading			
Listening to music			
Long, hot baths			
Gardening			
Needlework			
Working with wood			
Working with clay, pottery			
Drawing, painting			
Journal writing			
Writing poetry			
Writing letters			
Canoeing			
Horseback riding			
Shopping			
Relaxing in a meditative natural setting			
Playing a musical instrument			
Cleaning			
Watching television			
Watching videos, a movie, or a play			
Helping others			
Turning energy into creativity			

continues

Exhibit 22–3 continued

Support	Have Tried Successfully	Should Use More Often	Would Like To Try
Talking it out with an understanding person			
Getting emotional support from a person I trust			
Talking to a therapist or counselor			
Spending time with good friends			
Talking to staff at a crisis clinic or hotline			
Arranging not to be alone			
Reaching out to someone who understands			
Going to a support group			
Peer counseling			
Attitude	**Have Tried Successfully**	**Should Use More Often**	**Would Like To Try**
Changing negative thought patterns to positive ones			
Remembering that mania ends			
Focusing on living one day at a time			
Understanding what is happening			
Staying neutral			
Stopping regularly to ask myself, "How am I feeling right now?"; bringing my mind in touch with my body			

continues

Exhibit 22–3 continued

Management	Have Tried Successfully	Should Use More Often	Would Like To Try
Consulting with doctor			
Sleeping			
Eating a diet high in complex carbohydrates			
Avoiding caffeine and sugar			
Avoiding stimulating places and activities			
Using relaxation tapes and exercises daily			
Writing down a list of things to do and sticking to it			
Being in a quiet room with no outside stimuli			
Using self-control as much as possible			
Biofeedback			
Staying away from alcohol and illegal drugs			
Staying home			
Avoiding overextending myself			
Stimulating the left brain by paying attention to detail			
Surrendering all credit cards, checks, etc., to a responsible person			
"Tying" self down emotionally to familiar surroundings			
Staying away from groups of people			
Reducing environmental stress			

Source: Reprinted with permission from M. Copeland, *The Depression Workbook: A Guide for Living with Depression and Manic Depression*, pp. 80–82, © 1992, New Harbinger Publications, Inc.

Pollack said that "It was reported by a participant that if a person is feeling 'good' that person is not going to spend time thinking about whether what was being done was contributing to the good feeling. The good feeling would be accepted, without thought being given as to why it happened."[23(p.127)]

PATIENT EDUCATION

Patient education is very important, because the patient will need to manage the illness long term. One resource for information and support groups is the National Depressive and Manic Depressive Association. This organization can be contacted at Merchandise Mart, P.O. Box 3395, Chicago, Illinois 60654 and at (312) 939-2442. Patient education goals should be developed for each individual patient. The following are examples of typical education goals:

- The patient will identify medication(s), purpose, dosage and frequency, side effects, and need to monitor serum level if required.
- The patient will describe the phases of bipolar illness and relate to own cycle.
- The patient will identify indicators to self-monitor mood changes.
- The patient will identify strategies for seeking help
- The patient will identify critical elements of stress management and assertiveness related to self.
- The patient will identify the importance of exercise and nutrition in maintaining health.

FAMILY/SIGNIFICANT OTHERS: NEEDS AND STRATEGIES

Due to the manic behavior and the cyclic characteristic of the illness, family/SOs must cope with many problems. An ill family member who spends most of the family's money or exhibits other excessive behavior can cause much heartache for the family. The ill family member needs encouragement and support from family/SOs; at times this may be difficult for the family/SOs when they feel stress from experiencing the ill family member's behavior. Initially it may be the family/SOs who insist or force the ill family member to receive treatment.

SUMMARY

Caring for the patient with bipolar disorder who is manic is difficult in any setting. In the home with less structure, it is particularly problematic. Everyone who lives with the patient should become actively involved in the home care treatment. Home care staff are present for only a small part of the day. If the patient's behavior escalates and cannot be controlled, hospitalization may be required. If this occurs, the home care nurse must help the family/SOs express their feelings about the hospitalization and help them recognize that they are not to blame.

NOTES

1. G. Stuart, "Emotional Responses and Mood Disorders," in *Principles and Practice of Psychiatric Nursing*, ed. G. Stuart and S. Sundeen (St. Louis, MO: Mosby–Year Book, 1995), 413–451, at 421.
2. Stuart, "Emotional Responses and Mood Disorders," 417.
3. Agency for Health Care Policy and Research, *Depression in Primary Care*. Vol. 1. *Detection and Diagnosis* (Washington, DC: U.S. Department of Health and Human Services, 1993), 4.
4. Nurse Review, *Psychiatric Problems* (Springhouse, PA: Springhouse Corporation, 1990), 82.
5. Stuart, "Emotional Responses and Mood Disorders," 425.
6. B. Bower, "Manic Depression: Success Story Dims," *Science News* 139 (May 25, 1991): 7.
7. Nurse Review, *Psychiatric Problems*, 83.
8. Stuart, "Emotional Responses and Mood Disorders," 429.
9. Stuart, "Emotional Responses and Mood Disorders," 429.
10. American Psychiatric Association, *Diagnostic and Statistical Manual of Mental Disorders*, 4th ed. (Washington, DC: 1994), 351.
11. American Psychiatric Association, *Diagnostic and Statistical Manual of Mental Disorders*, 20.
12. Stuart, "Emotional Responses and Mood Disorders," 434.
13. Stuart, "Emotional Responses and Mood Disorders," 434.
14. North American Nursing Diagnosis Association, *Nursing Diagnoses: Definitions and Classification, 1995–1996* (Philadelphia: 1994), 13–14, 37–39, 42, 50, 63, 65–69, 74, 75, 79, 81–82, 86.
15. M. Copeland, *The Depression Workbook: A Guide for Living with Depression and Manic Depression* (Oakland, CA: New Harbinger Publications, Inc., 1992), 83.
16. Copeland, *The Depression Workbook: A Guide for Living with Depression and Manic Depression*, 103.
17. L. Pollack, "Striving for Stability with Bipolar Disorder Despite Barriers," *Archives of Psychiatric Nursing* 9, no. 3 (1995): 122–129, at 128.
18. M. Schou, "Relapse Prevention in Manic Depressive Illness: Important and Unimportant Factors," *Canadian Journal of Psychiatry* 36, no. 7: 501–504, at 502.
19. Pollack, "Striving for Stability with Bipolar Disorder Despite Barriers," 125.
20. Pollack, "Striving for Stability with Bipolar Disorder Despite Barriers," 126.
21. Pollack, "Striving for Stability with Bipolar Disorder Despite Barriers," 127.
22. Pollack, "Striving for Stability with Bipolar Disorder Despite Barriers," 127.
23. Pollack, "Striving for Stability with Bipolar Disorder Despite Barriers," 127.

SUGGESTED READING

American Psychiatric Association. 1995. *Diagnostic and statistical manual of mental disorders.* 4th ed. Washington, DC.

American Psychiatric Association. 1995. *Practice guidelines for treatment of patients with bipolar disorder.* Washington, DC.

Andreasen, N., and I. Glick. 1988. Bipolar affective disorder and creativity: Implications and clinical management. *Comprehensive Psychiatry* 29, no. 3: 207–217.

Coryell, W. et al. 1993. The enduring psychosocial consequences of mania and depression. *American Journal of Psychiatry* 150, no. 5: 720–727.

Dime-Meenan, S. 1995. Manic depression: Addressing family concerns. *Current Approaches to Psychoses: Diagnosis and Management* 4, no. 7: 7–8.

Goodwin, F., and K. Jamison. 1990. *Manic-depressive illness.* New York: Oxford University Press.

Gulesserian, B., and C. Warren. 1987. Coping resources of depressed patients. *Archives of Psychiatric Nursing* 1, no. 1: 392–395.

Horton, R., and C. Katona. 1991. *Biological aspects of affective disorders.* New York: Harcourt Brace Jovanovich.

Keitner, G. 1990. *Depression and families: Impact and treatment.* Washington, DC: American Psychiatric Press.

Keller, M., and L. Baker. 1991. Bipolar disorder: Epidemiology, course, diagnosis, and treatment. *Bulletin of the Menninger Clinic* 55, no. 1: 172–181.

Loomis, M. 1985. Levels of contracting. *Journal of Psychosocial Nursing* 23, no. 3: 9–14.

Maurin, J., and C. Boyd. 1990. Burden of mental illness on the family: A critical review. *Archives of Psychiatric Nursing* 4, no. 2: 99–107.

McEnany, G. 1990. Psychobiological indices of bipolar mood disorder: Future trends in nursing care. *Archives of Psychiatric Nursing* 4, no. 1: 29–38.

Pollack, L. 1995. Informational needs of patients hospitalized for bipolar disorder. *Psychiatric Services* 46, no. 11: 1191–1194.

Pollack, L. 1995. Striving for stability with bipolar disorder despite barriers. *Archives of Psychiatric Nursing* 9, no. 3: 122–129.

Pollack, L. 1995. Treatment of inpatients with bipolar disorders: A role for self-management groups. *Journal of Psychosocial Nursing* 33, no. 1: 11–16.

Schou, M. 1991. Relapse prevention in manic depressive illness: Important and unimportant factors. *Canadian Journal of Psychiatry* 36, no. 7: 502–506.

Simmons-Alling, S. 1990. Genetic implications for major affective disorders. *Archives of Psychiatric Nursing* 4, no. 1: 67–71.

Stuart, G., and S. Sundeen. 1995. *Principles and practice of psychiatric nursing.* St. Louis, MO: Mosby–Year Book.

Tardiff, K. 1989. *Assessment and management of violent patients.* Washington, DC: American Psychiatric Press, Inc.

23

Schizophrenia

INTRODUCTION

The seriously mentally ill, those patients with schizophrenia, are often admitted to the hospital for initial diagnosis and treatment or for severe, recurrent episodes; however, many are seen in the home either for treatment of schizophrenia or for treatment of medical problems in addition to schizophrenia. Many of these patients are young, which may cause home care staff to have many feelings about the chronicity of the illness in a young population. In the past, the prognosis for this disorder was the "rule of thirds": a third recovered, a third moderately improved, a third remained unimproved. Recently, this prognosis has changed. Torrey suggests that over the life course, 50 to 60 percent of patients may be "completely recovered" to "relatively independent."[1(pp.116–117)] In a research review, Malone noted that "professionals have little sense of what 'meaning' schizophrenia has for patients or their families [which] illustrates a lack of understanding of the human responses to mental illness."[2(p.6)] Hauk stated that "Home health nurses provide care in an ideal setting for such skill training because the home environment usually is less threatening to schizophrenic patients than anywhere else."[3(p.267)]

DEFINING CHARACTERISTICS

In recent years a biological model has been developed for schizophrenia. This has stimulated the growth of the discipline of neuroscience, which is a combination of related disciplines that share the common goal of understanding the relationship between brain structure and function and human thoughts, feelings, and behavior. Considerable evidence has been gained from research in the past 10 years that indicates schizophrenia is a brain disease with a likely pathological site in the limbic system. This system is the gate in the brain through which all incoming stimuli must pass. It is within this system that the individual selects, integrates, and unifies stimuli and experiences into organized reality. This site also contains most of the elements that define individual personality, cognitive style, and patterns of behavior.[4] Research indicates that in some patients there are changes in structure, particularly enlarged lateral and third ventricles and dilated cortical fissures and sulci.[5] In these locations, cells have been damaged, died, and the tissue has grown smaller with the ventricles enlarging to fill the empty space. These changes seem to relate more to severe symptoms or negative symptoms of schizophrenia.

Patients with schizophrenia exhibit problems related to inadequate processing of stimuli or information from the environment. These problems include difficulties in[6]

- selection of relevant stimuli
- direction and maintaining attention
- recognition and identification of stimuli
- integration, storage, recollection, and use of information appropriately

Schizophrenia is not split personality or multiple personality. This is a separate disorder, even though many laypersons think these are the same disorders.

Other biological factors that are important in schizophrenia are familial predisposition and biochemical stressors. Genetic theory has not yet been proven; however, there seems to be more and more evidence about the relevance of heredity as a factor that increases the vulnerability to schizophrenia. According to Kendler, "What is inherited is a predisposition . . . to schizophrenia. This predisposition interacts, in ways as yet largely unknown, with the environmental experiences of an individual, to govern whether or not that individual will eventually develop the disorder."[7(p.10)] Environment includes more than just psychological experiences, but also such factors as birth trauma, viruses, head injury, or excessive exposure to psychoactive drugs. In explaining the genetic factor to patients and family/ significant others (SOs), it is best to use the analogy of heart disease, which is easily understood by the lay public. Heart disease has a genetic factor; however, it does not mean that every family member will suffer from heart disease. It is a factor that increases the risk of illness.

Dopamine receptors are important biochemical stressors or neurotransmitters. The biochemical stressors theory focuses on an excess of these dopamine receptors in key areas of the brain, the limbic system. Dopamine receptors are blocked by neuroleptics, medications used to treat schizophrenia.[8] In schizophrenia norepinephrine is also increased, and serotonin is affected.[9] Even though there is no single conclusive theory about the etiology of schizophrenia, there is no doubt that biological alterations contribute to the pathological processes of the disorder.[10]

In the past, the etiological focus of schizophrenia was on family interactions; however, this is no longer considered an appropriate focus. It is now accepted that dysfunctional family interactions do not cause schizophrenia. Nor is stress a cause. Family interactions and stress may exacerbate an illness in a person who is at risk for the illness or make the illness worse, but they do not cause it. Schizophrenia is a brain disease, probably with multiple causes and different types of one illness. Its major symptoms are impaired thinking, hallucinations, delusions, and alterations in emotions and behavior. It is a chronic illness. The person will never return to premorbid functioning but may have periods of feeling better and then worse. Symptoms do not necessarily remain the same over time. There is still much research to be done in identifying cause(s) and treatment; however, at this time there is no firm acceptance of any single research theory.

Family members of an ill person have identified early warning signs of schizophrenia. They describe times when the ill person's thought patterns become illogical. The ill person may describe times when his or her sense of body boundaries is not clear. Auditory hallucinations and/or delusions may be experienced. The person appears to exhibit inappropriate emotions or a flat affect and distractibility/inattention. Productivity decreases. These signs may come and go for a period of time. Due to the serious nature of schizophrenia, diagnosis must be made carefully so as not to stigmatize a person with an inappropriate diagnosis— one that will be carried for life.

Schizophrenia is a disorder of remissions and relapses. It is a chronic illness. Exhibit 23–1 describes characteristics of the illness and their relationship to chronic illness. According to Freeman, "The most important cost-cutting measure in the treatment of schizophrenia is to avoid relapses. Hospitalization is the most expensive form of treatment."[11(p.5)] Patients tend to have fewer hospitalizations as the time passes; however, it always remains a possibility. With less money available for treatment, fewer patients are being hospitalized, even when hospitalization might be the best type of treatment for a specific situation. Psychiatric home care has a critical role to play in preventing relapse, and it begins with the home care admission assessment.

ASSESSMENT

Signs and Symptoms

Symptoms of schizophrenia are classified into positive and negative symptoms. These terms can be confusing; however, an understanding of these terms and their differences is important in understanding schizophrenia, its prognosis, and treatment.

Exhibit 23–1 Comparison of Chronic Medical Illness and Chronic Mental Illness

---

CHARACTERISTICS OF ALL CHRONIC ILLNESSES

- continuity in the relationship with the care provider
- education for the family unit so families may be informed, involved, and supportive
- early intervention and comprehensive treatment in order to avoid the worst outcomes of total disability and death

CHARACTERISTICS OF CHRONIC MENTAL ILLNESS: SCHIZOPHRENIA

- Impairments in brain function can produce changes in all areas of a person's life. Schizophrenia will impact on thought processes such as abstract reasoning, sequential tasks, and future planning. When these abilities are affected, the result is that overall intellectual functioning is impaired. We have seen our family members struggle to do routine tasks that they had mastered before getting sick. Judgment, including the ability to act in one's own self-interest, is often severely impaired. The person can be quite preoccupied with rushing, fragmented thoughts. Those who suffer from paranoia are particularly difficult to reach because of the fear that dominates each day.
- Almost unique to schizophrenia, is the profound lack of insight into the presence and nature of one's own illness. We have found this lack of insight to be the greatest single barrier to effective treatment and is only overcome with careful attention to establishing trust between patient and caregiver.
- Changes in mood and the loss of social skills affect ability to establish relationships with other people. Adding the impairment in social skills to the cognitive problems results in very limited job opportunities.

Source: Reprinted with permission from C. Knight, "President's Message," *Alliance for the Mentally Ill of Montgomery County, MD., Inc.*, Vol. 17, No. 7, pp. 1–2, © 1995, Alliance for the Mentally Ill of Montgomery County, Maryland.

- *Positive symptoms* are symptoms that are present but should be absent (such as anxiety, delusions, hallucinations). They develop over a short time and contribute little to overall prognosis.
- *Negative symptoms* are symptoms that are absent but should be present in a positive form (such as intellectual impairment, social withdrawal, blunt affect). They develop over a period of time and are more important in determining overall prognosis. Negative symptoms are the most troublesome symptoms for the staff and families/SOs as they are difficult to deal with effectively. In the past, these symptoms were thought to be a result of long-term

hospitalization; however, now they are considered to be a part of the illness process. These are the symptoms that led to the stereotype of "the state-hospital patient." Patients with negative symptoms may appear to be physical bodies with little emotion and connection to other people and the world around them. There is limited treatment for these symptoms. Most medications do not affect them; however, a new medication, clozapine, seems to affect these symptoms in some patients. Exhibit 23–2 compares these two types of symptoms. Breslin reports that "Clinicians have found that many patients have a mixture of symptoms. Thus the goal of treatment is to resolve not only the flagrant positive symptoms but also the more insidious deficit symptoms."[12(p.877)]

Critical signs and symptoms of schizophrenia include the following symptoms that affect daily function:

- *Disordered thinking.* The patient has illogical thoughts, rapid thoughts, decreased concentration, distractibility, fragmented thoughts, and decreased ability to identify relevant information. As a consequence of these symptoms, the patient feels overwhelmed with information. The patient has problems with concentration and attention. One patient has described it as "cannot keep to the point but 'there are so many points and all equally and insistently insignificant.'"[13(p.4)] Abstracting ability is inadequate. Blocking of thought occurs when the patient begins to speak but then stops and loses track of the meaning of the statement. *Loose associations* are statements that sound jumbled. The patient may exhibit concrete thought or the inability to generalize and the need to be extremely literal. Three speech patterns may be observed: (1) In *tangential speech* the patient begins to respond to a question but follows with a series of related topics that never really get to the point of the original statement. (2) In *circumstantial speech*, the patient does get to the point but only after adding many unnecessary details to the response. (3) *Perseveration* is a pattern of speech in which the patient repeats the same words or phrases over and over again.
- *Cognitive confusion.* According to Hatfield, patients have described "themselves as 'confused,' 'hazy,' 'bewildered,' and 'disoriented.' They have reported that they have suffered thought blocking and sometimes felt their minds going blank, and that they were unable to maintain control over their ideas. Patient reports reveal that the sense of time was often distorted during acute stages of the illness."[14(p.4)]
- *Impaired identity.* Hatfield states that "Alteration in the sense of self is common in schizophrenia. Most people have a clear sense of where their bodies end and the rest of the world begins. Without this capacity, orienting oneself in the world is extremely difficult."[15(p.4)]

Exhibit 23–2 Symptoms of Schizophrenia

Positive Symptoms	Negative Symptoms
• anxiety	• motor retardation
• delusions	• absence of pleasure
• hallucinations	• intellectual impairments
• agitation, pacing	• social withdrawal and isolation
• aggressiveness, hostility	• depressed mood
• somatic complaints	• apathy, disinterest
• suspiciousness	• poor grooming and self-care
• cognitive disorganization with	• lack of thoughts
poor concentration, loose	• lack of goal-directed behavior
associations	• blunt affect

- *Difficulty with relationships.* Buchanan states that "Social support is postulated to serve as a protective factor that facilitates coping and competence, thus modulating the deleterious effects of social and environmental stressors."[16(p.68)] Four functions of social support that are important to the patient and important for home care staff to understand are[17(p.69)]

  1. esteem support or information that one is esteemed, accepted, or affirmed
  2. informational support, sometimes referred to as advice or coping support
  3. affiliative support aimed at facilitating positive affective moods
  4. instrumental support or the provision of either tangible or intangible aid

  Coping with stress is not easy for the patient with schizophrenia, and it is suggested that a social network "buffers the individual against stress, which, in turn, may decrease symptomatology. An alternative hypothesis is that the development of reciprocal relationships may generate increased self-esteem and control. This may result in a perception of the environment as somewhat benign and manageable, which, in turn, may limit the development of serious symptomatology."[18(p.144)] Despite the importance of social support, the patient with schizophrenia has great difficulty with relationships. An assessment of this area of functioning assists in predicting future social functioning. Patients fear rejection and are very sensitive to it, often when others are not aware of their fear. They also have difficulty in assessing their own interactions with others, not recognizing when a relationship is not going well or what to do about it. Home care staff provide social support that might not otherwise be available to the patient.[19] Treatment goals are to help the patient move toward rehabilitation and away from disease and its symptoms; to help the patient focus on the here and now; and to assist the patient to learn social skills needed for daily living. A major factor related to these treatment goals is the patient's relationships with others.

- *Hallucinations.* A hallucination is a sensory perception that takes place without external stimuli. Hallucinations are very common in schizophrenia. There is an overacuteness of sensory activity: auditory, visual, olfactory, tactile, and taste. Auditory hallucinations are the most common. These can be a sound, a single voice, or multiple voices, which may be heard occasionally or continuously. When occasional, the hallucinations commonly occur at night before sleep. Most voices are unpleasant, directing the person to hurt the self or someone else. Even persons who have been deaf from birth have experienced auditory hallucinations. Visual hallucinations are less common and usually appear with auditory hallucination; hallucinations related to the other senses are not as common. Some patients are able to learn how to cope with daily hallucinations or occasional ones and are able to function on medications. Frederick and Cotanch stated that "Whether consciously or unconsciously, they develop ways of adapting to the hallucinatory experience through physiological, cognitive, and behavioral techniques."[20(p.223)] These authors identified self-help techniques from a study of 33 outpatients with schizophrenia.[21] Their results are consistent with other studies that have identified self-help techniques. A baseline assessment of hallucinations is important to provide comparison data that might be used later as hallucinations are monitored. The recommended techniques include the following:
  1. changing physiological arousal
     - reduction of physiological arousal: relax, lie down, sleep, calm music, drink alcohol, extra medication
     - increase physiological arousal: loud music, walk, pace, jog
  2. cognitive techniques
     - acceptance of voices: do as they say, talk to the voices
     - reduced attention to voices: ignore the voices, sing, pray
  3. behavioral techniques
     - Participate in leisure or work activities: reading, drawing, television, yardwork, shopping.
     - Seek interaction with others.
     - Isolate self.
     - Lie down.
- *Delusions.* A delusion is a false personal belief that is not subject to reason. Usually delusions involve themes of persecution and/or grandeur. Paranoid delusions are suspicious in nature. Grandiose delusions occur in schizophrenia but are found more in the manic episode of bipolar disorder. The patient may appear to have positive self-esteem; however, the patient really has a very low self-esteem and poor identity that is covered over. Typical delusions include the following:

1. delusion of persecution or a false belief that another person or others are persecuting the patient
2. delusion of grandeur or a false belief in which one views self with exaggerated importance
3. delusion of reference or a false belief that casual or unrelated remarks or behavior relate to oneself
4. delusion of influence or a false belief that others are controlling or influencing oneself
5. somatic delusion or a false belief related to one's body or physical functioning
6. erotic delusion or a false belief related to sexual or erotic content

Assessment Guidelines

What might the nurse encounter on the first visit? The patient often greets home care staff in a stilted and cold manner due to difficulties with social skills. The patient may not focus on staff when speaking and avoid contact. The patient may appear disheveled, with poor hygiene and grooming. Self-care needs may be identified as an immediate problem. The patient may exhibit strange mannerisms such as grinning, grimacing, or echopraxia (imitation of movements of another person). The patient may be quiet or agitated or constantly moving. With these behaviors the interview may be difficult. It should be short and focused on the here-and-now. The entire admission assessment may not be completed at the first visit.

Part of the home care assessment, either the initial admission assessment or ongoing assessment, is to determine if home care is the appropriate setting for the patient. There are times when more intensive treatment may be required. Criteria to determine if more intensive treatment is required include the following:

- safety (if the patient is a danger to self and/or others)
- medication assessment and intervention
- structure (due to decreasing ability to care for self)

During the assessment and as the home care nurse begins to make plans with the patient, the focus is on psychosocial rehabilitation. To accomplish this goal the assessment must include the patient's disability and functioning. Delving too deep into the patient's past is not appropriate. Home care staff who approach a patient who has serious mental illness with old treatment ideas and with expectations that cannot be met will quickly be frustrated. This frustration will be noticed by the patient and the family/SOs. The patient needs nursing staff who are caring in their approach and who recognize individuality with respect for each patient as a person.

As is true for all patients with mental illness, a physical assessment is very important. According to Holmberg, "People with mental illness are likely to have a physical disorder for which there is inadequate screening."[22(p.39)] The assessment should include screening for neurophysical illnesses, blood chemistry profiles, and urinary screening.

DIAGNOSIS

Medical diagnoses include five types of schizophrenia. These are paranoid, catatonic, disorganized, undifferentiated, and residual.[23] The nursing diagnoses are based on the North American Nursing Diagnosis Association (NANDA) and include the following possible diagnoses:[24]

- anxiety
- ineffective individual coping
- impaired verbal communication
- disturbance in self-concept
- impaired social interactions
- risk for injury
- alteration in thought processes
- alteration in sensory perceptions
- alteration in family processes
- self-care deficit

EXPECTED OUTCOMES

Establishing realistic goals within a realistic time frame can help both the patient and the staff. What is a good outcome for a patient with schizophrenia is yet to be defined; however, home care staff can help one another identify when goals are unrealistic. Intermittent short hospitalizations are becoming more common. These hospitalizations are not treatment failures but rather opportunities to achieve small goals. Using past medical records and information from family/SOs enhances the assessment data. From the very first contact, the nurse communicates to the patient verbally and nonverbally that the home care staff will protect the patient, be there when the patient needs help, and help the patient to prepare for discharge from home care.

Lacking confidence that they can succeed in the real world, many of these patients prefer to adopt the social role of "mental patient," which offers them some degree of support. Home care staff should work with the patient to prevent this from occurring by establishing realistic outcomes. The following are examples of desired patient outcomes.

- The patient will experience a reduction in symptoms (specify symptoms).
- The patient will focus on activities in the here and now.
- The patient will identify behaviors that interfere with functioning.
- The patient will develop strategies for changing behaviors that interfere with functioning.
- The patient will state rationale for medication in alleviating symptoms.
- The patient will identify name(s) of medications, purpose of taking, dosage and frequency, and side effects.
- The patient will exhibit appropriate activity level, sleep pattern, eating, and independent self-care within own limitations (specify for the individual patient).
- The patient will participate in treatment planning, assessment of progress, and discharge planning.
- The patient will develop a written contract for discharge from home care addressing responsibilities and schedule for postdischarge (who, what, when, where).
- The patient will exhibit coping behavior with family/SOs.
- The patient will comply with recommended medical treatment.
- The patient will not harm self or others.
- The patient will demonstrate relaxation exercises.

All of these may be difficult to achieve. Outcomes must be based on realistic expectations and the patient's strengths and limitations.

INTERVENTIONS IN THE HOME

When the patient is overwhelmed with stimuli, a relapse frequently occurs. Withdrawal from social situations may become the most effective coping method for reducing anxiety. The patient with schizophrenia is very sensitive to social situations that threaten self-esteem and anticipates rejection. Failure at work or with other tasks increases anxiety and the expectation of disapproval from others. As a coping mechanism, patients frequently avoid situations that might lead to more anxiety. This pattern of avoidance prevents the patient from developing living skills necessary for life, and his or her living skills soon atrophy.

Even with schizophrenia, there are different levels of acuity and individual differences in coping. Situations that embarrass the patient will decrease self-esteem. Home care staff may need to step in frequently and quickly, depending on the assessment of the patient's ability to cope. Limited problem-solving skills make the patient very vulnerable in most social situations.

The patient may not be able to handle another person's anger, joy, or sadness, even if the patient is not directly involved with the person or situation. Decoding the nonverbal behavior of others is often difficult and subject to misinterpretation. Teaching the patient how to interpret nonverbal communication is a valuable lesson. Exercises to practice decoding nonverbal facial communication can be a helpful activity, and these may be taught by an occupational therapist or other home care staff.

Aggressive and intimidating behavior is a common staff concern, as well as a concern for the family/SOs. A basic treatment principle is to keep the patient safe and to prevent the patient from interfering with or hurting others. A power struggle with the patient is not helpful. Nobody wins. A minority of patients with schizophrenia are aggressive. Assessing anxiety level, allowing for success in tolerating stimuli in increments, and setting limits before escalation are critical interventions. It does not help if the patient is allowed to become aggressive and intimidate home care staff or the family/SOs. This only increases the patient's anxiety. The reverse is also true. Staff need to protect the patient from intimidation from others. Because the patient has difficulty with social roles, it is the staff's responsibility to help the patient learn as much as possible about relating to others in a positive manner. This is not to say that staff should attempt to correct every annoying habit a patient exhibits. Staff should select one behavior at a time— preferably one that is most aberrant. The behavioral plan should emphasize positive behavior and communication while diminishing outlets for negative expression. Home care staff and family/SOs should communicate clear expectations to the patient. When something is promised, it should be met or, if not, an explanation should be given. Until symptoms diminish, it is best to limit the amount of time spent in situations that are difficult for the patient to manage.

Consistency is important, so it is critical that all staff apply the treatment plan. Treatment planning should be well thought out. It is critical to discuss the plan, work out the plan, and clearly communicate the plan to all concerned. It is very important to include family/SOs in the planning as they will have daily contact with the patient and may know the patient's early cues of lack of control. They will need to continue the plan after discharge from home care.

When communicating with the patient about the treatment plan, it is important to be very specific. Nagging or arguing with the patient is not productive. Stating clearly what must be done and the consequence if it is not done is the best approach (e.g., staff and family/SOs tell the patient the time for a shower and the consequence if the patient does not take the shower). The patient frequently interprets lengthy discussion as evidence of staff indecisiveness and ineffectiveness. The patient is afraid of losing control. Part of the treatment plan is to communicate expectations and consequences simply and nonpunitively. If external control is required, all efforts should be made to help the patient retain dignity. Staff need to follow through and should not make decisions about issues over which they have no power. Patients with increasing anxiety or in acute psychotic states cannot always identify relevant information. Staff and family/SOs can push any patient into a defensive escalated stance, but this is not the objective. Limits should be set firmly but kindly.

Specific interventions include the following:

- If patient resistance is viewed by staff and family/SOs as "the patient is uncooperative," this will result in nursing care that reinforces pathology, usually with subtle retaliation, coercion, control, or withdrawal.
- Interpersonal closeness often increases anxiety. It is best not to be too enthusiastic or impatient, or to approach the patient too directly or too verbally. With the patient's fear of closeness, care should be directed toward decreasing anxiety by assessing the patient's level of tolerance for physical and psychological closeness. Patients fluctuate in their ability to cope with closeness, depending on their affect/mood or symptom state.
- During the early stages of the staff-patient relationship, staff may need to use more nonverbal activity (e.g., listening to music, taking a short walk, preparing a meal, relaxation exercises).
- Verbal approaches should be nonprodding. To ask a question implies an expectation of a response. If the patient cannot respond, this may decrease self-esteem and possibly cause hostility. Staff may indicate that they do not understand the patient's anxiety and ask the patient to describe his or her feelings. This communicates that staff want to understand how the patient is feeling. Reflection may not be helpful with this patient. The more effective verbal approach is generalizing, which communicates acceptance and commonality.
- Patients with schizophrenia have some contact with reality and some capacity to relate to others. It is very easy to assume that all patients with this illness are hallucinating all the time and cannot relate to other people. This viewpoint, which is not productive for treatment, is often the result of stereotypes, myths, or prejudices. A major staff role is to keep the patient in contact with reality.
- Patient delusions and hallucinations can be difficult for staff, and they should not accept the patient's reality. However, arguing or trying to reason with the patient about the content of delusions or hallucinations is not helpful. Discussion of symptoms should refocus the patient on the here and now. Initially it may be best to approach the patient for frequent, short periods and then increase contact as the patient tolerates it. Verbal approaches should provide broad openings (e.g., "Tell me what is happening"). Words are said gently without confrontation. To reinforce reality, staff respond verbally to anything that is real with the following interventions:
  1. Ask the patient to describe what he or she is experiencing.
  2. Ask the patient to inform the staff when hallucinations begin during a conversation.

3. Validate with the patient the nature of the real situation before making a decision that the patient is hallucinating.
4. Avoid conveying to the patient that staff believe the voices are real or that they hear them too. Terms that are best to use are "the voices that you hear."
5. Help the patient to identify impersonal or universal pronouns. Staff should use personal or proper names with the patient, avoiding overuse of impersonal pronouns.
6. Increase the patient's social interactions gradually.
7. Teach the patient a variety of strategies to relieve anxiety.
8. Avoid demanding facts from the delusional patient about the delusions. In doing this, staff tend to ignore the patient as a person and the patient's feelings. The more facts requested, the more the patient feels obligated to give facts. This increases anxiety. The patient believes the delusion. Trying to convince the patient that the delusion does not exist only pushes the patient away; however, this does not mean that staff should say they believe the delusions. Staff may be fascinated with the patient's symptoms, but revealing this fascination is not helpful for the patient.
9. Recognize that problem solving may be difficult for the patient (e.g., following directions, planning the day, making decisions).

If hallucinations are commands to harm self or others, the patient may require more intensive treatment to protect self or others. Emergencies in the home are discussed in Chapter 29. Exhibit 23 3 describes additional strategies that might be used to help the patient cope with auditory hallucinations.

- The patient fears rejection, criticism, hostility and depreciation, and all these need to be avoided. Assisting the patient to understand feelings and behavior when the patient encounters these reactions from others is an important intervention to include in the treatment plan.
- When the patient asks questions, provide reassuring and honest replies.
- Home care staff establish contact with the patient by focusing the conversation on everyday topics and practical aspects of life. The patient's thinking is concrete with inadequate abstract thinking. Excessive stimuli, and for some patients even normal amount of stimuli, can make them very anxious. The patient cannot cut out the stimuli. For example, if staff give the patient several directions at once, this may increase the confusion. Directions must be simple, precise, and often repetitious; however, this can be frustrating for the home care staff. The patient may not be able to remove himself or herself from a situation appropriately when experiencing a loss or anxiety and may need help to do this. The patient will also need to learn how to do this for himself or herself.
- Silent patients are always difficult for staff because they make staff feel uncomfortable. It is best to show an interest in the patient; try to engage in some activity or sit quietly with the patient.

Exhibit 23–3 Self-Help Techniques for Auditory Hallucinations

---

CHANGE PHYSIOLOGICAL AROUSAL

- Reduction of physiological arousal: relax, lie down, sleep, calm music, extra medication
- Increase physiological arousal: loud music, walk, pace, jog

COGNITIVE TECHNIQUES

- Acceptance of voices: do as they say, talk to the voices
- Reduced attention to voices: ignore them, sing, pray

BEHAVIORAL TECHNIQUES

- Leisure or work activity: reading, drawing, television, yardwork, shopping
- Seek interaction with others
- Isolate self
- Lie down

Source: From *Issues in Mental Health Nursing*, Volume 16, pp. 219–220, J. Frederick and P. Cotanch, Taylor & Francis, Inc., Washington, D.C. Reproduced with permission. All rights reserved.

- The completion of simple tasks in the home can increase self-esteem and decrease time for focusing on hallucinations and/or delusions (e.g., making a bed, washing dishes, sorting laundry, gardening).
- Efforts should be made to increase the patient's self-esteem; however, feedback should be honest and appropriate. The patient will sense false or forced praise.
- The patient's hostility should not be taken personally. The patient needs to express anger appropriately; however, staff and family/SOs do not have to take abuse. There are times when limits must be set.
- The patient will test relationships, and this will frustrate staff. At these times, staff should step back and analyze what is occurring and why it is occurring. When the patient is able to listen, discuss the issue with the patient.
- Due to increased interest in biological factors, the patient may undergo testing such as electroencephalogram, computed tomography scan, or magnetic resonance imaging. These tests are explained to the patient and support is provided during the test. The patient may have concerns about what is being done to his or her brain. Assessment of the patient's response is important, as it may be difficult for the patient to cooperate due to fears. These fears and concerns should be discussed with the patient's physician and with staff at the testing site.

- Encouraging the patient to participate in family/SOs' activities will help the patient increase activities; however, an overly forceful approach only increases the patient's anxiety. Structure with flexibility is always a key element in any home visit, and should be part of the home environment 24 hours a day. Success for this patient may be experienced in very small amounts, but the patient still needs appropriate praise.
- Because the patient may not be able to inform staff or others about physical illness, assessment for physical illness and side effects from medications is important at every visit.
- Bowel and bladder elimination requires routine assessment. Medications can cause side effects in these areas. A diet that includes fruit, vegetables, and eight glasses of fluids daily are important to prevent problems. Some patients may benefit from the use of laxatives.
- Patient education should include information about medications and their side effects. The patient should report problems to the staff. Teaching the patient what to report is important, and this will be particularly important after discharge from home care.
- Assessment of nutrition and fluid intake on admission to home care and throughout treatment is part of the patient's treatment plan. The family/SOs may have developed strategies to resolve problems in these areas, and staff need to ask for their advice. The patient may have bizarre food and eating habits. If the patient and others are not harmed by these habits, it may be best not to intervene. A plan is developed and implemented consistently with the family/SOs.
- Assessment of sleep on admission to home care and periodically is standard for the patient with schizophrenia. Lack of sleep can exacerbate psychotic symptoms. At first, periods of rest to offset sleep deprivation may be necessary. Then home care staff help the patient to increase activity. Initially, the patient may be sedated by medications. This reality must be considered prior to encouraging the patient to increase activity. If lack of sleep is a problem, the patient needs assistance to get more sleep (e.g., provide calm environment, decrease caffeine, take medications later in the day, set specific bedtime, decrease sleep during the day, develop room plan as needed, do relaxation exercises, listen to quiet music, and decrease stimulating activity in the evening).
- Suicide does occur in schizophrenia. A bizarre method is often used, and it usually is in response to an auditory hallucination. Patients also may run away from home, which can be very frightening to family/SOs. Patients who have a history of suicidal behavior or running away may exhibit patterns that can be assessed early to prevent problems from occurring. The nurse discusses preventive measures with the family/SOs and with the patient. A no-harm contract or a contract related to running away may be developed with

the patient. The contract specifies early warning signs that indicate the patient has one of these problems and interventions to be taken by the patient and/or family/SOs. For patients who have overcome these behaviors in the past, the home care staff should remind the patient that they have overcome these feelings and can do so again. Emergencies in the home, such as suicidal feelings and behavior, are discussed in Chapter 29.

- Sharing information with the family/SOs will increase their participation and help them to feel more in control. Staff should focus on specific, practical advice (e.g., developing schedules, identifying interventions that work and those that do not, planning respite, coping with their own feelings, using support groups, giving medications, and discussing what to do in emergencies). The family/SOs of a newly diagnosed patient will have different needs from those who have dealt with the chronic illness for a longer period of time. Asking the family/SOs how home care staff can help will communicate that they are important and in control. The goal is to help the family/SOs interact constructively with the patient. This requires family/SO education as well as avoidance of a message of blaming the family/SOs.

- A room plan is a form of structure. Using a room plan helps the patient cope with people through the environment and helps the patient control his or her behavior. The purpose of the plan must be understood by the patient as well as by the family/SOs who will implement the plan daily. The patient, family/SOs, and home care staff should know the specific behavioral criteria for the use of the room plan, the length of time the plan should be used, and behavioral criteria for discontinuing the plan. A room plan is never used punitively. The patient is carefully assessed to determine if the plan might be helpful. After the plan is implemented, home care staff identify when a room plan is not effective. Families/SOs must be active in the planning. The plan is written with copies given to the patient, family/SOs, home care staff, and a copy placed in the medical record. If a patient is staying in his or her bedroom too much, a plan might be developed to have the patient stay out of the bedroom for a specified period of time. It may be necessary to lock the door to keep the patient out; however, this is an extreme intervention. The reverse can also be used—that is, the patient may be asked to spend specified time in the bedroom as a time-out. This is especially useful for patients who need a decrease in stimuli. At every home care visit, the room plan requires assessment. Is it being used? Why is it not being used? Is it being followed correctly? What problems are occurring? What can be done to make the plan more effective? The patient is given positive feedback about the plan from family/SOs and staff, even if it is for meeting only some part of the plan. If there is an excessive amount of activity in the home, the patient may not be able to say, "I've had enough," and remove himself or herself from the situation. Staff or family/SOs might say, "John, looks like you're having problems with being around others at this time and need a break. I will talk with you in 15 minutes and see how you are doing." If the patient is uncooperative and escalating, the room plan may not be enough and more intensive treatment outside the home may be required. Other interventions are included in Chapter 29. Room plans may also be used with patients who have diagnoses other than schizophrenia such as depression and bipolar disorder.

- The patient may be asked to keep a diary of behavior and feelings. The nurse should discuss how the diary is to be used with the patient so that the patient is clear about the purpose, what is to be written, and when it is to be written. The nurse or other home care staff then might discuss the diary entries at each visit with the patient.

- During the first six months of an evolving schizophrenic disorder, it is not uncommon for a patient to experience depressive symptoms. When psychotic symptoms are stabilized and the patient continues to have depressive symptoms, the physician may prescribe an antidepressant to be used with an antipsychotic.[25]

- Administration of medications is critical. The home care nurse should develop a method with the patient to remind the patient to take medications, teach the patient about the medication, develop methods with the patient to monitor medication response and side effects, and assess if the patient is taking the medication as ordered. If the patient requires serum level testing, this must be arranged and results reviewed with the physician as well as the patient. Some patients do better on depot neuroleptic medication. The nurse may administer this to the patient following the home care agency procedure. Weiden et al. studied the use of depot medications and found that "converting patients from an oral to a depot neuroleptic regimen before hospital discharge led to short-term improvement in outpatient medication compliance."[26(p.1053)] These authors found that there were higher rates of patient acceptance of depot medications while in the hospital where staff had more leverage. The patient could then continue receiving the depot medication after discharge. With a depot regimen, it is easier for staff to identify noncompliant patients, because it is immediately obvious when a patient refuses the medication. Staff can then begin interventions immediately to prevent further noncompliance. The half-life of depot medication is longer than oral medications, and thus psychotic symptoms will take longer to reoccur when the patient is noncompliant. Another advantage of depot medication is the family/SOs will experience less burden for supervising medication intake. At each visit, the nurse assesses the patient for side effects, particularly tardive dyskinesia and neuroleptic malignant syndrome. These side effects are discussed in detail in Chapters 18 and 19.

- Self-care or self-management is important for a patient with schizophrenia, but it is not easy for the patient. According to Connelly and Dilonardo, "Patients may wish to assume responsibility for their own care, but may not have the energy, confidence, or concentration to do so."[27(p.35)] Variables affecting self-care are related to the patient (particularly self-esteem, self-efficacy, and health beliefs) and to the nurse (e.g., accuracy of assessment, appropriate expectations of treatment outcomes, and support of patient autonomy).[28] These variables will be important to patient education and decision making. Environmental factors are also important to consider (e.g., interpersonal/family relationships, social demands, and/or socioeconomic conditions). As the patient progresses toward self-care and is successful, it is not uncommon for the patient to experience anxiety and symptoms of regression, rather than pride and the sense of improved well-being. After experiencing so many failures, the patient views new opportunities as more chances for failure. Many patients develop a pattern of avoiding failure. This can directly affect their participation in treatment and their motivation for self-care.
- Both internal and external stress can be very damaging to someone with schizophrenia. Internal stress has been identified by some patients as their altered perceptions, cognitive confusion, attention deficits, and impaired identity.[29] More problematic for home care staff is coping mechanisms that may appear to interfere with progress. According to Hatfield, "People with schizophrenia may appear rigid and unable to change directions without difficulty. This inflexibility is one way the patient maintains stability when the ground keeps shifting beneath the patient. Structure and predictability in the external world help compensate for the unpredictability of the inner world. Daily routines provide a pattern and a sense of order to life."[30(p.1143)]
- Communication is difficult with the patient who is withdrawn and hallucinating. It requires patience and a recognition that small steps are important. The patient needs time to feel comfortable with home care staff. When possible, the home care agency should assign consistent staff to this patient. Assessment includes the identification of patient behaviors that the patient uses to avoid relating, and then the staff must develop interventions to assist the patient to recognize that relationships are safe. Staff will be rejected, but they cannot take this personally. When the patient begins to avoid staff, the patient is probably experiencing anxiety. Staff should try to identify what happened or what was discussed before the patient began to avoid the staff. This will provide cues about what made the patient anxious. If the staff arrive at the home and the patient is not there, they should wait for a short while; they should then leave a note stating the time and date of the missed visit, the time and date of the next visit, and the expectation that the patient will be at home for the next visit. A telephone number should be left for the

patient with a request that the patient call the staff member. Some patients test the staff to see if they care enough to come back. When the patient and staff do meet, they must openly discuss the missed appointments.

Summary of critical points related to nursing interventions for the patient with schizophrenia include the following:

- During every home visit, home care staff must be willing to meet the patient on his or her ground and help develop skills necessary for functioning.
- Boundary awareness is a major problem for the patient with schizophrenia. When alone with the patient, it is best not to close the door as this may increase the patient's anxiety. Sitting closely to the patient is also not recommended. Standing directly in a doorway may cause the patient to feel that there is no escape, and the patient's anxiety may increase. The patient may then try to get through the door regardless of who is standing in it. If the patient's anxiety is increasing, staff or family/SOs may quietly ask the patient to leave the area or may tell the patient that someone will sit next to him or her and help the patient cope with increasing anxiety.
- Arguing with the patient about the patient's view of reality increases the patient's anxiety.
- Staff feelings of helplessness and inadequacy may be communicated to the patient. Developing a clear picture of realistic goals for the patient will help staff have more realistic reactions toward the patient and the patient's illness. When staff are unable to deal with their feelings about a patient, it is useful to talk with other home care staff to gain a more objective perspective.
- Lack of patient motivation is a major problem in all areas of treatment. After experiencing repeated failures, the patient may view new experiences not as opportunities for growth but as opportunities for more failure. The patient may avoid situations that may lead to failure and thus refuse to try new experiences due to fear. Staff should consider whether they are setting up the patient to fail when they ask the patient to do something that he or she has no chance of accomplishing.
- Activities of daily living are important skills for each patient to learn to do as independently as possible. These skills are based on the patient's living situation, strengths, and limitations.
- Failure to keep appointments or take medication are characteristics of the illness, not indications of a "bad patient." According to Knight, "It is more appropriate to suspect a bad treatment plan than to label a patient as bad."[31(p.2)] Compliance must be assessed on admission and throughout home care; however, it must be approached positively. The nurse and the patient should discuss the patient's responses to and views of the illness and the treatment. Listening is very important. There are many possible

reasons for noncompliance, including side effects from the medications, poor understanding of the illness and its treatment, paranoid delusions about medications, conflicts with the family/SOs about appropriate treatment, and lack of engagement with the home care staff and other health care providers.[32]

PATIENT EDUCATION

Patient education is a major component of the treatment plan for the patient with schizophrenia. Patient education and psychiatric rehabilitation are inseparable interventions for this patient. Examples of patient education goals include the following:

- The patient will identify name(s) of medications, purpose of taking, dosage and frequency, and side effects (as well as blood tests required, frequency, and how to obtain).
- The patient will identify early warning signs that indicate more support is required.
- The patient will identify and apply strategies to decrease early warning signs.
- The patient will identify relevant stress management techniques.
- The patient will use relaxation exercises as needed.
- The patient will identify the potential harmful effects of using alcohol/drugs to decrease anxiety or depression.

Rehabilitation is very important with schizophrenia, particularly emphasizing social and vocational training. Programs such as vocational counseling, job training, problem solving, money management skills, and use of public transportation should be developed specifically for each patient. Rehabilitation is discussed in more detail in Chapter 2.

HOME CARE STAFF: RESPONSES TO THE
HOME CARE PATIENT

Patients have identified external factors that affect their recovery, and some of these relate to staff. Patients have identified caring staff who reinforce the patient's autonomy, respect the patient as a person, and show confidence in the potential for recovery.[33] It is easy for staff to view the noncompliant patient as "difficult" and with limited commitment to improve; however, staff must see patient's behavior as part of the illness, its process, and its symptomatology. The home care staff's view of the illness and its symptoms will affect their responses to the patient and to the family/SOs.

FAMILY/SIGNIFICANT OTHERS: NEEDS AND STRATEGIES

Families/SOs often experience stigma, secrecy, and shame due to mental illness. They frequently blame themselves, which causes them great pain. Schizophrenia and its relationship to the family/SOs has had a long and troubled history. This history has included painful incidents of health care professionals blaming parents for the illness and/or criticizing parents for being overinvolved or neglecting their children. This has led to parents being very suspicious of health care professionals and has helped parents to develop their own support systems, such as the National Alliance for the Mentally Ill (NAMI). This organization has helped many patients and their families/SOs, publishes useful literature, and lobbies for research funds and for improvement in treatment. Home care staff should work with family/SOs and with NAMI. Parents who have adult children with schizophrenia usually have been through health care system after health care system, have talked about their history to death, know the pros and cons of various treatments, and recognize quality care. Each encounter with a health care professional, institution, or agency feels like starting all over again rather than another phase of treatment that uses what has been learned in the past to build a better treatment approach or to maintain treatment that is helpful. In their experience, few professionals have really listened to family members. This is a sad commentary. Home care nurses can learn from parents who have cared for their adult children in the their home or supported them elsewhere. Parents usually provide helpful information about symptoms, patterns of behavior and likely end results, response to medications and other treatments, and effective and ineffective communication methods.

This is not to say that families do not need support; they do. Often hospitalization offers a respite, but not if it becomes a time of more accusations and criticisms that do not recognize family members' contributions, frustrations, hopelessness, and concerns (such as, "Who will be there for my son or daughter when I am gone?"). Families may need help in reaching a balance between allowing their adult child as much as independence as possible and maintaining their own personal lives. A family may become overwhelmed with caring and forget about themselves or not know how to care for themselves. This is due, in part, to the difficulties that patients with schizophenia have with relationships. The patient may try to force the family to take over and provide structure, and then resent it and rebel. This cycle can be repeated over and over again. The hopelessness that the family feels can also be experienced by the patient and home care staff. It is very contagious. This hopelessness can lead families to be very desperate for a cure, regardless of risk. Families of patients with schizophrenia pushed for the use of clozapine in research trials prior to U.S. Food and Drug Administration approval, and families are now pushing for a decrease in the cost of clozapine and other expensive drugs.

Families may encounter another problem when the ill family member improves. The family/SOs may have both positive and negative reactions. The patient may want more independence, and the family/SOs may find this difficult to accept after having control for many years. Najarian states that "A common concern for families is, 'My child is better, now what?' Even though patient concentration, initiative, and social skills may improve with clozapine treatment, many patients may not feel ready for major changes such as a job or a romantic relationship. Functional improvement often brings new challenges with it."[34(p.19)]

Family therapy should be used with families who need and want it to help the family support the patient, to give the family support, and to help the patient learn how to relate to his or her family in a more productive way. It should be reality oriented, with a practical focus and a focus on problem solving. The therapy should not be used to point to the family as the cause of the illness. Many families refuse family therapy as a result of negative past experiences or lack of a real need. This may be particularly true for the family who has experienced multiple hospitalizations. Since patients with schizophrenia often live with their families/SOs or in close proximity, the family/SOs are frequently the caregivers. This leads to long-term stress for them. According to Malone, this can "strain a marriage, interfere with normal social life, take an emotional toll on siblings, and drain the family's resources."[35(p.7)] Ultimately, the family/SOs must decide how much direct assistance they want, and this must be respected.

SUMMARY

Nursing care for the patient with schizophrenia is complex, but it can be rewarding. The important factor is to recognize that schizophrenia is a chronic illness, but patients can be helped within their limitations. Goals should be of shorter range, very specific, and realistic for the individual patient, and they should have a psychosocial rehabilitation focus. Hauk summarizes the nurse's role as follows: "For an hour or so, with each visit, nurses share that life with their patients and in doing so have the opportunity to assist in the process of implementing change so that patients' lives may be fuller and their trips to the hospital less frequent."[36(p.268)]

NOTES

1. E. Torrey, *Surviving Schizophrenia: A Family Manual* (New York: Harper & Row, 1988), 116–117.
2. J. Malone, "Schizophrenia Research Update: Implications for Nursing," *Journal of Psychosocial Nursing* 28, no. 8 (1990): 4–9, at 6.
3. D. Hauk, "The Acutely Depressed or Schizophrenic Patient," in *Home Health Nursing Practice: Concepts and Application*, ed. R. Rice (St. Louis, MO: Mosby–Year Book, 1992), 260–272, at 267.

4. N. Andreasen, *The Broken Brain: The Biological Revolution in Psychiatry* (New York: Harper & Row, 1985), 71.

5. Torrey, *Surviving Schizophrenia*, 138–140.

6. Andreasen, *The Broken Brain: The Biological Revolution in Psychiatry*, 71.

7. K. Kendler, "Genetics, Not Environment, Is Major Factor in Schizophrenia," *NAMI Advocate* 13, no. 6 (1992): 10.

8. Andreasen, *The Broken Brain: The Biological Revolution in Psychiatry*, 222–225.

9. E. Garza-Trevino et al., "Neurobiology of Schizophrenic Syndromes," *Hospital and Community Psychiatry* 41, no. 9 (1990): 975–976.

10. Garza-Trevino et al., "Neurobiology of Schizophrenic Syndromes," 978.

11. H. Freeman, "Preventing Relapse: Key to Cost-Effectiveness in the Treatment of Schizophrenia," *Current Approaches to Psychoses: Diagnosis and Management* 3, no. 10 (1994): 5–6.

12. N. Breslin, "Treatment of Schizophrenia: Current Practice and Future Promise," *Hospital and Community Psychiatry* 43, no. 9 (1992): 877–885, at 877.

13. A. Hatfield, "The Internal Stress of Schizophrenia," *Alliance for Mentally Ill of Maryland, Inc., Newsletter* 8, no. 3 (1990): 4.

14. Hatfield, "The Internal Stress of Schizophrenia," 4.

15. Hatfield, "The Internal Stress of Schizophrenia." 4.

16. J. Buchanan, "Social Support and Schizophrenia: A Review of the Literature," *Archives of Psychiatric Nursing* 9, no. 2 (1995): 68–76, at 68.

17. Buchanan, "Social Support and Schizophrenia: A Review of the Literature," 69.

18. L. Gillies et al., "Differential Outcomes in Social Network Therapy," *Psychosocial Rehabilitation Journal* 16, no. 3 (1993): 142–145, at 144.

19. H. Nieminen, "Life Circumstances and the Use of Mental Health Services: A Five Year Follow-Up," *Social Psychiatry* 21, no. 3 (1986): 123–128.

20. J. Frederick and P. Cotanch, "Self-Help Techniques for Auditory Hallucinations," *Issues in Mental Health Nursing* 16, no. 3 (1995): 223.

21. Frederick and Cotanch, "Self-Help Techniques for Auditory Hallucinations," 213.

22. S. Holmberg, "Physical Health Problems of the Psychiatric Client," *Journal of Psychosocial Nursing* 26, no. 5 (1988): 35–42, at 39.

23. American Psychiatric Association, *Diagnostic and Statistical Manual of Mental Disorders*, 4th ed. (Washington, DC: 1994), 19.

24. North American Nursing Diagnosis Association, *Nursing Diagnoses: Definitions and Classification* (Philadelphia: 1994), 29, 37, 38, 43, 50, 65–69, 77, 79, 86.

25. J. Feighner, "Treatment for Schizophrenic Patients with Depression," *Current Approaches to Psychoses: Diagnosis and Management* 4 (January 1995): 10–11.

26. P. Weiden et al., "Postdischarge Medication Compliance of Inpatients Converted from an Oral to a Depot Neuroleptic Regimen," *Psychiatric Services* 46, no. 10 (1995): 1049–1054, at 1053.

27. C. Connelly and J. Dilonardo, "Self-Care Issues with Chronically Ill Psychotic Clients," *Perspectives in Psychiatric Care* 29, no. 4 (1993): 31–36, at 35.

28. Connelly and Dilonardo, "Self-Care Issues with Chronically Ill Psychotic Clients," 32.

29. A. Hatfield, "Patients' Accounts of Stress and Coping in Schizophrenia," *Hospital and Community Psychiatry* 40, no. 11 (1989): 1141–1145.

30. Hatfield, "Patients' Accounts of Stress and Coping in Schizophrenia," 1143.

31. C. Knight, "President's Message," *Alliance for the Mentally Ill of Montgomery County, MD, Inc.* 17, no. 7 (1995): 2.

32. Breslin, "Treatment of Schizophrenia: Current Practice and Future Promise," 882.

33. E. Leete, "The Treatment of Schizophrenia: A Patient's Perspective," *Hospital and Community Psychiatry* 38, no. 5 (1984): 486–491.

34. S. Najarian, "Family Experience with Positive Client Response to Clozapine," *Archives of Psychiatric Nursing* 9, no. 1 (1995): 11–20, at 19.

35. Malone, "Schizophrenia Research Update: Implications for Nursing," 7.

36. Hauk, "The Acutely Depressed or Schizophrenic Patient," 268.

SUGGESTED READING

American Psychiatric Association. 1988. *Rights of the mentally disabled: Statements and standards.* Washington, DC.

Andreasen, N., and M. Flaum. 1990. Schizophrenia and related psychotic disorders. *Hospital and Community Psychiatry* 41, no. 9: 954–956.

Awad, A. 1992. Quality of life of schizophrenic patients on medications and implications for new drug trials. *Hospital and Community Psychiatry* 43, no. 3: 262–265.

Bachrach, L. 1988. Defining chronic mental illness: A concept paper. *Hospital and Community Psychiatry* 39, no. 4: 383–388.

Beebe, L. 1990. Reframe your outlook on recidivism. *Journal of Psychosocial Nursing* 28, no. 9: 31–33.

Boyd, M. 1994. Integration of psychosocial rehabilitation into psychiatric nursing practice. *Issues in Mental Health Nursing* 15, no. 1: 13–26.

Breir, A., and J. Strauss. 1984. The role of social relationships in the recovery from psychotic disorders. *American Journal of Psychiatry* 141, no. 8: 949–955.

Breslin, N. 1992. Treatment of schizophrenia: Current practice and future promise. *Hospital and Community Psychiatry* 43, no. 9: 877–885.

Buchanan, J. 1995. Social support and schizophrenia: A review of the literature. *Archives of Psychiatric Nursing* 9, no. 2: 68–76.

Conley, R., and R. Baker. 1990. Family response to improvement in a relative with schizophrenia. *Hospital and Community Psychiatry* 41, no. 8: 898–901.

Connelly, C., and J. Dilonardo. 1993. Self-care issues with chronically ill psychotic clients. *Perspectives in Psychiatric Care* 29, no. 4: 31–35.

Dillon, N. 1992. A screening system for tardive dyskinesia: Development and implementation. *Journal of Psychosocial Nursing* 30, no. 10: 3–7.

Dzurec, L. 1990. How do they see themselves? Self-perceptions and functioning for people with chronic schizophrenia. *Journal of Psychosocial Nursing* 28, no. 8: 10–14.

Field, W. 1985. Hearing voices. *Journal of Psychosocial Nursing* 23, no. 1: 9–14.

Field, W., and W. Ruelke. 1973. Hallucinations and how to deal with them. *American Journal of Nursing* 73, no. 4: 638–640.

Garza-Trevino, E. et al. 1990. Neurobiology of schizophrenic syndromes. *Hospital and Community Psychiatry* 41, no. 9: 971–980.

Geller, J. et al. 1992. A practitioner's guide to use of psychotropic medication in liquid form. *Hospital and Community Psychiatry* 43, no. 10: 969–971.

Gillies, L. et al. 1993. Differential outcomes in social network therapy. *Psychosocial Rehabilitation Journal* 16, no. 3: 141–146.

Hamilton, D. 1990. Clozapine: A new antipsychotic drug. *Archives of Psychiatric Nursing* 4, no. 4: 278–281.

Hatfield, A. 1989. Patients' accounts of stress and coping in schizophrenia. *Hospital and Community Psychiatry* 40, no. 11: 1141–1145.

Hatfield, A., and H. Lefley. 1993. *Surviving mental illness*. New York: Guilford Press.

Holmber, S. 1988. Physical health problems of the psychiatric client. *Journal of Psychosocial Nursing* 26, no. 5: 35–39.

Jaretz, N. et al. 1992. Clozapine: Nursing care considerations. *Perspectives in Psychiatric Care* 28, no. 3: 19–26.

Junginger, J. 1995. Command hallucinations and the prediction of dangerousness. *Psychiatric Services* 46, no. 9: 911–914.

Kraus, J., and A. Slavinsky. 1982. *The chronically ill psychiatric patient and the community*. Boston: Blackwell Scientific Publications.

Lefley, H. 1987. Aging parents as caregivers of mentally ill adult children: An emerging social problem. *Hospital and Community Psychiatry* 38, no. 10: 1063–1070.

Loomis, M. 1985. Levels of contracting. *Journal of Psychosocial Nursing* 23, no. 3: 9–14.

Malone, J. 1990. Schizophrenia research update: Implications for nursing. *Journal of Psychosocial Nursing* 28, no. 8: 4–9.

Mason, S. et al. 1990. Patients' and caregivers' adaptation to improvement in schizophrenia. *Hospital and Community Psychiatry* 41, no. 5: 541–544.

Maurin, J. 1989. *Caring for the chronically mentally ill*. Thorofare, NJ: SLACK, Inc.

Maurin, J., and C. Boyd. 1990. Burden of mental illness on the family: A critical review. *Archives of Psychiatric Nursing* 4, no. 2: 99–106.

Minkoff, K. 1987. Beyond deinstitutionalization: A new ideology for the postinstitutional era. *Hospital and Community Psychiatry* 38, no. 9: 945–950.

Moller, M., and J. Wer. 1989. Simultaneous patient/family education regarding schizophrenia: The Nebraska model. *Archives of Psychiatric Nursing* 3, no. 6: 332–337.

Segal, S., and D. VanderVoort. 1993. Daily hassles of persons with severe mental illness. *Hospital and Communtiy Psychiatry* 44, no. 3: 276–278.

Spiegel, D., and T. Wissler. 1987. Using family consultation as psychiatric aftercare for schizophrenic patients. *Hospital and Community Psychiatry* 38, no. 10: 1096–1099.

Sullinger, N. 1988. Relapse. *Journal of Psychosocial Nursing* 26, no. 6: 20–23.

Thompson, E. 1988. Variation in the self-concept of young adult chronic patients: Chronicity reconsidered. *Hospital and Community Psychiatry* 39, no. 7: 771–775.

Torrey, E. 1988. *Surviving schizophrenia*. New York: Harper & Row.

Turnbull, J. et al. 1990. Turn it around: Short-term management for aggression and anger. *Journal of Psychosocial Nursing* 28, no. 6: 7–11.

CHAPTER

24

Dual Diagnosis

INTRODUCTION

Patients with serious mental illness have a high risk, approximately 50 percent, of abusing or becoming dependent on alcohol or other drugs.[1] Because of this risk, it is very important that home care staff assess every psychiatric home care patient for substance abuse problems to determine if specific interventions are required.

DEFINING CHARACTERISTICS

The first question that usually arises when discussing mental illness and substance abuse (*dual diagnosis*) is why they occur together so frequently. There is no firm answer to this question, but several theories have been proposed. One proposal is that those with mental illness use alcohol and/or drugs to self-medicate for symptoms that are very disturbing to them. There is some evidence that the biological elements of substance abuse might be important. According to Zauszniewski, "The serotonergic deficits in alcoholism, the endorphin deficits of opioid dependence, and the dopamine depletion might all predispose one to depression."[2(p.56)] In some patients, drug intoxication or withdrawal may mimic psychiatric symptoms and thus make assessment very difficult. When a psychiatric problem and a substance abuse problem coexist, the patient has a dual diagnosis. The patient has "two separate chronic illnesses. While each illness exacerbates the other, they are driven by different genetic, biochemical, and social factors."[3(p.196)]

When assessing patients, it is important to be aware of the following characteristics of patients with dual diagnosis:[4]

- Dual-diagnosis patients are usually young.
- The psychiatric diagnoses found in these patients are heterogeneous.
- Polysubstance abuse is frequent.
- Some dual-diagnosis patients have some positive elements in their lives, while others have a variable medical history and progressive deterioration.

Vulnerability of patients with psychiatric problems to substance abuse is high. In addition, these patients tend to be very sensitive to the effects of alcohol and other drugs. This is one reason that patients with psychiatric problems, regardless of whether they have a substance abuse problem, are told to abstain from alcohol and other drugs. According to Drake, "Moderate doses of alcohol, nicotine, or caffeine can induce psychotic symptoms in a person with schizophrenia; and small amounts of marijuana, cocaine, or other drugs can precipitate prolonged psychotic relapses."[5(p.5)] In addition, there are many adverse interactions between alcohol and prescribed drugs, and substance abuse can interfere with medical treatment.

ASSESSMENT

Generally, patients with dual diagnosis deny that they have substance abuse problems, are noncompliant with treatment (particularly prescribed medications), and avoid rehabilitation. These patients usually provide inadequate information during assessment, which makes it necessary to use other resources to obtain data. In addition, they may have cognitive impairments that prevent them from providing complete or accurate information. The assessment process itself may be difficult, due to the patient's need to develop trust and inability to tolerate long interviews. The following guidelines may be helpful as the patient is interviewed:[6]

- The focus of the interview is on the patient, to communicate staff support and interest. Listening to the patient is important.
- Discussions that focus on the patient's rationalizations about the use of alcohol or drugs are not productive.
- The nurse asks simple questions about the frequency and amount of substances used.
- "Why" questions are not asked.
- Questions about substance abuse are approached as any other health care–related questions. Judgment is not helpful. Substance abuse is an illness, just as a psychiatric problem is an illness.
- The patient's self-deception is part of the illness and must be considered as questions are answered. The patient may try to convince home care staff that there is no problem.
- Specific, factual questions, particularly open-ended questions, will provide more information and less opportunity for the patient to be evasive.
- If the patient is vague, questions should be repeated.

- Staff and the patient must accept that the patient has multiple problems and that focusing only on some of them will not be successful in the long run.

The assessment includes routine screening that should be used for all psychiatric patients to identify patients who might have a substance abuse problem and initial assessment for those who do have a problem. The following components are important to include in the assessment.[7]

Screening

Screening is an assessment method that focuses on the effects of substance use rather than the consumption level, with the goal of identifying problems. It includes the following:

- questioning the patient about the use of alcohol or drugs
- inquiring about the consequences of alcohol or drug use from the patient's perspective and the family/significant others' (SOs') perspective
- observing for signs of drug-seeking behavior (e.g., seeking medications for anxiety or depression by pretending to experience these symptoms; frequently requesting refills with unusual excuses; displaying disinterest in diagnosis or treatment other than to obtain medication; making staff feel manipulated).

Initial Assessment

Initial assessment occurs when there is an identified problem, and further assessment is required of the following factors:

- substances abused
- pattern of use; frequency; amount per use; number of times per week; circumstances around use; amount required to feel effect
- preoccupation and efforts to control usage; changes in circumstances of usage; periods of abstinence; attempts to decrease amount of substance or to stop its usage
- family/SOs' views of the abuse (Have they noticed the use of alcohol or drugs? What have they said or done? What effect did it have?)
- memory lapses (e.g., blackouts with alcohol use)
- problems that have resulted from use of alcohol or drugs (e.g., marital, employment, follow-through with treatment, medical, financial, or legal problems)
- family/SO history (who; abused substance; abstinence; present use in the home)
- past treatment (type; success; abstinence period; patient's feelings about the treatment and progress)
- dual-diagnosis factor or how the patient views substance abuse affecting other symptoms

- drug testing and screening to determine use of alcohol and drugs (When specimens are collected, the patient must be supervised due to the risk of the patient substituting a "clean" specimen.)

Exhibit 24–1 describes signs and symptoms of intoxication and withdrawal that should be assessed during each home visit.

DIAGNOSIS

Diagnosis is difficult, due to the complex nature of substance abuse and psychiatric problems. The patient may have any of the diagnoses discussed in previous chapters, as well as diagnoses related to the substance abuse. These have been identified in the *Diagnostic and Statistical Manual of Mental Disorders (DSM-IV)*.[8]

- alcohol use disorders
- alcohol-induced disorders
- amphetamine use disorders
- amphetamine-induced disorders
- caffeine use disorders
- caffeine-induced disorders
- cannabis use disorders
- cannabis-induced disorders
- cocaine use disorders
- cocaine-induced disorders
- hallucinogen use disorders
- hallucinogen-induced disorders
- inhalant use disorders
- inhalant-induced disorders
- nicotine use disorders
- nicotine-induced disorders
- opioid use disorders
- opioid-induced disorders
- phencyclidine use disorders
- phencyclidine-induced disorders
- sedative, hypnotic, or anxiolytic use disorders
- sedative, hypnotic, or anxiolytic-induced disorders

Nursing diagnoses are similar to those found in psychiatric illness, including the following:[9]

- ineffective individual coping
- anxiety
- impaired social interaction

Exhibit 24–1 Substance Abuse: Intoxication and Withdrawal

Drug	Signs and Symptoms of Intoxication	Signs and Symptoms of Withdrawal
Opioids	Euphoria Dysphoria Apathy Pupillary constriction, but dilation if major overdose Drowsiness Slurred speech Impaired attention or memory Impaired social judgment Decreased temperature Decreased respiration Decreased blood pressure	Rhinorrhea Lacrimation Sweating Diarrhea Yawning Mild hypertension Tachycardia Pupillary dilation Insomnia Fever Gooseflesh Anxiety Muscle jerks
Cocaine	Elation Grandiosity Depression Suicidal thoughts Delusions Hallucinations Tachycardia Pupillary dilation Increased blood pressure Perspiration or chills Nausea and vomiting	Muscular aches Chills Tremors Anxiety Prolonged sleep Depression/suicidal thoughts
Barbiturates	Decreased respiration Decreased blood pressure Disinhibition of sexual and aggressive impulses Uncoordination Unsteady gait Impaired social judgment Impaired attention or judgment Slurred speech	Nausea and vomiting Sweating Anxiety Depressed mood or irritability Orthostatic hypotension Tremulousness Hallucinations Disorientation Convulsions Cardiovascular collapse Shock
Hallucinogens	Increased temperature Increased blood pressure	None known

continues

Exhibit 24–1 continued

	Euphoria	
	Psychomotor agitation	
	Anxiety or panic	
	Paranoia	
	Visual hallucinations	
	Muscle rigidity	
	Gait ataxia	
	Grandiosity	
	Emotional lability	
	Suicide attempts	
	Sweating	
	Palpitations	
	Uncoordination	
	Impaired judgment	
Marijuana	Euphoria	None known
	Tachycardia	
	Sensation of slowed time	
	Increased appetite	
	Dry mouth	
	Excessive anxiety	
	Impaired judgment	
	Conjunctival injection	
	Orthostatic hypotension	

- disturbance of self-esteem
- risk for self-injury
- alteration in thought processes
- sleep pattern disturbances
- sensory-perceptual alteration
- risk for violence

EXPECTED OUTCOMES

Clearly, a major desired outcome for any patient with a dual diagnosis is long-term abstinence. As the patient works toward long-term abstinence, short-term goals should be identified. This approach is less anxiety provoking for the patient who has additional psychiatric problems. The patient's commitment to treatment for substance abuse as well as for mental illness may be difficult to obtain. Ideally, both illnesses should be dealt with concomitantly; however, if the psychiatric symptoms are so severe that they interfere with substance abuse treatment, then they must be dealt with first. According to Drake, "Because many [substance abuse treatment] programs make no attempts to integrate treatment approaches, the patient, with impaired cognitive capacity, is entirely responsible for the integration. Not surprisingly, the patient often fails in this situation and is considered difficult or labeled as 'treatment resistant.'"[10(p.6)] Some treatment programs have combined treatment approaches for patients with dual diagnosis; however, the home care nurse will be working with the patient in the home without elaborate structured programs. Eventually, the patient should be directed to seek further treatment outside the home and appropriate support groups. As the nurse helps the patient to make this transition, the nurse must determine if the programs are appropriate for dual diagnosis and the patient.

HOME CARE STAFF: RESPONSES TO THE PATIENT

The dual-diagnosis patient is not an easy patient to care for, because of the patient's complex needs and often frustrating behavior. Staff may have negative or prejudicial reactions to substance abuse and may not recognize it as an illness. This makes it even more difficult to provide care, because staff cannot treat only half of the patient's problems. In addition, the patient may have medical problems that have been caused by substance abuse. In fact, the medical problems may be the reason the patient has been referred to home care. Staff need supervision and opportunity to discuss in a nonthreatening environment their reactions to this patient. Staff education should provide information about the dual-diagnosis patient and substance abuse.

INTERVENTIONS IN THE HOME

According to Drake, "Although people with co-occurring mental illness and substance abuse desperately need help with both problems, the service system's organization structures and financing mechanisms often provide barriers to obtaining treatment. The crux of the problem is that the mental health and substance abuse treatment systems are parallel and quite separate."[11(p.5)]

The focus of the interventions described below is on substance abuse. Interventions for specific psychiatric problems are described in previous chapters.

- Assess the patient routinely for intoxication and withdrawal.
- Provide educational material about substance abuse and time to discuss this information.
- Identify with the patient the negative consequences of drug interactions with prescribed medications.
- Assess the home environment for increased risk of alcohol and drug availability and discuss this with the patient and family/SOs to encourage changes in the environment.

- Reinforce the need for abstinence. Abstinence goals must be reasonable.
- Discuss with the patient all incidents of alcohol and drug use that occur during the time the patient is in home care, focusing on the behavior and consequences.
- Identify with the patient alternative methods for anxiety reduction and implement them.
- Provide education about the human immunodeficiency virus (HIV).
- Assess the patient for suicidal feelings and take appropriate steps.
- Remind the patient about the dangers of alcohol and drug use when driving or using equipment.
- Discuss potential and actual substance abuse problems with the family/SOs as well as provide education.

FAMILY/SIGNIFICANT OTHERS: NEEDS AND STRATEGIES

Family/SOs find that the combination of psychiatric problems and substance abuse problems is very difficult to cope with on a daily basis. They experience secretiveness, disruptive behavior, and violence with the ill family member. Dual diagnosis brings additional burdens to the family/SOs, who are already strained. In some cases, a patient's family members/SOs abuse alcohol or drugs or have abused them in the past. In these situations, there is a greater risk of alcohol and drug availability in the home, as well as an environment that condones their use. If the family/SOs are not in treatment for this problem, it will be very difficult to help the patient.

SUMMARY

The two major hurdles in caring for the patient with a dual diagnosis in the home are the home care staff's reactions to substance abuse and the availability of alcohol and drugs in the home or nearby community. If staff are not realistic about their expectations, they will easily become frustrated, and this will decrease the effectiveness of home care. The patient with dual diagnosis is a challenge. Success is highly variable.

NOTES

1. R. Drake, "Substance Abuse and Mental Illness: Recent Research," *NAMI Advocate* 16 (January/February 1995): 5–6.

2. J. Zauszniewski, "Severity of Depression, Cognitions, and Functioning among Depressed In-patients with and without Coexisting Subtance Abuse," *Journal of the American Psychiatric Nurses Association* 1, no. 2 (1995): 55–60, at 56.

3. F. Osher, "Dual Diagnosis," in *Clinical Manual of Substance Abuse*, ed. J. Kinney (St. Louis, MO: Mosby–Year Book, 1991), 195–201, at 196.

4. Osher, "Dual Diagnosis," 197.

5. Drake, "Substance Abuse and Mental Illness: Recent Research," 5.

6. P. Whitmer and J. Kinney, "Routine Screening and Initial Assessment," in *Clinical Manual of Substance Abuse*, ed. J. Kinney (St. Louis, MO: Mosby–Year Book, 1991), 34–48, at 44.

7. Whitmer and Kinney, "Routine Screening and Initial Assessment," 37–44.

8. American Psychiatric Association, *Diagnostic and Statistical Manual of Mental Disorders*, 4th ed. (Washington, DC: 1994), 16–19.

9. North American Nursing Diagnosis Association, *Nursing Diagnoses: Definitions and Classifications, 1995–1996* (Philadelphia: 1994), 5, 29, 38, 63, 73, 75, 79, 82, 86.

10. Drake, "Substance Abuse and Mental Illness: Recent Research," 6.

11. Drake, "Substance Abuse and Mental Illness: Recent Research," 5.

SUGGESTED READINGS

American Psychiatric Association. 1993. *Dual diagnoses of mental illness and substance abuse: Collected articles from HC & P.* Washington, DC.

American Psychiatric Association. 1995. *Practice guideline for treatment of patients with substance use disorders: Alcohol, cocaine, opioids.* Washington, DC.

Kinney, J., ed. 1991. *Clinical manual of substance abuse.* St. Louis, MO: Mosby–Year Book.

Tsuang, J., and J. Lohr. 1994. Effects of alcohol on symptoms in alcoholic and nonalcoholic patients with schizophrenia. *Hospital and Community Psychiatry* 45, no. 12: 1229–1230.

Zauszniewski, J. 1995. Severity of depression, cognitions, and functioning among depressed impatients with and without coexisting substance abuse. *Journal of American Psychiatric Nurses Association* 1, no. 2: 55–60.

CHAPTER

25

AIDS: Neuropsychiatric Complications

INTRODUCTION

Acquired immune deficiency syndrome (AIDS) and its neuropsychiatric problems are complex and require intensive home care nursing. According to Flaskerud, "It is important for mental health nurses working in the community, and mental health nurse consultants in general hospitals, to be aware of the high incidence of central nervous system (CNS) complications in this group of patients. The symptoms of neurologic dysfunction are very similar to those seen in depressive or anxiety syndromes and may also imitate those of bipolar illness and schizophrenia."[1(p.17)] Some of the problems that may occur are[2(p.24)]

- progressive symptoms leading to increased dependence
- emotional resistance to intervention
- unstable or transient lifestyle
- absent or unreliable caregivers
- lack of appropriate residential facilities
- limited trained attendants and mental health home care professionals

These problems occur in addition to psychological responses to a terminal illness and neurological changes that cause major problems for the patient. The home care nurse cannot ignore this patient's psychological needs, as they will affect the patient's daily care. According to Lasalle and Lasalle, "HIV [human immunodeficiency virus] disease presents the patient and loved ones with a series of stressors, sometimes occurring simultaneously, sometimes sequentially. Nurses need to pay special attention to the psychosocial needs of HIV patients because these stressors may directly affect the patient's health and the patient's willingness and ability to fully utilize the health-care system."[3(p.970)]

DEFINING CHARACTERISTICS

The diagnosis of HIV infection is clearly a devastating diagnosis, and many patients respond with maladaptive coping. Carwein and Longley report that "It is estimated that anywhere from 30 to 90 percent of individuals with HIV infection will suffer some form of dementia; in approximately 25 to 30 percent of patients, neurologic dysfunction is the first manifestation of the disease."[4(p.21)] Treatment itself can cause psychiatric changes. Understanding the psychosocial aspects of HIV infection and AIDS and the phases and crises of the illness is helpful in providing care to the patient with neuropsychiatric complications in the home.

PSYCHOSOCIAL ASPECTS OF HIV INFECTION AND AIDS

HIV infection and AIDS directly assault the patient's psychosocial needs. Uncertainty is always with the patient. With this illness of remissions and exacerbations and many possible complications, the patient will never be able to experience a secure life again. Coping with uncertainty is not easy and requires support from others; however, support from others may be a problem with this illness. AIDS is an illness of losses, and one loss is relationships. Many fear the illness and fear contact with those who have it. Due to alternative lifestyles, the patient may already experience isolation. The family/significant other (SO) may withdraw from the patient at the news of the illness, often due to stigma and fear of contracting the illness. Some families draw closer. As the patient becomes sicker, there are fewer and fewer opportunities for contact with others. The patient may experience the loss of self-esteem, dignity, body image, and losses in practical areas of living such as employment or even housing. No areas of the patient's life are unaffected, and the patient's quality of life changes. As the patient experiences more stress, he or she may exhibit alcohol and/or drug abuse and promiscuity. The patient may feel guilt about sexuality, use of drugs, and number of sexual partners. Patients who contract the illness through means other than drug use or homosexual behavior may be tremendously angry about their fate. They are stigmatized, as others wonder how they got the illness. Some try to keep their illness a secret, which causes more stress.

The patient who has a substance abuse problem may frequently use denial to cope.[5] The patient may use the illness to justify increased use of drugs in order to cope with the feelings about the diagnosis and/or the illness's symptoms. Continuing drug abuse may help the patient feel "healthy," and thus the presence of illness is denied. The patient who does not use drugs may also experience denial. Other typical emotional responses are anger, hopelessness, and anxiety, as well as clinical depression and anxiety disorders. Anger may make the patient noncompliant with treatment and recommendations about lifestyle changes (e.g., stopping drug use, changing sexual behavior).

PHASES OF ILLNESS AND CRISES

The patient with AIDS experiences several phases of the illness and many crises during the illness.[6] The first phase and initial crisis occurs at the time of diagnosis. Some patients are diagnosed as HIV-positive, with no assurance that AIDS will develop. Others are diagnosed with AIDS. Both types of patients should receive information about the test results as soon as possible. They will have to learn to live with the uncertainty as well as make lifestyle changes in order to decrease the risk of transmitting the virus to others. Those with AIDS usually respond with disbelief, numbness, and denial, followed by anger, extreme anxiety, depression, and perhaps suicidal ideation.[7] They will need to learn to live with a terminal illness. After the initial diagnosis, there usually is a quiet period in which the patient focuses on learning about the illness; during this period, patients often change to a more healthy lifestyle (e.g., emphasizing nutrition, exercise, rest).[8]

The next phase begins when the first opportunistic infection occurs. The patient again experiences a range of feelings accompanied by symptoms of the illness and the treatment (such as weakness). It is now more difficult to deny the illness, so this phase may be more difficult than the time of diagnosis. The illness becomes real. The patient may experience fear of pain, debilitation, disfigurement, and isolation. After treatment is completed, the patient is left with new fears and anxiety related to disease progression. The patient becomes very concerned with every change in the body, fearful that new symptoms indicate more problems. According to Flaskerud, "Hypervigilance with bodily functions and the appearance of new symptoms can result in hypochondriacal concerns, demanding behavior towards medical personnel and excessive dependence on health care givers."[9(p.10)] This can be draining for all concerned—the patient, home care staff, and family/SOs. When a relapse occurs, the patient feels hopeless and helpless. Home care staff may observe signs of sadness, low self-esteem, loss of control, and suicidal ideation. Dependency increases, and the patient fears that health care staff will abandon him or her.

The final phase is the terminal one. The symptoms of the illness are most severe, and the patient feels ambivalence, dependence, disinterest, and/or resolution.[10] The patient tires easily. The nurse may be involved with a review of the patient's life and preparations for death with the patient. It is a difficult time for all. Some patients are at peace at this time; they have worked through many of their feelings and are able to be open with others. There is a sense of relief for many—relief from pain, the remission and relapse cycle, and the constant fears. Family/SOs and staff may have similar feelings.

Throughout the illness, home care staff must help the patient and family/SOs with many physical, psychological, and social crises. Patients and family/SOs need help in coping with practical issues such as finances, housing, and meals.

General interventions include allowing time for the patient to discuss feelings, listening to the patient, providing routine assessment of psychological status, encouraging attendance at support groups when appropriate, and using community resources to provide services as needed. Accessing community support services can lead to further anxiety, because the risk of being denied these services is a realistic concern for many patients.

DEPRESSION

Depression is a common response to the diagnosis. It can occur due to the many losses the patient experiences and to the feelings of isolation, changes in body image, guilt over sexual or drug-related behavior, and fear of death.[11] In addition, depression may be caused by brain lesions induced by the HIV infection.[12] Depression interferes with functioning and affects the patient's overall response to the illness. It is important that the patient receive treatment for it. Supportive relationships and interventions to increase self-esteem are helpful. The patient's sadness and maladaptive grieving can be manifested by the following symptoms:[13]

- tearfulness
- expressions of worthlessness, hopelessness, and helplessness
- slumped posture
- withdrawal
- projection of guilt and anger by blaming others
- suspiciousness
- verbal and physical abuse
- frequent, often unrealistic demands
- suicidal and homicidal ideation and attempts

It is important to differentiate between depression and dementia, because apathy and psychomotor retardation can be seen in both. When a clear diagnosis is made, however, depression can be treated with medications. The following characteristics and methods are helpful in differentiating the two:[14]

- A depressed patient is morose and expresses feelings of hopelessness and worthlessness.
- A depressed patient may admit suicidal feelings.
- A patient with dementia has difficulty drawing. The home care nurse can ask the patient to draw simple figures (e.g. square, triangle). The depressed patient does not have difficulty doing this drawing.

- A patient with dementia has difficulty producing a list of words that begin with a specific letter of the alphabet when asked to do so. The depressed patient has no difficulty doing this exercise.

NEUROPSYCHIATRIC COMPLICATIONS

AIDS and its treatment can cause many neuropsychiatric complications. The most common is AIDS-dementia complex. The symptoms of central nervous system complications can be confusing; they can resemble the symptoms of a patient who has been informed that he or she has a terminal diagnosis or one who has clinical anxiety or depression. In many cases, the patient is not aware of the initial symptoms. The symptoms can be categorized as initial complaints, early symptoms, and later symptoms.[15,16]

- initial complaints
    1. forgetfulness
    2. recent memory loss
    3. poor concentration
    4. decreased spontaneity
    5. poor cognitive flexibility
    6. bilateral leg weakness
    7. poor coordination with handwriting changes
    8. psychomotor slowing
- early symptoms
    1. unsteady gait
    2. uncoordination
    3. loss of interest in work
    4. loss of libido
    5. blunted affect
    6. agitation
    7. organic psychosis
    8. withdrawal
- later symptoms
    1. total personality change
    2. increased leg weakness with myoclonic jerking
    3. cerebellar ataxia
    4. confusion
    5. disorientation
    6. seizures
    7. mutism
    8. incontinence
    9. hemiparesis/paraparesis

10. blindness
11. delirium
12. coma

The typical differentiation between dementia and other problems is in the patient's cognition. The rate at which patients deteriorate is highly variable. During the early stages, some patients have symptoms that mimic bipolar disorder and schizophrenia. Again, impairment of cognitive functioning can help to differentiate between these mental illnesses and central nervous system complications of AIDS.[17] Because medications can be used for bipolar disorder and schizophrenia, it is important to diagnose the problem in order to select the correct treatment. Nervous system complications worsen. According to Swanson, "In the final stages of AIDS-dementia complex, patients may become immobile, unable to speak, profoundly confused, and incontinent."[18(p.35)]

ASSESSMENT

Observations made while providing care are extremely helpful in assessing the patient's mental status and behavior. Assessment methods might include the following:[19]

- Short-term memory is assessed by asking the patient to repeat a list of numbers. Healthy persons can repeat five to seven numbers. Anxiety affects successful completion of this test. Inability to complete this test indicates that the patient requires written or verbal direction to complete routine tasks.
- Sensation is assessed by asking the patient to identify, with eyes shut, numbers written on his or her fingertips with a capped pen. Problems doing this indicate that the patient has sensory deficits and, consequently, the patient's safety may be compromised (e.g., the patient may not recognize the temperature of water).
- Assessment of upper-extremity functioning is done by asking the patient to alternately supinate and pronate his or her hands. The patient may be unable to do this, appear clumsy, or be unable to maintain the sequence of movements. Occupational therapy interventions may be helpful for this patient. Lower extremities are assessed by observing the patient's gait.
- Abstract thinking is assessed by asking the patient to explain common proverbs. If the patient experiences problems doing this, he or she will have difficulty learning new behaviors and problem solving.
- Problem solving is assessed by asking the patient to respond to a hypothetical problem.

As care is provided, home care staff are able to assess many aspects of the patient's emotions and behavior.[20] They might notice that the patient loses his or her train of thought in the middle of a sentence or needs lists to complete daily tasks; both of these behaviors indicate problems with concentration and memory. The patient may be unable to transfer learned information to new situations, indicating problems with abstracting and ability to form concepts. Impaired impulse control and emotional lability may be seen in the patient who is agitated, combative, or experiences panic attacks. Impaired motor coordination may be a problem when the patient is clumsy, ataxic, or has slurred speech. The patient may become confused easily and become angry about it. The patient may display poor social judgment and overreaction. Observations about dress, grooming, and personal hygiene can indicate possible problems. Are buttons fastened? Is the patient wearing appropriate clothing? Is the patient clean? Speech can be assessed by observing the volume, rate, rhythm, articulation, and fluency of the patient's speech.[21] None of these behaviors are difficult for staff to observe, and they require no special testing. To help the patient cope with these changes, home care staff will have to adjust their plan of care. As staff observe that the patient's behavior and condition are changing, they should document these observations and communicate them to the patient's physician.

A comprehensive assessment for the patient with neuropsychiatric complications should include the following:[22]

- general appearance/behavior
- mood and emotions
- intellectual level
- orientation and memory (immediate and delayed)
- ability to follow simple to complex commands
- ability to perform motor tasks when requested to do so
- judgment
- speech (slurred, dysarthria, aphasia)
- thought content (preoccupation, perseveration, confabulation)
- thought patterns (incoherence, delusions, hallucinations)
- attention and concentration
- ability to recognize the form of a solid object by touch; stereognosis
- changes in sensory and perceptual functioning
    1. pupillary reflexes; reaction to light
    2. ocular movements; follow finger
    3. vision acuity (blurred, presence of floaters)
    4. taste (sugar, salt, etc.)
    5. facial movement (frown, wink, etc.)
    6. pharynx and tongue movements
    7. smell (lemon, peppermint, etc.)
    8. hearing
    9. vestibular alterations; vertigo, nystagmus

10. arms (finger-nose, finger-finger, pronation-supination, patting or tapping tests)
11. legs (heel-knee, heel-toe walking)
12. trunk (gait, station)
13. touch (cotton wisp)
14. pain (pin prick)
15. temperature (heat and cold)

Other areas that require assessment focusing more on psychologial and sociological issues are social isolation; alteration in quality of life; change in self-esteem; intensity of emotions; issues of control; denial; financial stressors; and ethical issues such as power of attorney, living will, and decisions about life-sustaining treatment. These areas of assessment may take more time than the usual initial assessment; however, they are very important to the patient's care and the patient's daily life.

HOME CARE STAFF: RESPONSES TO THE PATIENT

Home care staff who work with AIDS patients must confront many challenges. Fear of contagious disease is present, even for those who are educated about the illness. AIDS education is critical for all home care staff, and they must apply this information in the home environment for all patients. Staff prejudices about the patient's lifestyle or use of drugs may also interfere with care. According to Lasalle and Lasalle, "Although a nurse is entitled to have private views, there is an obligation to provide the best nursing care available to each patient. Disapproval of the patient's past behavior is the nurse's prerogative. The challenge is to keep that view from interfering with care while accepting the patient as a person."[23(p.979)] Caring for any dying patient is difficult and stressful, particularly if staff are caring for many of these patients. Often these patients are young, which adds to the pain for all. Some staff may blame the patient's behavior for the outcome and become unable to focus on the patient as a person who is dying. Staff who have this problem will need supervision to cope with the problem; in some cases, a staff member may not be appropriate to care for a particular patient. All home care staff who care for AIDS patients need a safe place to express their feelings and work through them so that the feelings do not interfere with the care that is needed.

INTERVENTIONS IN THE HOME[24–26]

Providing care for the patient who has AIDS is complex and intensive and consumes staff energy. Developing a plan with interventions to meet the patient's ever-changing needs is critical. Example interventions follow.

Overall Care Needs

Interventions to meet the overall needs of the patient include the following:

- A structured program is developed for the patient to help the patient feel secure.
- The environment should be kept as familiar and consistent as possible.
- Consistent staff should be used whenever possible.
- Staff must explain care to the patient using short, simple explanations and recognizing that repetition may be required.
- Preparation for changes is critical to decrease the patient's anxiety.
- When the patient is asked to perform a task, allow enough time to complete the task.
- Time is required to listen and talk with the patient.
- Confidentiality is a major issue and should be discussed with the patient.
- Staff need to work with family/SO caregivers to help them provide care that meets the patient's needs while understanding their own needs and providing support to them.

Problems with Intellectual and Cognitive Dysfunction

Problems with intellectual and cognitive dysfunction (e.g., impaired concentration, memory deterioration, impaired abstracting ability, slowing of mental capabilities, psychomotor retardation, delirium, and late stage akinetic mute state may be a major focus of care. Interventions include the following:

- When teaching the patient, make sure that the environment is free of distraction. The patient should be taught simple ideas or tasks and provided written information. Home care staff should also teach the patient's caregivers.
- Use the following strategies to help the patient with memory problems: provide written information; have the patient repeat important information; write down appointments and schedules; provide similar information for family/SOs; and avoid confronting patient about loss of memory.
- Provide structure and consistency.
- When trying to include the patient in decision making, identify only a limited number of options. This will help to decrease the patient's anxiety about choices.
- Divide tasks into small steps.
- Encourage the patient to identify pros and cons when solving problems.
- Identify with the patient factors that might interfere with decision making.
- Let the patient know that it is acceptable to make mistakes and support the patient during these times.

- Assist the patient in implementing decisions.
- While considering the patient's limitations, encourage independence at all times. However, allow the patient more time for activities of daily living and other activities.
- Prevent isolation by encouraging some socialization as long as the patient can tolerate it.
- Limit abrupt changes in schedule, home care staff, environment, and treatment.
- Reorient the patient as needed (e.g., use large calenders, large-faced clocks, medication reminder system; write out medication schedule and all other treatment instructions; label rooms; use reflective tape to direct the patient to the bathroom and other important areas; provide extra lighting in the environment).
- Provide time to discuss the patient's concerns about memory loss.
- If the patient has a tendency to wander, instruct caregivers to check the patient frequently at night.
- Before the patient deteriorates, encourage an open discussion about the patient's wishes for life-sustaining treatment, etc.

Problems with Sensorimotor Dysfunction

Problems with sensorimotor dysfunctioning will affect the patient's daily functioning. Interventions focusing on these problems include the following:

- Safety is very important. Provide assistance with activities of daily living as required to ensure safety. Use skid-resistant decals or mats in the shower/bathtub. Avoid use of razors and sharp instruments without help. The patient may need assistance with hazardous tasks such as cooking, smoking, and driving. Remove scatter rugs and limit furniture in high-traffic areas. Numb areas of body need to be protected from harm (e.g., extreme temperatures, sharp objects).
- Problems with mobility are monitored routinely for complications, particularly skin breakdown, deep vein thrombosis, and pneumonia.
- The patient should ambulate when possible and perform range-of-motion exercises. It is best to do these exercises at the same time each day. Physical therapy may be used at this time.
- If the patient cannot speak, staff should develop methods for communicating with the patient and work with family/SOs to use the same methods.
- Rest periods are very important and will increase as the patient's condition deteriorates.
- If the patient cannot do activities of daily living for self, the patient should be encouraged to direct these activities.

- Bladder and bowel incontinence is very difficult for the patient because of fear of dependency, lowered self-esteem, body-image changes, fear of response from others, physical problems such as skin breakdown, odor, etc. The patient will need support and information about why incontinence is occurring.

Problems of Personality and Behavioral Disturbances

Problems of personality and behavioral disturbances (e.g., impaired impulse control, emotional lability) will disturb the patient and everyone who has contact with the patient. Interventions include the following:

- Redirect behavior rather than trying to control it. Remove the object or person who may be causing agitation in the patient.
- Protect the patient from self-injury. Assess suicidal ideation and feelings routinely.
- Encourage the patient to participate in treatment and to remain in as much control of the treatment as possible.
- Decrease environmental stimuli when necessary.
- Provide medications (e.g., antidepressant, antianxiety) when ordered. Assess carefully for side effects that may be harmful.
- Limit caffeine.
- Teach the patient and those who care for the patient stress management techniques such as relaxation.
- Help the patient to set realistic goals.

Depression

Depression is a common occurrence requiring interventions.

- Utilize interventions identified in Chapter 21.
- Provide time to discuss losses, death, and AIDS.
- Recommend that the patient participate in an AIDS support group when this is appropriate and the patient is able. Encourage family/SOs to do this, as well.

FAMILY/SIGNIFICANT OTHERS: NEEDS AND STRATEGIES

Family/SOs must cope with all of the problems that home care staff encounter with the patient who has AIDS. They, however, also experience personal loss and pain as they watch someone they love slowly die. Home care staff cannot care for this patient without caring for the family/SOs. Clearly, the spouse, parent if the patient is a child, or the patient's partner are the most affected. Family/SOs may experience guilt, particularly a partner or parent who believes he or she transmitted the illness. Family/SOs may experience anxiety and depression, and staff may need to refer them for help to resolve these problems. The family/SOs will experience problems with changes in relationships, social stigma, fear of contagion, burden of caring for a very ill loved one, financial burden, as well as the common feelings associated with having a loved one die. Home care staff should help family/SOs do the following:

- cope with stress
- problem solve practical issues regarding the care of the loved one
- learn about the illness, treatment, and the care that is required
- discuss their feelings and reactions to the illness and the changes in their lives
- identify and use methods for support (e.g., support groups, reading material about the illness, respite)
- prepare for death and its aftermath (e.g., emotional responses, advance directives, durable power of attorney, funeral plans)

SUMMARY

The AIDS patient is a complex patient who is experiencing overwhelming physical problems and psychosocial responses to the illness. Everyone who cares for the patient and the family/SOs experiences strong emotions about the illness and the patient. Home care staff must provide time to discuss and cope with these feelings and reactions while providing quality physical care and support.

NOTES

1. J. Flaskerud, "Neuropsychiatric Complications," *Journal of Psychosocial Nursing* 25, no. 12 (1987): 17–20, at 17.
2. V. Carwein and C. Longley, "AIDS Dementia: Assessment and Interventions for Home Hospice Care," *Caring* 8, no. 6 (1989): 21–27, at 24.
3. P. Lasalle and A. Lasalle, "Psychological Care of the Patient with HIV/AIDS," in *Principles and Practice of Psychiatric Nursing*, ed. G. Stuart and S. Sundeen (St. Louis, MO: Mosby–Year Book, 1995), 969–982, at 970.
4. Carwein and Longley, "AIDS Dementia: Assessment and Interventions for Home Hospice Care," 21.
5. S. Batki et al., "Psychiatric Aspects of Treatment of IV Drug Abusers with AIDS," *Hospital and Community Psychiatry* 39, no. 4 (1988): 439–441.
6. J. Flaskerud, "Psychosocial Aspects," *Journal of Psychosocial Nursing* 25, no. 12 (1987): 9–16, at 10–11.
7. Flaskerud, "Psychosocial Aspects," 10.
8. Lasalle and Lasalle, "Psychological Care of the Patient with HIV/AIDS," 972.
9. Flaskerud, "Psychosocial Aspects," 10.

10. Flaskerud, "Psychosocial Aspects," 10.

11. Lasalle and Lasalle, "Psychological Care of the Patient with HIV/AIDS," 973.

12. B. Swanson et al., "Dementia and Depression in Persons with AIDS: Causes and Care," *Journal of Psychosocial Nursing* 28, no. 10 (1990): 33–39, at 35.

13. Swanson, "Dementia and Depression in Persons with AIDS: Causes and Care," 37.

14. Swanson, "Dementia and Depression in Persons with AIDS: Causes and Care," 38.

15. Flaskerud, "Neuropsychiatric Complications," 19.

16. Carwein and Longley, "AIDS Dementia: Assessment and Interventions for Home Hospice Care," 22–23.

17. Flaskerud, "Neuropsychiatric Complications," 18.

18. Swanson, "Dementia and Depression in Persons with AIDS: Causes and Care," 35.

19. Swanson, "Dementia and Depression in Persons with AIDS: Causes and Care," 37–38.

20. Swanson, "Dementia and Depression in Persons with AIDS: Causes and Care," 35.

21. Carwein and Longley, "AIDS Dementia: Assessment and Interventions for Home Hospice Care," 26.

22. Flaskerud, "Neuropsychiatric Complications," 19.

23. Lasalle and Lasalle, "Psychological Care of the Patient with HIV/AIDS," 979.

24. Carwein and Longley, "AIDS Dementia: Assessment and Interventions for Home Hospice Care," 23.

25. Swanson, "Dementia and Depression in Persons with AIDS: Causes and Care," 36–37.

26. Lasalle and Lasalle, "Psychological Care of the Patient with HIV/AIDS," 975–978.

SUGGESTED READING

Batki, S. 1988. Psychiatric aspects of treatment of IV drug abusers with AIDS. *Hospital and Community Psychiatry* 39, no. 4: 439–441.

Carwein, V., and C. Longley, 1989. AIDS dementia: Assessment and interventions for home hospice care. *Caring* 8, no. 6: 21–27.

Durham, J., and F. Cohen, eds. 1991. *The person with AIDS: Nursing perspectives.* New York: Springer.

Durham, J. 1994. The changing HIV/AIDS epidemic: Emerging psychosocial challenges for nurses. *Nursing Clinics of North America* 29, no. 1: 9–19.

Flaskerud, J. 1987. AIDS: Neuropsychiatric complications. *Journal of Psychosocial Nursing* 25, no. 12: 17–19.

Flaskerud, J. 1987. Psychosocial aspects. *Journal of Psychosocial Nursing* 25, no. 12: 9–16.

Forstein, M. 1984. The psychosocial impact of the acquired immunodeficiency syndrome. *Seminars in Oncology* 11, no. 1: 77–82.

Govini, L. 1988. Psychosocial issues of AIDS in the nursing care of homosexual men and their significant others. *Nursing Clinics of North America* 23, no. 4: 749–765.

Korniewicz, D. et al. 1990. Coping with AIDS and HIV. *Journal of Psychosocial Nursing* 28, no. 3: 14–21.

Landau-Stanton, C., and C. Clements. 1993. *AIDS: Health and mental health.* New York: Brunner/Mazel, Inc.

Marzuk, P. et al. 1988. Increased suicide risk of suicide in persons with AIDS. *Journal of American Medical Association* 259, no. 9: 1333–1337.

Ostrow, D. et al. 1988. Assessment and management of the AIDS patient with neuropsychiatric disturbances 49, no. 5: 14–22.

Pessin, N. 1993. Integrating mental health and home care services for AIDS patients. *Caring* 12, no. 5: 30–34.

Pfeifer, W., and C. Houseman. 1988. Bereavement and AIDS: A framework for intervention. *Journal of Psychosocial Nursing* 26, no. 10: 21–26.

Salisbury, D. 1986. AIDS: Psychosocial implications. *Journal of Psychosocial Nursing* 24, no. 12: 13–16.

Servellen, G. et al. 1989. Coping with a crisis: Evaluating psychological risks of patients with AIDS. *Journal of Psychosocial Nursing* 27, no. 12: 16–21.

Shilts, R. 1987. *And the band played on.* New York: St. Martin's Press.

Swanson, B. et al. 1990. Dementia and depression in persons with AIDS: Causes and care. *Journal of Psychosocial Nursing* 28, no. 10: 33–39.

26

Psychological Care of the Medically Ill Patient in the Home

INTRODUCTION

The experience of illness requires all the resources a patient can pull together. Most patients are very successful and survive the experience with minimal if no psychological damage; however, other patients need more help. According to Strain and Grossman, "The vulnerability of a given patient to such stress, and the kind of psychological response it gives rise to, will depend on many variables, including (1) the nature of the stress the patient is experiencing (special meaning the illness and hospitalization hold for the patient), (2) the patient's characteristic mode of coping with stress, and (3) the patient's previous experiences with doctors, illness, and hospitalization."[1(p.24)] To apply the appropriate interventions for psychological responses to medical illness, home care staff must understand stress, as well as how patients with specific medical illnesses respond to the stress of being ill.

STRESS

Stress and coping are common topics today; however there are no generally accepted definitions for *stressor*, *stress*, or *coping*. Stress theories are divided into four categories: physiological, psychosocial, cognitive, and biopsychosocial.

1. *Physiological theories*[2] focus on generality versus specificity of response. Selye was the first to work extensively in this area. He identified the general adaptation syndrome or GAS, which is a nonspecificity model. It includes three phases; alarm, resistance, and exhaustion. Research today on psychoendocrinology has disputed his nonspecificity model, as researchers have noted that the neuroendocrine response differs for different

stressors. The neuroendocrine response can be affected by subtle psychosocial stimuli. Selye proposed that diseases of adaptation can occur if stress is prolonged or severe or if adaptation is ineffective. He believed that illnesses such as rheumatoid arthritis, hypertension, and peptic ulcer were diseases of ineffective adaptation. Today there is less support for the role of maladaptation in the development of these diseases; however, the theory has not been totally discarded.

2. *Psychosocial theories*[3] focus on life events versus personality variables. This research has produced results such as the relationship of critical life events to stress. The Holmes and Rahe Social Readjustment Scale is based on this idea. A person identifies which of the life events on the scale are personally relevant and, based on these events, the person identifies his or her stress rating. Examples of items on the scale are change of job, marriage, divorce, death, and childbirth. Identification of the Type A personality is another example of the application of psychosocial theories. This type of personality has been associated with a coping pattern that is most commonly identified with coronary heart disease. Psychosocial theories have led to disagreements about the possibility of identifying a disease-prone personality.

3. *Cognitive theories* focus on the "dynamic, mutually reciprocal relationship or the transaction, between the person and the environment."[4(p.223)] Lazarus presented what may be the most widely used psychological definition of stress, which resulted from his research. He defined *stress* as "a particular relationship between the person and the environment that is appraised by the person as taxing or exceeding his or her resources and endangering his or her well-being."[5(p.19)] According to this definition of stress, *coping* describes the process the person uses to manage stress and its impact on psychosocial functioning, quality of life, and somatic health. This theory has been expanded by others to include appraisal of the stress experience and identification of assets and liabilities or resources and deficits.[6] Appraisal and transactional models are based on cognitive theories.

4. *Biopsychosocial theories* support the need for an integrative approach with a more holistic view. These theories express the idea that "stress must be understood in terms of the biological processes which mediate adaptation as well as the psychosocial processes underlying appraisal and coping."[7(p.223)]

More recently researchers have focused on the study of neuroendocrine-immune system interactions and stress, particularly the influence of psychosocial factors on immune functions and health. Studies have indicated that the stress response has a simultaneous effect on the sympathetic-adrenomedullary system, which releases epinephrine and norepinephrine, and the hypothalmic-pituitary-adrenocortical system leading to the elaboration of endogenous opioid peptides, corticotropin, and cortisol.[8] Cortisol is an immunosuppressive, reducing lymphocyte numbers and functions and natural killer cell activity. Inhibited production of cytokines by cortisol interferes with virtually all components of the immune system. This may have important implications for illness and stress, but it is necessary to conduct more research.

STRESS ADAPTATION MODEL

How can knowledge about stress theories be useful for the home care nurse? Stuart has developed a model of stress adaptation that incorporates many of the ideas presented in stress theories and applies these ideas to nursing care.[9] This model includes five components: predisposing factors, precipitating stressors, appraisal of stressor, coping resources or strategies, and coping mechanisms. Each factor plays an important role in the continuum of coping responses—some adaptive and others maladaptive—that the patient experiences. The goal is to assist the patient toward growth and goal achievement by strengthening these five components.

1. *Predisposing factors.* Predisposing factors are biological, psychological, and sociocultural. They are "conditioning factors that influence both the type and amount of resources the person is able to use to handle stress."[10(p.84)]
2. *Precipitating stressors.* Precipitating stressors are "stimuli that the individual perceives as challenging, threatening, or demanding. . . . [They] require energy and produce a state of tension and stress with the individual."[11(p.84)] Stressors may be biological, psychological, or sociocultural, and for each patient they are internal and external.
   - For each patient, the timing of the experience is a critical factor—particularly when the stressor occurs, its duration, and its frequency.
   - The number of stressors is also a critical factor. Some patients can tolerate many stressors at one time or over a period of time; however, if the patient is in pain or confused, the patient may have less ability to cope with stress.
3. *Appraisal of stressor.* The appraisal of the stressor is the assessment of the stress experience. How the patient appraises the event is the key to understanding the patient's coping and the nature and intensity of the stress response. There is a danger in presuming to know how the patient is appraising a stressful event. This may lead to mistakes in the selection of interventions, and the patient may feel that the home care nurse is not really listening to the patient and including the patient in the treatment process. Typically, responses fall into the following categories:
   - *Cognitive responses.* The patient's decision making is influenced by many factors such as emotions, physiological status, and beliefs and values. Generally, the patient views a stressful event as a loss, a threat, or a challenge.

- *Affective responses*. The most frequent affective response to stress is anxiety. Depression and anger may also be experienced.
- *Physiological responses*. The fight-or-flight physiological response stimulates the sympathetic division of the autonomic nervous system and increases activity of the pituitary-adrenal axis. For patients with some medical problems (e.g., cardiac or respiratory), these responses may have a direct effect on their physical status.
- *Behavioral responses*. These responses are varied and usually relate to the patient's affective response.
- *Social responses*. The patient looks for the meaning of the stressful event. The patient may compare the event with others, seek information, and search for cause. These responses are important as the patient evaluates his or her need for support.
4. *Coping resources or strategies*. There are several critical questions related to coping resources: What options are available? What will they accomplish? Can the patient use resources or strategies successfully? These coping resources include personal abilities, social support, material assets, positive beliefs, social skills, problem solving, health, and energy.
5. *Coping mechanisms*. Coping mechanisms can be constructive or destructive. The home care nurse should help the patient use constructive coping mechanisms. It is important to remember that different patients respond to different interventions. Examples of simple interventions that might be used to increase constructive coping include the following:[12]
   - assertiveness training
   - time management
   - anger management
   - conflict management
   - social problem solving
   - relaxation training

Another intervention approach is to use several types of interventions that combine behavioral, cognitive, and relaxation techniques. Diversion and relaxation might be used to cope with chemotherapy, cancer, pain management, preparation for surgery or with a stressful medical procedure. Other techniques that might be used are teaching healthy eating and exercise, enhancing health-related treatment adherence, and controlling smoking and substance abuse.

BASIC STRESSORS OF ILLNESS AND TREATMENT

The following are examples of basic stressors experienced by patients during illness and treatment:[13]

- *Basic threat to narcissistic integrity.* Illness, hospitalization, and potential of death pose a threat to the common but irrational belief that the patient is always capable, independent, self-sufficient, indestructible, and in control. The patient is confronted with dependency and often treated like a child; however, it is not acceptable to act like one (e.g., demanding, complaining, irritable). The patient is told when and how to do things the patient normally does for himself or herself. Staff expect that the patient will comply. Autonomy and control are lost.
- *Fear of strangers.* The patient must put self and his or her care into the hands of strangers with limited knowledge of staff competence. The patient may be assigned inconsistent staff in the home, increasing the fear of who is coming each day.
- *Separation anxiety.* The patient may be separated from important persons and things or lose privacy and important personal possessions—particularly if the patient's room must be changed in the home due to the patient's needs (such as changing to a room on the ground floor without steps). Separation is not just physical but also psychological (e.g., change in relationships).
- *Fear of the loss of love and approval.* A change in body image or a loss of time at work where the patient usually receives approval can be very stressful. The patient may fear that illness and dependency may drive away loved ones.
- *Fear of loss of control of developmentally achieved functions.* The loss of physical and mental functions, even temporary loss, is stressful. There is always the fear of not regaining them.
- *Fear of loss of or injury to body parts.* The patient fears the loss of body parts or function or injury to body parts. These fears are in addition to fears about diagnostic procedures, treatment, and outcomes.
- *Guilt and fear of retaliation.* Some patients may feel that illness is related to punishment. The inability to cope with pain only affirms this loss of control.

Patients respond to stress with loss of self-esteem, which is accompanied with effects such as anxiety, shame, guilt, degrees of "normal depression," and helplessness. If these effects continue or become very intense, some patients may replace them with inappropriate pleasant affects (such as euphoria or mania) or use of inappropriate defense mechanisms. Physiological responses to these affects may cause further medical problems or limit recovery. Typical responses are fear, anxiety, loss of control, sensory overload, regression, loneliness, demanding/complaining behavior, anger, noncompliance, increased sleep, and lack of appetite.[14] According to Strain and Grossman, "The nature and magnitude of the patient's response to these stresses will depend on what illness and hospitalization mean to the patient in terms of his past experiences and development, and in terms of his current psychological resources."[15(p.29)]

COMMON RESPONSES TO ILLNESS AND TREATMENT

The most common responses to illness and treatment are loneliness, demanding and complaining behavior, anger, anxiety, and depression. Each of these responses should be considered in the home care treatment plan.

- *Loneliness.* Illness leads to separation from family, friends, work, and usual social outlets. This occurs even in the home as the illness causes separation from usual routines and relationships. The amount of separation varies, depending on the patient's routines and relationships prior to illness, the nature and duration of the illness, caregivers' responses to the illness, home care staff, and the patient's strengths and limitations. Most patients do not find loneliness a positive experience and want to avoid it. Loneliness usually results in increased anxiety. Sometimes bringing the problem out in the open helps the patient feel less lonely. Mentioning that it is a common feeling may make the patient feel more comfortable. However, it is not helpful to approaching it by saying, "Everybody feels it. It's alright." Listening to the patient will prevent this staff attitude.
- *Demanding and complaining behavior.* This patient frustrates most home care staff and family/significant others (SOs) because the patient makes others feel incompetent and unappreciated. The staff/family/SOs' responses are helplessness, anger, frustration, impatience, and a feeling that they are unable to meet the patient's needs no matter what is done. The patient may compare one staff member with another, which only increases staff negative feelings. If staff cannot cope with their feelings and reactions toward the patient, they will find themselves in a crisis. Staff will withdraw from the patient or feel jealousy when the patient praises another staff member; staff conflict may develop about the patient and the care; staff may treat the patient inappropriately; and staff may criticize the patient while ignoring his or her needs. It is easy to forget that the demanding, complaining patient usually feels lonely, frightened, and anxious, and may have a very low self-esteem. This patient may be confused about the illness, treatment, and the responses from those who are important to the patient. As the patient's anxiety increases, so does the irritating behavior. The patient wants to feel secure; however, the methods chosen to feel secure do not help.
- *Angry behavior.* The angry patient has expectations and is frustrated when expectations are not met. This is viewed as a threat to self. Feeling completely overwhelmed, anxious, powerless, and insecure, the patient copes by using anger, unconsciously; changes anxiety to aggression; and seeks the feeling of power rather than powerlessness. The patient can express anger directly or indirectly.

- *Anxiety*. Anxiety, as discussed in Chapter 20, affects the patient both physiologically and psychologically. Some anxiety is beneficial; however, severe or panic levels of anxiety are unhealthy. The patient who is experiencing anxiety at these high levels will need immediate interventions.
- *Depression*. For some patients the response to medical illness is depression. This depression may or may not require medical interventions. Nursing interventions, however, will be helpful. Chapter 21 provides more information about interventions for depression.

What can the home care staff do in response to a patient's psychological responses to illness? Staff must recognize their own feelings and behaviors toward the patient. Withdrawing is not helpful. Withdrawal can be physical or psychological. In the latter case, home care staff provide care for the patient without relating to the patient as a person. The patient will perceive this as rejection and will be devastated—even the patient who does not seem to care. Interventions that might be used to help the patient cope with illness and treatment include the following:

- Provide consistent care.
- Meet needs before requested.
- Offer the patient choices when possible.
- Involve the patient in decision making and care.
- Communicate in an open and clear manner.
- Set limits on inappropriate behavior.
- If the patient is angry, help the patient to see the situation as an opportunity to learn and then use his or her energy to learn.

CHRONIC ILLNESS

Chronic Illness versus Acute Illness

Home care patients are seen for chronic illness, for an acute illness with a concomitant chronic illness, and psychiatric illness with a concomitant chronic medical illness. Strauss defined chronic illness as "all impairments or deviations from normal which have one or more of the following characteristics: are permanent, leave residual disability, are caused by nonreversible pathological alteration, require special training of the patient for rehabilitation, may be expected to require a long period of supervision, observation, or care."[16(p.1)] Chronic illness is very common in all age groups, but particularly for patients over 60.

How is acute illness different than chronic illness? The most critical element is that in acute illness, treatment focuses on *curing* the patient. In chronic illness, treatment focuses on *caring* for patients for whom staff can "only" make comfortable or assist with adaptation to their illness. Curing has always been more satisfying for the patient, home care staff, and family/SOs. Another critical difference between acute and chronic illness is that with acute illness, treatment usually focuses primarily on physical needs with some attention given to psychological and social concerns. In chronic illness, the psychological and social problems are more critical. To develop a better understanding of chronic illness, it is important to understand the patient's day and functioning. The overall goal with a patient who has a chronic illness is to improve the quality of the patient's life.

Chronic Illness Framework

Any chronic illness can potentially cause multiple problems of daily living for the patient. Strauss developed a framework for chronic illness to help others better understand the experience for the patient and the effects the chronic illness has on daily living. This framework is helpful for home care staff as it provides guidance about the focus for interventions.

- *Prevention and management of medical crisis.*[17] The prevention and management of a medical crisis focuses on the identification of the signs of the crisis and organizing for the crisis. Education of patient and family/SOs is very important in order to accomplish prevention and management. For example, a diabetic patient is taught the signs of hypoglycemia and what must be done for self-management, such as carrying candy at all times or having enough insulin during a trip. The cardiac patient is taught the signs of chest pain and shortness of breath and the importance of the availability of nitroglycerin. Even with the most prepared patients, there are breakdowns in the organization. When a crisis is not foreseeable, there is a greater chance of a crisis. The longer the period between medical crises, the less prepared the patient will be. Family/SO stress may lead to decreased alertness to the needs. A temporary or permanent loss of a family member or significant other (such as a trip, divorce, or death) will weaken the patient's support resources. If the patient in crisis requires medical attention, particularly hospitalization, the patient and the family/SOs must then give up some responsibility to the hospital. This may be a relief to them, but some will see it as a failure. Home care staff should avoid emphasizing family/SO failure to monitor symptoms or follow through on treatment. As soon as possible, the patient and family/SOs should be brought back into the care process. Patients with multiple hospitalizations or medical crises tend to frustrate staff, and the patient soon realizes this reaction. When a crisis does occur after a period of recovery, the patient should review what happened with the home care staff and family/

SOs when appropriate. The focus is not on blame, but rather on development of better methods for prevention and management of medical crises.

- *Symptom control.*[18] Symptom control is very important for a patient with a chronic illness. The patient will need to learn his or her symptom pattern. (For example: What are the consequences for bodily movements, abilities, work, his or her moods, family/SOs, social relationships, diet, and independence? What are the patient's strengths? What are the patient's limits?) The patient may need to redesign his or her lifestyle due to symptoms. This is referred to as *normalizing*. Some examples of normalizing might be to stop smoking, move to a one-level house, change diet, begin exercising, or adapt past exercises. Symptoms and what the patient must do to control the symptoms may change the patient's interactions with others. Not only may the patient withdraw from others, but family/SOs may withdraw from the patient, especially if the patient becomes demanding and unpleasant or if the consequences of the illness are difficult to watch (e.g., paralysis, shaking).
- *Management of the treatment plan.*[19] Management of the treatment plan requires certain social and financial conditions, particularly the following:
  1. initial and continuing trust in health care professionals (The patient needs someone who listens and believes that there is a problem. Patients who experience a long period without a clear-cut diagnosis frequently have less trust in home care staff.)
  2. belief that the treatment chosen is the best (This is a difficult condition, and one that is not always fully met. Patients may ask if there are other treatments available or if there is a folk remedy that is better.)
  3. evidence that the treatment either controls the disease itself or its symptoms
  4. no frightening side effects
  5. symptom relief or fear of the illness outweigh risks of side effects
  6. limited interference with important daily activities
  7. limited negative impact on the patient's sense of identity

It is easy to see that these conditions are ideal and difficult to maintain for most patients; however, they indicate for home care staff the areas of concern for the patient with chronic illness. In addition, characteristics of the treatment plan that will be of great concern to the patient include the following:[20]

  1. patient's knowledge about the treatment plan including accepting the treatment, administering it, and making adjustments for it (such as eliminating something or adding something)
  2. time, particularly how much time is involved and how much is taken from family/SOs, work, and personal life
  3. amount of discomfort, effort, energy, visibility, and stigma

4. efficiency or how quickly the treatment becomes effective, especially in relationship to the patient's expectation
5. expense of the treatment and its effects on other financial issues such as income
6. knowledge of the disease and its deterioration pattern
7. normalizing

Normalizing

The most important goal for the patient with a chronic illness is not just to stay alive or keep symptoms under control, but also to live as normally as possible despite the symptoms and the disease. When the treatment, symptoms, or knowledge of the disease turn out to be intrusive, then the patient must work very hard to create some semblance of a normal life for himself/herself and for those around the patient. Even when this is accomplished, there will be ups and downs.

Intrusiveness of symptoms varies depending upon the illness and the symptoms. Some symptoms are not visible, some are very visible, and others affect relationships more than others. For example, angina is not visible unless the patient responds to it in some way that can be observed; however, it is still very intrusive on the patient's life. Serious scars from surgery for neck cancer are very visible and can affect relationships and casual encounters with others. The patient who cannot normalize his or her life will find that symptoms become the focus of interactions. In normalizing, the patient tries to keep symptoms invisible or at least decrease them. If the patient is unsuccessful, there is greater potential for isolation (e.g., the patient with Parkinson's disease whose trembling causes him or her to withdraw into isolation).

For some patients, trying to normalize may increase anxiety instead of decreasing it. This can occur if the patient is worried about what others might see or if there is disagreement with others about the extent of the illness. Even with successful normalizing, there will be down times. How will the patient accept these times? Will the patient be able to adapt? If the fear of a relapse dominates the patient's life, it can be very destructive; however, denying the possibility is also unrealistic. The patient must reach a balance.

Psychological Responses to Chronic Illness

The typical initial responses to chronic illness are experiencing denial and repression, giving up control and regressing, clinging to hope that life will return to the way it was in the past, and viewing the physician as omnipotent. The goal is to help the patient to acknowledge the reality and to learn the required information to be as independent as possible and yet cope with the illness daily. Other reactions the patient may have are anxiety, depression, anger, hopelessness, and guilt. The patient might experience guilt if he/she feels that he/she did something or failed to do something that might have led to the illness. In most cases, this is an unrealistic view, but if it interferes with treatment and normalizing, it needs to be identified.

SPECIFIC MEDICAL ILLNESSES AND PSYCHOLOGICAL RESPONSES

Pain

The patient's view of pain is important. Some anxiety helps the patient cope with the anticipation of pain. As anxiety increases, pain increases, and as pain increases, anxiety increases. It is important for the patient to learn about pain and anxiety. Patient education may accomplish the following:

- prevent the patient from using fear-producing fantasies for the lack of knowledge
- help the patient feel more in control of pain and treatment
- increase the patient's communication with staff and family/SOs about anxiety, pain, and needs
- decrease the element of surprise and thus make the patient feel less victimized

Factors that affect the patient's response to pain are powerlessness, the attitudes of others, the patient's information, degree of threat from the pain, past experiences with pain, and pain used for secondary gain. Pain used for secondary gain is when the patient uses the pain to illicit sympathy; this is done to prevent or decrease loneliness, to control the actions of others, or to allow the patient to be dependent on others and to avoid responsibility.

Coronary Heart Disease[21,22]

Typically a patient who has coronary heart disease experiences fear and anxiety as well as periods of depression. Lifestyle changes are required such as cessation of smoking, diet changes, and addition of an exercise program. Emotions, particularly anxiety, increase cardiac work. According to Strain and Grossman, "The relationship between physiological and psychological factors persist during the convalescent phase of coronary heart disease, and now manifests itself in mood disorders and phobias and inhibitions surrounding sex and work."[23(p.155)]

The patient may be fearful of being alone, particularly soon after discharge from the hospital. Hypochondriacal fears may arise, and they may not be related to the heart. The patient may somatize anxiety and experience palpitation, dyspnea, excessive fatigue, and chest pains, and fear that another heart attack is occurring. It is difficult for home care staff to recognize hypochondriacal symptoms, as these symptoms can be serious and related to further coronary problems. Decreasing stress will help the patient, and the patient needs to learn about stress management and apply it. During home care, the patient should be given as much control as possible, because loss of control and fear of this loss will increase anxiety. The patient may also use anger to help feel in control. Some patients may deny there is a problem, particularly when coronary symptoms first occur. The home care nurse should help the patient adapt, but the adaptation needs to be based on realistic limitations. Some patients may feel that they have unrealistic limitations.

Questions that might be considered in the assessment of a patient with coronary heart disease include the following:

- Has the patient experienced significant losses in the past year?
- Has the patient experienced any recent psychosocial stress that revived earlier unresolved losses?
- Is the patient perceiving the current illness as a loss (loss of function, self-worth, interpersonal relationship, economic resources)?
- Does the patient use coping skills that are appropriate and effective?
- Is the patient future oriented?
- How realistic are the patient's goals and the means for attaining them?
- How realistic is the patient's view of his or her limitations?
- How logical is the patient's thinking?
- What are the patient's personal resources?
- What environmental conditions are influencing the patient's ability to cope?
- Is the patient willing to learn about the illness and its treatment?

The Agency for Health Care Policy and Research (AHCPR) reports that "The prevalence of various forms of depression in patients who have had a myocardial infarction is estimated at 40 to 65 percent. High prevalence rates have also been found in patients undergoing coronary artery or heart transplant surgery."[24(p.61)] Patients who experience depression and myocardial infarction tend to have more social problems in the first year of recovery, take more time to return to work, and experience more stress. Some studies have indicated that there is a link between depression and noncompliance with treatment.

The common causes of anxiety in the cardiac patient include the following:

- fear of death or chronic illness
- uncertainty of etiology of illness and prognosis
- development of complications

- threat to self-image
- misinterpretation of information and misconceptions of experience such as perceiving that general weakness means there is permanent heart damage

Consistent and knowledgeable home care staff can help decrease anxiety. Patient involvement in care and sharing information with the patient are also important. If the patient's anxiety increases, it may be necessary for staff to repeat information.

Schizophrenia and Medical Illness

Patients with schizophrenia have a low tolerance of anxiety, and it can make their symptoms worse. If home care staff are afraid of the patient or feel uncomfortable with the patient's behavior, the patient senses this fear. This is not helpful for treatment. There is no reason to be fearful if staff care for the patient's needs and assess the patient's anxiety and intervene as needed. The patient may be terrified by the sense of powerlessness felt as he or she experiences a medical illness and treatment. Helping the patient increase control over the situation may help to decrease anxiety that might exacerbate psychotic symptoms. Routines may help staff anxiety and for some patients routines help their anxiety. However, the patient will need some flexibility; knowing when to be more flexible is important. Staff should not speak to the patient as if the patient does not understand; they should speak clearly, avoid vague language, and ask only one question at a time. If the patient seems confused, gently repeating the message will help. If the patient is delusional or hallucinating, arguing with the patient about these experiences only increases patient anxiety. Although hallucinations and delusions exist for the patient, it will frighten the patient if others agree with the delusion or hallucination and imply that they experience the same thing. It is best for staff to say that they have not seen or heard the hallucination or felt the delusion, and that it must be frightening to the patient. If the patient has auditory hallucinations and the voices are telling the patient to harm the self or others, this can be very dangerous. It is important to discuss these concerns with the patient. As with any patient, it is important to treat the patient with respect and to involve the patient in treatment decisions, treatment, and self-management. The patient may have had bad experiences in hospitals, particularly psychiatric hospitals, and may assume that all hospitals are the same. If the patient's behavior is inappropriate, it may be necessary for staff to set limits. This should be done simply, informing the patient that the particular behavior is not acceptable. If the patient cannot stop the inappropriate behavior, staff must help the patient. If the patient's behavior escalates, home care staff or family/SOs may need to call for help. This is discussed in Chapter 29.

Borderline Personality Disorder and Medical Illness

A patient with a borderline personality disorder does not have an anxiety disorder but does experience higher levels of anxiety and causes increased anxiety in others. Most staff find this patient to be demanding, manipulative, hostile, and very difficult. The patient manages to affect everyone's morale and certainly interferes with his or her own care. A patient with borderline personality disorder feels he or she is a victim, expects mistreatment, and expects to be misunderstood. A medical illness is not uncommon in this patient, who may complain about physical problems and may not care for himself or herself. Many patients with borderline personality disorder are admitted to hospitals for suicide attempts, injuries due to accidents, and problems with substance abuse. Hospitalization increases the patient's anxiety and may affect the patient's tenuous grasp of reality.

Patients with borderline personality disorder use the defense mechanisms of projection and identification. Examples of projection are "It's your fault, not mine. You're angry, not me." The patient reacts to people as he or she expects them to behave. The slightest hint of rejection leads to anger. With identification, the patient sees himself or herself as powerless over authoritative figures and has little trust that needs will be met, so the patient demands that these needs are met.

Due to these defense mechanisms, the patient has a sense of entitlement and uses splitting or views the world as "owing him and he plans to make it pay." With splitting, the patient praises some staff and criticizes others. Home care staff may begin to feel the way they are described, and this causes staff conflict. The patient complains to everyone about the incompetent staff. This patient easily provokes staff or any caregiver's anger, and the result is often inappropriate behavior in staff and caregivers. If staff are aware of this behavior, they can be alert to it, prevent inappropriate responses toward the patient, and avoid counterattacking. Goals for treatment might include the following:[25(pp.1646–47)]

- Reduce the patient's anxiety to a tolerable level and decrease impulsivity.
- Defuse the power struggle between patient and home care staff so that they are able to deliver optimal care.
- Manage the patient's behavior purposefully—that is, by staff acting and not reacting.
- Collaborate with other disciplines to stop disruptions and follow the plan.

Cancer

Depression may worsen as physical health improves, and a patient is never too weak to attempt suicide. Because many of the symptoms of depression are the same as for physical illness, it is easy to miss depression. Some "red flags" are[26]

- difficulty in making decisions, frequent crying, and feelings of dissatisfaction (These symptoms usually indicate a mild depression.)
- feelings of failure, loss of interest in people, seeing one's illness as a punishment, and suicidal ideas (These symptoms are usually associated with severe depression.)

Cancer and suicide have been associated with the following risk factors:[27(p.46)]

- prior suicide attempts
- substance abuse
- single status
- severe emotional distress
- exhausted social resources
- family/SOs conflict
- poor prognosis
- pain, nausea, or other negative effects of the illness or treatment

Patients with cancer who are most at risk for suicide have gastrointestinal, head or neck, or metastasized cancer. Interventions that might be used with these patients include the following:

- If the patient tells the staff/family/SOs that he or she is depressed or suggests it, they should take time to talk with the patient about these feelings. Appropriate interventions must be taken to ensure that the patient is safe.
- It is not helpful to say, "You'll feel better." It only makes light of what the patient is feeling.
- Relief of physical problems will help to decrease depression.
- Encouragement of self-care communicates to the patient that he or she continues to be a responsible person. Sympathizing with the patient's fatigue and excusing the patient from all self-care is not helpful. It is best to say, "I know you are tired, but it is best if you do part of your bath."
- Physical activity that is broken into small parts will aid the patient in accomplishing tasks and increasing the patient's self-esteem. Giving positive feedback to the patient is important as the depressed patient tends to focus on the negative or what was not done.
- This patient tends to interpret information from a negative point of view (e.g., a borderline laboratory test result is viewed as proof of a complication; patient misinterprets what is heard; patient misinterprets sounds that are heard from medical equipment).
- Staff should help the patient identify alternatives to negativism and despair.

Exhibit 26–1 provides additional suggestions for communication with patients who have cancer and their family/SOs.

Exhibit 26–1 Communication Skills with Patients with Cancer and Their Families/Significant Others

- Always question your assumptions.
  - Don't assume you know what people need or why they are behaving as you observe.
- Attending behaviors.
  - Give attention and actively listen.
  - Listen and observe.
  - Make eye contact (may vary with different cultures).
  - Posture should indicate interest and readiness to listen.
  - Verbal responses should accurately reflect what was said.
- Encourage verbal communication.
  - Ask open questions (only use closed questions if the patient is anxious or you need specific information).
  - Avoid leading questions.
  - Avoid "why" questions.
  - Give minimal nonverbal and verbal leads, e.g., nodding head, "I see."
- Paraphrase the content of what was said.
  - Communicate understanding.
  - Validate your understanding.
  - Allow the person to hear what was said.
- Reflect feelings—express your perception of what the person feels—to
  - Communicate that feelings are accepted.
  - Allow recognition that feelings are normal.
  - Permit statements of feelings the person is finding hard to verbalize.
  - Validate your judgment of the feelings. Reflection of feelings is often helpful with angry patients who may not even realize their angry behavior.
- Summarize to
  - Show your effort to accurately understand.
  - Verify content and feelings.
  - Clarify meaning.
  - Encourage further exploration once a central theme is identified.
  - Close discussion of topic to open way for new topics.
  - Terminate the session.
- Self-disclosure—sharing your own feelings, attitudes, experiences for the benefit of the patient/family.
  - Should relate directly to the patient's sitation—am I wanting to reveal this for the patient/family or my own needs?
  - Should be short and to the point.
  - Do so only on a level of intimacy you're confortable with—how will I feel later about having disclosed these feelings/expressions? Remember this in regard to patients also. Have them reflect on whether they really want to disclose intimate information to you.

continues

Exhibit 26–1 continued

- Confrontation
  - Stimulate exploration of something the person is uncomfortable with or avoiding.
  - Assess the need for confrontation by identifying discrepancies between behavior and verbal communication.
- Problem solving (for those things that can be changed)
- Support and reassurance
  - Demonstrate acceptance and understanding
  - Do not have to respond verbally—staying with the patient is just as important.
  - Reassurance should always be realistic. Don't make blanket statements such as, "Everything will be alright."
- Humor
  - Can relieve stress.
  - Laughter is therapeutic.
  - Assess appropriate timing and content and patient receptiveness.

Source: Reproduced by permission of the National Association for Home Care, from *CARING* Magazine XII, no. 2 (February 1993).

Stroke[28,29]

Psychiatric complications related to stroke are recognized stroke complications; however, they are often overlooked in treatment. There is a high prevalence of these problems, and they do affect recovery and increase long-term mortality. Patients with mental illness can have movement disturbances that mimic certain strokes, and this should be considered when an assessment is done. In addition, personality changes that result from a stroke are sometimes diagnosed as a mental illness. This can lead to inappropriate treatment. A clear diagnosis is very important. Typical psychological responses to a stroke include depression, anxiety, apathy, catastrophic reaction, and emotional lability. Psychoses and mania are rare.

- *Depression.* Depression is the most common response, with a rate of 40 percent. It affects recovery, intellectual impairment, and activities of daily living. Depression occurs more in patients with left frontal and left basal ganglia lesions. Tricyclic antidepressants can be helpful, but in the elderly there is a higher risk of causing delirium.
- *Anxiety.* There is a 27 percent rate of anxiety with a stroke. It is more common with lesions of the right hemisphere, and there often is a history of alcoholism.
- *Apathy.* Apathy is "the absence or lack of feeling, emotion, interest, or concern."[30(p.466)] It can occur with or without depression and occurs at a rate

of 20 percent. It is seen more with lesions of the posterior limb of the internal capsule as well as in older patients and those with deficits in activities of daily living.

- *Catastrophic reaction.* A catastrophic reaction is seen in 20 percent of patients with a stroke. Its symptoms are inability to cope with physical or cognitive deficits, anxiety, tears, aggressive behavior, swearing, displacement, refusal, and renouncement. These patients may boast that they are able to perform a task, and when they fail say it is due to fatigue and lack of concentration. Often these patients have a family history of psychiatric disorders. According to Starkstein and Robinson, "The catastrophic reaction may not represent an independent clinical syndrome, but may be a behavioral and emotional expression of depressed patients with anterior subcortical damage."[31(p.470)]
- *Emotional lability.* Emotional lability is very common in the stroke patient. It may coexist with depression. The patient exhibits sudden, easily provoked crying in appropriate situations. Some patients, however, experience pathological laughing and crying in inappropriate situations.

Parkinson's Disease[32]

Distinguishing between Parkinson's disease and mental illness is not always easy. Alterations in mental function are a part of the disease process, and this can be misleading. The patient may have cognitive dysfunction, sleep disturbances, and/or clinical psychiatric illness. Primary degenerative dementia that occurs is very similar to that found in Alzheimer's dementia, which can further complicate the picture. Dysfunctions might be observed in memory, language, visuospatial function, and complex cognition (e.g., abstraction, calculation, judgment, affect).

According to Koller and Megaffin, "The psychiatric manifestations of Parkinson's disease may be as or more disabling than the motor dysfunction. They may occur as a complication of pharmacotherapy for the motor symptoms or result from the disease itself."[33(p.442)] The typical psychiatric problems are depression and anxiety, with mania and delusions less common. Depression occurs in 40 to 50 percent of patients with Parkinson's. It is important to distinguish symptoms of depression from those of dementia. The following is a comparison of these symptoms:[34]

- *Level of consciousness*: With depression, the patient is alert; the patient with dementia is also alert.
- *Mood/affect*: The patient with depression is sad and appears depressed; with dementia, the mood/affect depends upon the content.
- *Behavior*: The patient with depression has psychomotor retardation and decreased energy; with dementia, the patient experiences "sundowning" or confusion at night.

- *Hallucinations and delusions*: The patient with depression may have mood-congruent hallucinations and/or delusions; with dementia, the patient may be delusional.
- *Orientation*: The patient with depression has no problems with orientation; with dementia, the patient may not have problems but may tend to confabulate.
- *Memory*: Memory is normal in depression; with dementia, there are changes in recent and remote memory and loss of common knowledge.
- *Level of functioning*: Both depression and dementia have a slow deterioration in level of functioning.
- *Onset*: Both depression and Parkinson's disease occur slowly.
- *Thinking*: The patient with depression may have thought blocking and delusions; with dementia, thinking is impoverished.
- *Perception*: The patient with depression has normal perception; with dementia, misperceptions are present.

Depressive symptoms with Parkinson's disease are mild to moderate, and suicide is rare. Medications used to treat Parkinson's, particularly levodopa, can cause problems. This medication may cause symptoms of psychoses and may predispose the patient to depression. Patients with Parkinson's disease are usually very sensitive to the side effects of antidepressants. Electroconvulsive therapy may be used if the patient is unable to take antidepressants.

Anxiety is seen in 35 to 40 percent of patients with Parkinson's. Anxiety may coexist with depression. Benzodiazepines may be used with antidepressants, and buspirone is used for anxiety. Sleep disturbances may be experienced. Predictors of this problem are older patients, multiple drug therapy history, premorbid history of psychiatric illness, and use of anticholinergics. As many as 20 percent of patients experience visual hallucinations, seeing formed objects such as people and animals. This usually occurs at night, and those with the highest risk for hallucinations are those on dopaminergic agents who are not experiencing delirium. Delusions have a broader range of potential, from 30 to 50 percent. They may be self-persecutory, and older patients with dementia are more susceptible.

Diabetes[35,36]

Diabetes requires that the patient make important lifestyle changes, some of which are not easy to do. The patient's premorbid personality, past problems and problem solving experience, and attitudes will affect how the patient responds to this chronic illness. At first the patient may experience denial. The patient may want to prove that he or she is in control and may do this by refusing to learn about the illness and treatment or refusing treatment. The consequences of this response and behavior can be life threatening. It may take a medical emergency to change the patient's response. Some patients become very dependent, almost immobilized by the disease. They may experience regression and increased anxiety and demanding behavior. When things do not go as the patient hopes, depression may occur. Suicidal feelings and behaviors are possible, and a common suicidal method is refusal to follow treatment recommendations. Monitoring these feelings is important. Other patients may feel that they are being punished; then the patient feels hostile and resentful resulting in overeating, which can be dangerous. Dietary restrictions provide a method for the patient to act out feelings rather than to talk about them and try to resolve them. When the patient with diabetes experiences stress, it may increase blood glucose; thus, stress needs to be managed. The day-to-day management of diabetes can affect self-image and lead to embarrassment, fatigue, and frustration. As some pleasures are denied, such as by dietary restrictions, the patient needs to find new pleasures. Patients' strengths need to be supported so that they can manage their illness. Opportunity to discuss feelings and fears are very important; however, it is not helpful to argue with the patient about noncompliance. The focus should be on behavior and results. Patient education is critical to put the patient back in control.

When a patient with diabetes is also taking psychotropic medications, serious problems can occur that need monitoring. Phenothiazines have endocrine and metabolic effects that may lead to high or low blood sugar and alteration of glucose tolerance curves. Tricyclic medications change gastric emptying, and this can affect blood sugar levels and interfere with adequate blood sugar control. Patients who have mental illness may have difficulty monitoring their symptoms and following the treatment.

Respiratory Diseases[37]

Respiratory diseases, particularly chronic obstructive pulmonary disease (COPD), are chronic illnesses that often leave the patient feeling hopeless. Many patients respond to this illness with resentment, anger, anxiety, fear, and depression, all of which interfere with treatment. Some patients use defense mechanisms, such as repression and denial, to cope with the illness. Patients with severe respiratory problems cannot afford to become angry, anxious, or depressed, because these responses can contribute to physiological decompensation. Some patients protect themselves from these responses by becoming isolated and decreasing interactions with others. Loss of energy can lead to further isolation. Activities of daily living must be carefully planned to allow for the most efficient use of the patient's minimal energy and tolerance of emotions. As the illness progresses, dependency increases, which cause the patient to fear alienating those who are important. Previous behavior may have caused problems in relationships that are important now that the patient is more dependent. This can make the patient anxious. When the patient keeps feelings inside, the patient will feel more isolated. The patient may be described as living in an "emotional straitjacket."

Medications used to treatment psychiatric disorders can also affect the physiological status of respiratory disorders.[38] These medications can cause respiratory suppression by increasing viscosity of pulmonary secretions. The patient exhibits changes in sputum, increased frequency of coughing, increased severity of cough, increased breathing problems, increased respiratory rate, and increased use of chest wall muscles to aid in breathing. The patient may not notice these changes immediately or may not report them, but they are very important. When the patient has respiratory problems, the home care nurse should consider the medications that the patient may be taking for psychiatric illnesses.

End-Stage Renal Disease

End-stage renal disease affects all parts of the patient's life. Biological, psychological, and social adaptation are required. When the patient begins dialysis, there usually is a honeymoon period lasting about six months. Prior to dialysis the patient was very sick, and when dialysis begins the patient feels better. The patient will feel hopeful and confident but lack a real perception of the physical limitations and problems that are brought on by dialysis. Following this stage, the patient experiences discouragement. This usually begins abruptly as the patient experiences the stress of planning and trying to get routine back into his or her life. The patient feels helpless and sad. At this time, many patients experience medical complications. The third stage is the period of long-term adaptation. The goal is for the patient to become more accepting of the limitations.

Depression is frequent in patients with renal disease. The home care nurse should assess for it routinely. Suicidal feelings and behavior may occur. It is easy for the patient to harm the self directly, or indirectly by not following the treatment plan. Loss of self-esteem and changes in body image occur throughout the illness. As the patient becomes more dependent on a machine, he or she experiences increased loss of control and independence. The time taken for treatment further isolates the patient, which is not helpful for depression. The patient should make the time that is available for social contacts as effective as possible. As the patient is monitored routinely, it is important to remember that uremia can cause bizarre behavior; interventions for this problem would be different than for patients with bizarre behavior that is not caused by a medical problem. The medical problem will need to be resolved.

Many patients with end-stage renal disease are waiting for transplants, which is an additional source of stress.[39] If family members cannot provide a kidney, they may feel guilty. Family/SOs may resent the demands placed on them by the patient. This can be destructive to family/SO interactions and communication, with the family/SO covering over feelings of displeasure, resentment, anger, and disappointment. Some family/SOs may be overly protective and treat the patient like a child. The patient may then feel guilty when he or she feels angry toward a family member, and displace this anger onto the staff. Home care staff can support the family/SOs by encouraging them to discuss their feelings and develop methods to decrease the disruption of the family life. The nurse helps to identify the patient's capabilities and to emphasize the need for the patient to be as independent as possible. If the patient is waiting for a transplant, the patient and family/SOs will need someone to speak with them about their feelings and to provide accurate, up-to-date information.

Rheumatoid Arthritis

Rheumatoid arthritis (RA) is a chronic illness in which physiological changes can occur quickly, even from hour to hour. According to Lambert and Lambert, "The rheumatoid arthritic person is likely to live a life filled with unpredictability because of not knowing when pain may occur, when stiffness may result, whether deformities may set in, or whether disability will occur."[40(p.555)] These changes have a direct effect on the patient's activity level. Stress seems to aggravate the disease, but it is not the cause of the disease. Rehabilitation is very important for this patient. Patient education plays an important role in this process. With the prognosis uncertain, the patient may feel that health care professionals are being evasive. This may increase the patient's anxiety and decrease trust in caretakers. Denial may also occur, but with time this usually resolves. It is important that the home care nurse communicates a positive attitude about self-management to the patient and family/SOs. Providing the patient with interventions that can help to control symptoms is part of the treatment plan. This will help to decrease the patient's feelings of hopelessness. The patient always has to live with the dread of where the disease will strike next and the fear of increasing dependency. When the patient sees others with more severe RA, there is the relief that the illness is not as bad; however, there is always the fear that the patient could get worse. It is important to offer opportunities for the patient to discuss these mixed feelings.

How does a patient with RA normalize his or her life in face of the disease's uncertainty? The patient may use strategies related to covering up, keeping up, justifying inaction, pacing, and renormalizing.[41]

- *Covering up.* This is the main strategy used to cope with a chronic illness. It involves concealing the disability and/or pain; however, this is not denial. It is the rejection of the social significance of the handicap but not of the handicap itself. Certainly, the more visible the illness, the less chance that covering up will be successful (e.g., the patient with RA who has hand deformities or who is unable to walk well). If covering up is successful, there is a price to pay: the strategy can deplete the patient's energy. For the RA patient, it is important to conserve energy.

- *Keeping up.* Keeping up with what is perceived to be normal activities is another important strategy. These efforts may be irrational, but the goal is to maintain a self-image. As the patient tries to keep up, the pain tolerance threshold may be raised. As a result, the patient may be slow to recognize the signs of body dysfunction. This can create additional problems, because the RA patient should decrease activities when pain increases.
- *Justifying inaction.* Patients with RA may at times have difficulty justifying inaction due to the uncertainty of their illness. Many of the symptoms are not visible to others, such as pain and stiffness, and the patient may work hard to appear healthy. In such a case, the patient has convinced others that there is no problem, and it works against the patient when symptoms are worse.
- *Pacing.* Pacing requires that the patient identify activities that can be done, how often they can be done, and under what circumstances. As the patient's status changes, so does the pacing. When the patient is in remission, more activities may be accomplished; however, as symptoms become worse, activities need to be changed. This may be difficult for others to understand.
- *Renormalization or adaptation.* Renormalization requires the patient to lower expectations and develop new norms for action. This directly relates to the intensity and change in symptoms. If the patient must change expectations, this can lead to depression, anger, regression, and anxiety. To accomplish renormalization, the patient must ask for and accept help (which carries with it the fear of dependency and being a burden) and balance options related to daily life and treatment.

SUMMARY

Home care staff encounter many patients with medical illness who either have a psychiatric diagnosis or psychological responses associated with their medical illness. Some patients may not have a psychiatric diagnosis but should have one identified. Home care for the patient with medical and psychological problems is complex. Home care staff must be able to assess the patient thoroughly and identify multiple problems. Interventions must be planned to support one another and meet the physical and psychological needs of the patient. Priorities must be set. This very challenging home care patient needs staff who believe that total patient care is critical. If staff consider these additional problems and intervene appropriately, they can provide more comprehensive care for this patient.

NOTES

1. J. Strain and S. Grossman, *Psychological Care of the Medically Ill: A Primer in Liaison Psychiatry* (New York: Appleton-Century-Crofts, 1975), 24.

2. N. McCain and J. Smith, "Stress and Coping in the Context of Psychoneuroimmunology: A Holistic Framework for Nursing Practice and Research," *Archives of Psychiatric Nursing* 7, no. 4 (1994): 221–227, at 222.

3. McCain and Smith, "Stress and Coping in the Context of Psychoneuroimmunology: A Holistic Framework for Nursing Practice and Research," 222–223.

4. McCain and Smith, "Stress and Coping in the Context of Psychoneuroimmunology: A Holistic Framework for Nursing Practice and Research," 223.

5. R. Lazarus and S. Folkman, *Stress, Appraisal, and Coping* (New York: Springer, 1984), 19.

6. J. Smith, *Understanding Stress and Coping.* (New York: Macmillan, 1993).

7. McCain and Smith, "Stress and Coping in the Context of Psychoneuroimmunology: A Holistic Framework for Nursing Practice and Research," 223.

8. McCain and Smith, "Stress and Coping in the Context of Psychoneuroimmunology: A Holistic Framework for Nursing Practice and Research," 224.

9. G. Stuart, "A Stress Adaptation Model of Psychiatric Nursing Care," in *Principles and Practice of Psychiatric Nursing*, eds. G. Stuart and S. Sundeen (St. Louis, MO: Mosby–Year Book, 1995), 79–101.

10. Stuart, "A Stress Adaptation Model of Psychiatric Nursing Care," 84.

11. Stuart, "A Stress Adaptation Model of Psychiatric Nursing Care," 84.

12. McCain and Smith, "Stress and Coping in the Context of Psychoneuroimmunology: A Holistic Framework for Nursing Practice and Research," 224–225.

13. Strain and Grossman, *Psychological Care of the Medically Ill: A Primer in Liaison Psychiatry*, 24–27.

14. Strain and Grossman, *Psychological Care of the Medically Ill: A Primer in Liaison Psychiatry*, 22–23.

15. Strain and Grossman, *Psychological Care of the Medically Ill: A Primer in Liaison Psychiatry*, 29.

16. A. Strauss, *Chronic Illness and the Quality of Life* (St. Louis, MO: The C.V. Mosby Company: 1975), 1.

17. Strauss, *Chronic Illness and the Quality of Life*, 13–20.

18. Strauss, *Chronic Illness and the Quality of Life*, 34–43.

19. Strauss, *Chronic Illness and the Quality of Life*, 21–33.

20. Strauss, *Chronic Illness and the Quality of Life*, 58–65.

21. G. Lipkin and R. Cohen, *Effective Approaches to Patients' Behavior* (New York: Springer Publishing Co., 1992), 205–213.

22. Strain and Grossman, *Psychological Care of the Medically Ill: A Primer in Liaison Psychiatry*, 151–170.

23. Strain and Grossman, *Psychological Care of the Medically Ill: A Primer in Liaison Psychiatry*, 155.

24. Agency for Health Care Policy and Research, *Depression in Primary Care, Volume 1. Detection and Diagnosis* (Washington, DC: U.S. Department of Health and Human Services, 1993), 61.

25. N. Runyon et al.; "The Borderline Patient on the Med-Surg Unit," *American Journal of Nursing* 88, no. 12 (1988): 1644-1649, at 1646.

26. S. Valente and J. Saunders, "Dealing with Serious Depression in Cancer Patients," *Nursing* 89 no. 2 (1989): 44–47, at 46.

27. Valente and Saunders, "Dealing with Serious Depression in Cancer Patients," 46.

28. S. Starkstein and R. Robinson, "Neuropsychiatric Aspects of Stroke," in *Textbook of Geriatric Neurospsychiatry*, ed. C. Coffey and J. Cummings (Washington, DC: American Psychiatric Press, Inc., 1994), 457–477.

29. A. Esser and S. Lacey, *Mental Illness: A Homecare Guide* (New York: John Wiley & Sons, 1989), 85.

30. Starkstein and Robinson, "Neuropsychiatric Aspects of Stroke," 466.

31. Starkstein and Robinson, "Neuropsychiatric Aspects of Stroke," 470.

32. W. Koller and B. Megaffin, "Parkinson's Disease and Parkinsonism," in *Textbook of Geriatric Neurospsychiatry*, ed. C. Coffey and J. Cummings (Washington, DC: American Psychiatric Press, Inc., 1994), 434–456.

33. Koller and Megaffin, "Parkinson's Disease and Parkinsonism," 442.

34. Z. Lipowski, "Transient Cognitive Disorders in the Elderly," *American Journal of Psychiatry* 140, no. 11 (1983): 1426–1432, at 1432.

35. Lipkin and Cohen, *Effective Approaches to Patients' Behavior,* 189–194.

36. Esser and Lacey, *Mental Illness: A Homecare Guide*, 85–87.

37. Esser and Lacey, *Mental Illness: A Homecare Guide*, 85.

38. Esser and Lacey, *Mental Illness: A Homecare Guide*, 85.

39. Lipkin and Cohen, *Effective Approaches to Patients' Behavior,* 214–220.

40. V. Lambert and C. Lambert, "Coping with Rheumatoid Arthritis," *Nursing Clinics of North America* 22, no. 3 (1987): 551–558, at 555.

41. C. Wiener, "The Burden of Rheumatoid Arthritis," in *Chronic Illness and the Quality of Life*, ed. A. Strauss (St. Louis, MO: C.V. Mosby, 1975), 71–80.

SUGGESTED READING

American Psychiatric Association. 1993. *Practice guidelines for major depressive disorder in adults.* Washington, DC.

Burckhardt, C. 1987. Coping strategies of the chronically ill. *Nursing Clinics of North America* 22, no. 3: 543–549.

Christenson, J. 1993. Chronic pain: Dynamics and treatment strategies. *Perspectives in Psychiatric Care* 29, no. 1: 13–17.

Depaulo, J., and K. Ablow. 1989. *How to cope with depression.* New York: McGraw-Hill.

Dye, C. 1985. *Assessment and intervention in geropsychiatric nursing.* New York: Grune & Stratton.

Falvo, D. 1991. *Medical and psychosocial aspects of chronic illness and disability.* Gaithersburg, MD: Aspen Publishers, Inc.

Gorman, L., and M. Luna-Raines. 1989. *Psychosocial nursing handbook for the non-psychiatric nurse.* Baltimore, MD: Williams & Wilkins.

Klein, D., and P. Wender. 1988. *Do you have a depressive illness?* New York: New American Library.

Lambert, C., and V. Lambert. 1987. Psychosocial impacts created by chronic illness. *Nursing Clinics of North America* 22, no. 3: 527–533.

Lambert, V., and C. Lambert. 1987. Coping with rheumatoid arthritis. *Nursing Clinics of North America* 22, no. 3: 551–558.

Lewis, S. et al. 1989. *Manual of psychosocial nursing interventions: Promoting mental health in medical surgical settings.* Philadelphia: W.B. Saunders Company.

Lipkin, G., and R. Cohen. 1992. *Effective approaches to patients' behavior.* New York: Springer Publishing Co.

Lorig, K., and J. Fries. 1990. *The arthritis helpbook.* New York: Addison-Wesley Publishing Co.

McCain, N., and J. Smith. 1994. Stress and coping in the context of psychoneuroimmunology: A holistic framework for nursing practice and research. *Archives of Psychiatric Nursing* 8, no. 4: 221–227.

McPherson, M. 1990. Drug-induced mental status changes. *Journal of Home Health Practice* 2, no. 3: 69–73.

Morris, D. 1995. Why my pain is not your pain. *Arthritis Today* 9, no. 6: 23–24.

Neese, J. 1991. Depression in the general hospital. *Nursing Clinics of North America* 26, no. 3: 613–622.

Okoon, M., and S. Morrow. 1995. When rhematology meets psychology. *Arthritis Today* 9, no. 6: 28–33.

Pollin, I. 1995. *Medical crisis counseling: Short-term therapy for long-term illness.* New York: W.W. Norton & Company.

Shang, A., and S. King. 1991. Parkinson's disease, depression, and chronic pain. *Hospital and Community Psychiatry* 42, no. 11: 1162–1163.

Thobaben, M. 1990. Depression in the medically ill homebound patient. *Journal of Home Health Care Practice* 2, no. 3: 33–38.

Witter, D. 1995. A family in pain. *Arthritis Today* 9, no. 6: 34–39.

PART VI

Psychiatric Care of the Elderly Patient in the Home

Principles of Geropsychiatric Treatment in the Home

INTRODUCTION

The elderly patient is the most common patient found in home care. One survey estimated that 50 to 70 percent of elderly patients who receive home care have behavioral, emotional, and mental disorders.[1] This is a very high percentage. Many of these patients are referred for home care primarily for medical problems and not for psychiatric problems; however, psychiatric home care can be a viable treatment option.[2] The home is the most realistic environment for care. Elderly patients are complex, with medical and psychological problems that affect all aspects of their lives. According to Harper, "Health for the elderly may be conceptualized as the ability to live and function effectively in society and to exercise maximum self-reliance and autonomy; it is not necessarily the total absence of disease. Mental illness occurs at that time when a cluster of behavioral signs and symptoms come together and become overly disruptive of the elderly person's ability to function effectively in the mainstream of his or her family and community."[3(p.5)] The psychiatric home care nurse must enter the home of the elderly patient with an understanding of the psychiatric disorders, neurological diseases, medical illnesses, as well as the multiple factors that affect the patient's daily life and functioning. According to Buckwalter and Stolley, "the demand for mental health home services will increase because the number of frail, mentally impaired elders who live at home is predicted to increase."[4(p.139)] Thus, the need for psychiatric home care for the elderly will be expanding.

GEROPSYCHIATRY

Definition of Geropsychiatry

Geropsychiatry focuses on the diagnosis and treatment of psychiatric or behavior disorders in aging patients who have disturbances of brain structure or function. The nursing specialty in this area is becoming more important due to the size of the patient population and these patients' complex needs. Elderly psychiatric patients often exhibit different symptoms and etiologies from younger adult patients and, consequently, they may require different interventions. Continuity of care is a critical component of this care, as well as the need to minimize fragmented care. There are four dimensions important to the continuity of care.[5]

1. *Longitudinal access*. Services must be available over long periods.
2. *Psychological access*. Systems of care must be easily accessible, helpful, and leave elderly patients and their families/significant others (SOs) with positive feelings about their use.
3. *Financial access*. Elderly patients and their families/SOs must be able to pay for needed services.
4. *Geographical access*. Elderly patients and their families/SOs must be able to get to places where the care is provided or the services must be taken to them.

Goals of Geropsychiatry in the Home

Goals of geropsychiatric care in the home include the following:

- to maintain the patient in the home as long as possible
- to maintain the patient's maximum functioning
- to support the patient's family/SOs and any other caregivers in their caregiving and their own needs
- to enhance the patient's self-esteem and personal integrity
- to provide for the patient's medical needs
- to maintain activities of daily living
- to provide education to the patient and family/SOs/caregivers as required by the patient's needs
- to provide care that minimizes fragmentation and emphasizes continuity of care

POTENTIAL GEROPSYCHIATRIC PATIENTS FOR HOME CARE

Psychiatric home care can be provided to patients with geropsychiatric problems and to elderly patients with medical problems accompanied by geropsychiatric problems. All elderly patients referred for home care should have an assessment of their mental status to rule out these problems. Risk factors for developing emotional problems include chronic illness, functional decline, change in social contacts, and death of a spouse or close friend/change in interaction with a significant other.[6] Elderly home care patients who tend to be more problematic are those with delirium; suicidal ideation and attempts; wandering, pacing, and restlessness; Alzheimer's; hostile or agitated behavior; depression; and psychotropic interactions resulting in confusion.[7] Common psychiatric disorders and neurological diseases for the elderly home care patient include depression, anxiety, late-life-onset psychosis, delirium, sleep disorders, substance abuse, nondegenerative dementing disorders, Alzheimer's disease, drug-induced neuropsychiatric syndromes, and neuropsychiatric aspects of a stroke. Depression is the most frequent diagnosis.

DISCHARGE PLANNING AND PSYCHIATRIC HOME CARE

An important consideration with elderly patients who have been referred to psychiatric home care from a medical or psychiatric inpatient setting is the discharge planning process. With today's short lengths of stay, discharge planning should be a critical element of inpatient care, and it should be developed from the time of admission. However, with less hospital staff, more stress, and less time, discharge planning may be inadequate. What does this mean to the psychiatric home care nurse? Patients may be referred to home care who need more intensive care than can be provided in the home. Patients may be referred for one problem when they have additional, more pressing problem(s). The referral source may not have considered the home environment and adequacy of caregivers in the home. The patient usually has received minimal education and instructions about the illness and treatment. The patient who has already tried home care and has been noncompliant may not be fully identified in the discharge plan. Factors that should be considered during the predischarge assessment are formal and informal supportive networks, social issues, mental health and cognitive status, legal and financial factors, environmental variables, safety issues, and ability to perform maintenance activities.[8] Discharge planning should be evaluated carefully by the home care nurse. The nurse should ask whether the discharge plan meets the needs of the patient at the time the home care nurse visits the patient and conducts the admission assessment.

NEUROPSYCHIATRIC ASSESSMENT

The assessment for the elderly patient includes much of the information described in Chapter 10 on assessment in the home; however, there are some differences. The physical assessment is critical for any elderly psychiatric patient, due to the organic causes for many psychiatric problems for the elderly. Problems may be encountered even in conducting the assessment. Sensory problems, such as hearing and sight, may interfere with the process. The elderly may have concerns about stigma related to psychiatric problems and particularly to substance abuse. Due to this fear, they may deny such problems. Often elderly patients are not accustomed to discussing their private feelings. They may have problems concentrating and remembering. The accuracy of the data must be evaluated. Other sources may need to be used, particularly family/SOs. The environment in which the assessment is conducted is very important. If it is too stimulating, the patient may not be able to focus on the assessment. The patient may tire easily and not be able to sit through a complete assessment during one visit. In addition, the patient may not understand why the home care nurse is in the home, who the home care nurse is, and what the assessment is. It is easy to label the patient as noncompliant when there are reasons for noncompliance other than refusal to accept treatment. It may be very difficult for the patient to admit that he or she is changing and unable to function as before. All of these factors make assessment of the elderly patient a challenge.

In addition to a physical assessment and psychiatric history, components of the assessment for the elderly patient include the following:[9,10]

- *Functional assessment.* The major concerns are physical and instrumental activities of daily living, nutrition, mobility, sleep, sensorium, and medication behavior. The following information is important to maintain for the patient in the home:
  1. *Functional ability.* This is the patient's independence or the amount of partial or complete assistance in performing activities of daily living that the patient requires.
  2. *Nutritional status.* The nutritional status is very important, because malnutrition is a common problem in the elderly. Dementia, depression, and other problems can be a consequence of nutritional deficiencies. If possible, the cause of poor nutrition should be identified (e.g., medications such as digoxin and theophylline; emotions such as depression; anorexia nervosa; late life paranoia; swallowing difficulties; oral problems; poverty; wandering and other dementia-related behaviors; hyperthyroidism and hyperparathyroidism; malabsorption; eating problems such as tremors; low-salt or low-cholesterol diet; and problems with shopping or meal preparation.[11] Hydration should be part of this assessment, because the elderly develop an inability to recognize and respond to the need for fluids or hypodipsia. This can lead to dehydration, which can cause delirium.
  3. *Mobility.* Can the patient move about his or her home or leave the home? Does the patient use aids for mobility? How has the patient adapted to any mobility problems?
  4. *Sleep.* Sleep disorders are common in the elderly, and thus sleep needs to be assessed. What is the patient's sleep pattern? Is the patient tired

during the day? A review of the patient's medications is also relevant to the patient's sleep. Does the patient take sedative-hypnotic agents? Sleep apnea can be worsened by benzodiazepines. If the patient has a mood disorder, intermittent awakening and terminal insomnia may be present. Patients with dementia also tend to have sleep disturbances.

5. *Hearing and vision.* Both hearing and vision have physical and psychological ramifications for the patient. Patients with impaired hearing or vision have greater risks for falls, limits on movement, limits on interactions, and limits on daily activities. At times, these patients may even appear to be demented.

6. *Medication behavior.* Usually the elderly patient is taking many medications that require careful assessment and monitoring.

7. *Mental assessment.* Cognition, speech, comprehension, insight, affect, and mood are important parts of the mental assessment. Memory impairment and amnestic disorders are common in the elderly. During the assessment, the nurse should determine if the patient has insight or an ability to understand his or her problem or condition and the need for treatment. Suicidal ideation and behavior must be assessed. Exhibit 27–1 provides an example of a mini-mental status exam, which can be used to quickly assess the elderly patient or any home care patient.

8. *Geriatric behaviors.* Geriatric behaviors include dress, cooperation or resistance, aggressive behavior, sexual behavior, repetitive behaviors, hallucinations, and delusions.

9. *Substance abuse.* Substance abuse is not uncommon in the elderly and must be considered with each patient. Typical substances abused are alcohol, caffeine, prescription drugs, and over-the-counter drugs. The nurse should learn about the patient's past history of substance abuse.

10. *Caregiver assessment.* Because many elderly patients who live at home have a family member/SO who provides some or all of the caregiving, it is important to assess the caregivers and their coping strategies. The assessment includes general appearance, general health, perceived burden, coping strategies, knowledge about resources, and functional status. Is the caregiver able to care for the patient without compromising his or her own health?

11. *Family functioning assessment.* Is the family functioning in a healthy manner? What are its strengths and resources? What are its limitations?

12. *Home environment assessment.* The home environment assessment is discussed in Chapter 10. Safety is an important concern, as well as the need to adapt the home to meet the needs of the patient and yet allow for the needs of other family/SOs.

One approach to the assessment is to ask the patient to describe a typical day, which will provide data about lifestyle, activities of daily living, functioning, and

Exhibit 27–1 Short Portable Mental Status Questionnaire (SPMSQ)

1. What is the date today?   (month)   (day)   (year)
2. What day of the week is it?
3. What is the name of this place?
4. What is your telephone number?
5. What is your street address? (Ask only if the patient does not have a telephone.)
6. When were you born?
7. Who is the President of the United States now?
8. Who was the President before him?
9. What was your mother's maiden name?
10. Subtract 3 from 20 and keep subtracting 3 from each new number all the way down.

Indicate total number of errors =
  0–2 errors = intact intellectual functioning
  3–4 errors = mild intellectual impairment
  5–7 errors = moderate intellectual impairment
  8–10 errors = severe intellectual impairment

Source: Reprinted with permission from E. Pfeiffer, "A Short Portable Mental Status Questionnaire for the Assessment of Organic Brain Deficit in Elderly Patients," *Journal of the American Geriatric Society*, Vol. 23, No. 10, p. 433, © 1975, Williams & Wilkins.

social interactions. This is called storytelling, and elderly patients usually respond favorably to it. The following questions might be asked:[12(p.96–97)]

- What is your typical day like from the time you get up until you go to bed?
- What is your night like from the time you go to bed until you get up the next morning?
- What do you eat in a 24-hour period?
- How many times a day do you eat?
- What changes have you noticed in your life?
- What type and how much exercise do you get?
- How do you feel about yourself?
- What changes have you noticed in your health?
- Have you noticed changes in your response time? In your ability to react? In your coordination?
- How do you feel about yourself sexually?
- Have you experienced any problems with urination or changes in your bowel movements?

- What changes have you noticed in your body?
- How do you use your leisure and recreation time?

The overall goal of the assessment is to identify strengths and resources so that they may be incorporated into the treatment plan. The question of how the elderly patient is adapting and coping on a daily basis should be answered at the conclusion of the assessment, and the same question should be asked about the family/SOs as caregivers. Nursing problems or diagnoses should be identified after the assessment is completed and analyzed. Examples of possible diagnoses that might be identified are[13]

- self-care deficit: feeding/bathing/hygiene/dressing/grooming/toileting
- altered nutrition: less than body requirements
- sleep pattern disturbance
- altered patterns of urinary elimination
- constipation
- diarrhea
- sensory-perceptual alteration: visual, auditory, kinesthetic, gustatory, tactile, olfactory
- impaired physical mobility
- altered thought processes
- anxiety
- impaired verbal communication
- altered health maintenance
- impaired home maintenance
- knowledge deficit
- potential for injury
- activity intolerance
- potential for violence
- potential for self-harm

GERONTOLOGICAL PSYCHOPHARMACOLOGY

Medications can be used very successfully with the elderly psychiatric patient in the home; however, there are special considerations in using psychotropic medications with the elderly when treatment is initiated and throughout treatment. The choice of medication will be influenced by the medication's side effects and the elderly patient's physical and psychological problems. Side effects that may cause additional medical problems or exacerbate existing medical problems should be avoided. According to Keltner and Folks, "Competent administration of psychotropic agents depends on the knowledge of the processes that determine the intensity and duration of a drug's effect."[14(p.34)] Pharmacokinetic factors include the following:

- *absorption*: the process by which a drug enters the circulatory system
- *distribution*: the process by which drugs reach body sites distant from the gastrointestinal tract
- *metabolism*: the process by which drugs are transformed into active or inactive metabolites
- *excretion*: the process by which drugs are eliminated from the body

Exhibit 27-2 describes the effects of pharmacokinetics on the elderly patient.

Factors that are considered in the selection and administration of medications for the elderly psychiatric patient include the following:[15–18]

- The elderly are particularly susceptible to anticholinergic-induced constipation.
- Decreasing the dose or taking the medication at bedtime helps to decrease anticholinergic side effects.
- The elderly and particularly those with cardiovascular disease are more susceptible to orthostatic hypotension.
- The elderly respond better to drugs for anxiety that are shorter-acting (e.g., oxazepam; lorazepam; and, for chronic anxiety, buspirone).
- The sedative effects of benzodiazepines are increased in the elderly.
- Lithium should be used carefully with patients who have dementia.
- Benzodiazepines can increase confusion in patients with organic mental disorder.
- Patients with organic mental syndromes usually respond more quickly to low doses of antipsychotic medications than patients with schizophrenia, often within several hours. "After-sundowning" agitation may also be relieved. Large doses may lead to sedation.
- Tacrine has been used in the early stages of Alzheimer's disease; however, the results are inconclusive.
- Drug toxicity is a major concern in the elderly; these patients are more prone to it due to impaired absorption, metabolism, and excretion of drugs.
- Double dosing or taking medications from several physicians is not uncommon.
- Use of over-the-counter drugs is of concern with the elderly because this may cause drug interaction problems.
- Self-medication is always a risk.
- The elderly tend to make medication administration errors or have medication administration problems (e.g., omission of drug or doses; self-prescribing; incorrect dose, time, or frequency; memory problems; inability to open container; inability to read label; discontinuation of drugs; continuation of drugs after recommended).
- Patients who are taking more than three medications, which is true for many elderly patients, have a greater risk of overmedicating or experiencing toxicity.

Exhibit 27–2 Pharmacokinetics and the Geropsychiatric Patient

Focus	Changes
Decreased absorption in gastrointestinal tract	Increased gastric pH Delayed gastric emptying Diminished blood flow Impaired intestinal motility *Few psychotropic drugs have any delayed rates of gastrointestinal absorption.
Distribution	Decrease in total body water Decrease in lean body mass Proportional increase in body fat *Lipid-soluble drugs (e.g., benzodiazepines) have an increased distribution due to increase in body fat and prolonged action due to increased elimination half-life.
Metabolism	Decrease in hepatic mass Decrease in blood flow Metabolism affected by smoking, alcohol, diet, other drugs, illness, and caffeine *The clearance of many drugs is decreased. *Drugs eliminated primarily by the kidneys have increased risk of toxic effects (e.g., amantadine, lithium, beta blockers, and clonidine).

Source: Reprinted with permission, Nursecom, Inc.

- Lithium must be titrated carefully based on serum levels. Therapeutic effects occur at lower levels for elderly patients due to prolonged half-life and changes in their renal glomerular filtration.
- Lithium side effects of decreased awareness and clouding of sensorium require a decrease in dosage.
- Dosage must initially be low and carefully increased due to complex needs of the elderly.
- Cardiovascular side effects (e.g., tachyarrhythmia, orthostatic hypotension, and congestive heart failure) are very dangerous for elderly patients.

- Antipsychotic drugs interact with many drugs taken by elderly patients (e.g., antihypertensives, anticonvulsants, antacids, and antiparkinsonian drugs). Nonessential prescriptions as well as caffeine, over-the-counter medications, and alcohol should be stopped.
- Most elderly patients require one-third of the usual adult dose of antipsychotics initially; if it is necessary to increase medications, dosage must be increased slowly.
- Increased extrapyramidal side effects occur with the more potent antipsychotic drugs. The less potent drugs cause anticholinergic, sedative, and orthostatic hypotension effects.
- The best antipsychotics to use with the elderly are the intermediate drugs (e.g. loxapine, molindone).
- The injectable antipsychotic tolerated best by the elderly is haloperidol decanoate.
- Psychotropic drugs can cause memory problems for the elderly.
- The symptoms for which these medications are prescribed (e.g., decreased concentration, decreased attention span, fatigue, apathy and indifference, feelings of helplessness and hopelessness, decreased memory) interfere with patient education about medications.
- The elderly may fear that psychotropic drugs are "mind-altering" and these patients may also have concerns about stigma. The best approach is to discuss the chemical changes in the patient's body and the importance of helping the body adjust to these changes.
- It is best to do an electrocardiogram for patients with borderline conduction defects prior to beginning treatment on an antidepressant and weekly for the first month.
- A typical clinical trial period is 4 weeks, but some patients may require as long as 12 weeks.
- Plasma levels are important for desipramine, imipramine, and nortriptyline to determine their therapeutic window.
- To prevent additional problems with orthostatic hypotension, elderly patients should sit and dangle their legs before standing. They are most at risk at night when they get up to void.
- Patients should be told not to take these medications on an as-needed basis unless there is a specific order to do this.

CLINICAL MANAGEMENT STRATEGIES

Clinical management strategies for the elderly psychiatric patient in the home vary, depending on the patient's problems, resources, and home environment. Chapter 28 discusses strategies or interventions for specific illnesses. The following clinical management strategies are general strategies that might be used for a variety of problems or illnesses:

- *Education.* Patient and family/SOs/caregiver education is a critical component of care for every elderly patient in the home. Elderly patients need to know about their illnesses, medications, treatment, home safety, and skills required for self-care. This is all dependent on each patient's ability to learn. The patient's symptoms might not make it easy for the patient to understand or remember. Caregivers must also be taught about the ill family member's problems, medications, treatment, home safety, behavioral management strategies, coping skills, problem solving, and communication with the ill family member. This takes time and requires repetition and reinforcement.
- *Caregiver services.* The caregivers need support. They need to be assessed for burnout. Their health is critical to the health of the ill family member. Services include education, collaboration with treatment planning, support, and, when required, respite.
- *Supportive telephone contact.* The patient and family/SOs/caregivers are given a telephone number to be used when they have questions or there is an emergency. Home care staff may also call between visits to ask how things are going and to assess future needs. This also communicates that the patient and family/SOs/caregivers are not alone.
- *Reduction or elimination of environmental stress.* If stimulation is a problem for a patient, stimulation can be decreased by decreasing noise, even for short periods of time; turning off the television or radio (which may be confusing for the patient); decreasing the number of people visiting at one time; and decreasing the intake of caffeine.
- *Problem-solving difficulties.* If the patient has problem-solving difficulties, emphasizing problem solving will increase the patient's anxiety and decrease self-esteem. Routines are helpful and provide support for the patient. It is best not to reason with the patient or to force the patient to do something he or she cannot do. If the patient has memory problems, learning new ways of doing something may be very difficult. When the patient is given choices, it is best to limit the choice to two. The patient should not be rushed, and staff and caregivers should provide care in an unhurried manner.
- *Attitude toward patient.* All elderly patients should be respected and spoken to as adults. There will be times when staff and caregivers are frustrated and need a break. The patient may not always be appreciative; but verbal and physical abuse from the patient does not have to be tolerated. Staff should communicate that the patient is important by using appropriate praise, encouraging the patient to do as much as possible for self, and asking for the patient's opinion as well as participation in treatment planning and evaluation.

- *Fatigue and stress.* The elderly patient has less energy and a low stress threshold. Care and activities should be planned with these in mind. Plan for rest periods, and introduce change slowly.
- *Communication.* Communication is part of the care provided in the home. During the admission assessment, the home care nurse assesses the patient's communication skills as well as the family/SOs/caregivers' skills. Problems are identified and included in the treatment plan. Depending upon the patient's condition, speech may need to be slower, with shorter sentences; it may be necessary to say the words more clearly to adjust for the patient's hearing. Questioning should include only one question at a time, and the patient must be given time to answer the question. Questions may need to be repeated, but repeated exactly as asked initially. It is best to be in front of the patient and to use eye contact. Listening is critical to get information and to communicate interest to the patient.
- *Reality orientation.* Reality orientation is focusing the patient on the here and now in regard to time, place, person, and thing; however, this is not helpful for all patients. Patients who have a memory problem and are intellectually impaired, especially those with dementia, will not be able to remember. Pressuring them to remember when they cannot only will increase everyone's stress.
- *Validation.* Validation can be helpful with the elderly patient who is having problems with reality, confused, or disoriented.[19] Confrontation or trying to force the patient back to reality is not always helpful. If the patient is experiencing anxiety, talking about the past may make it easier for the patient to become more oriented to the present.
- *Delusions and hallucinations.* Confrontation about delusions and hallucinations is not helpful, nor is trying to prove that a hallucination or delusion is wrong. With the elderly, the best intervention is to try to distract the patient.

FAMILY/SIGNIFICANT OTHERS

Often the family/SOs/caregivers want to be told what to do. Some of this may be due to their expectation that the health care provider knows what to do, and some may be due to fatigue and stress. They want someone to take over for them, and it is a mistake for staff to take over. Family/SOs should participate in the planning and decision making. The first step is to clarify their expectations of the ill family member as well as expectations of themselves as caregivers. Having an ill family member at home will affect the entire environment 24 hours a day. Questions that the home care nurse might ask include the following:[20(p.40)]

- Has the family care partner attained an adequate understanding of the patient's medical condition and become competent to carry out the prescribed therapeutic regimen?
- Does the family realistically balance self-confidence with the need to accept true limitations?
- Is the family dealing constructively with stressful situations and life changes?
- Are the family members continuing to fulfill their expected roles in the household and in the community?
- Are the patient's expectations of the care partner reasonable?
- Have sufficient outside resources been identified that can be called upon when additional help is needed?
- Do the patient and family communicate well and share decision making as a mutually supporting venture?

The caregiver may experience denial as a part of grieving for a relationship that has changed. According to Collins et al., denial "allows individuals to manage multiple and often overwhelming feelings and to control noxious emotions until resources are adequate for the task of processing details."[21] Often, elderly spouses or caregiver plan that this time in life will be different, and this is painful. "Extraordinary coping resources are often required to maintain psychosocial equilibrium over the long, changing, and unpredictable course of . . . [a family member's] disease."[22(p.64)] It is important to remember that initially denial is helpful. It is a protection for the individual. Most family members will pass through denial to confronting the reality of the illness and the changes it has brought to the family. Then caregivers need to be assessed for depression. Signs of depression in caregivers include the following:[23]

- loss of energy or fatigue
- difficulties with concentration
- neglect of vital physical needs
- uncharacteristic crying or agitation
- difficulty sleeping at night
- increased use of sleeping pills, alcohol, or caffeine
- decreased resistance to illness
- marked changes in appetite
- signs of impatience in giving care

Due to the responsibilities of caregiving, family members of the ill person may experience social isolation and actual or perceived lack of social support. This will only make their situation worse and affect their emotional status. Home care staff can assist them by listening, identifying coping strategies, teaching care skills, encouraging and helping the caregivers to find ways to take time for themselves, and encouraging them to participate in appropriate support groups.

There may come a time when some patients require care in a long-term care facility. The family will need support and guidance from the home care nurse. It is difficult to make the decision about the best alternative care to meet the ill family member's needs. It is a very emotional experience, and families will experience anxiety, depression, loss, guilt, and anger. The patient should be involved in the decision as much as possible. Exhibit 27–3 provides some guidelines for choosing a long-term care facility. The more informed the family, the better the decision making.

ELDER ABUSE

Elder abuse is not a topic that most people want to discuss, but it does occur. The home care staff must be alert to the possibility of abuse. This abuse may include physical injury; unrealistic confinement; unreasonable punishment; sexual offenses; exploitation by taking unfair advantage—particularly in financial areas; and deprivation of minimum food, shelter, clothing, supervision, and physical and mental health care.[24] Other examples of abuse are verbal abuse, threats, and violation of rights such as privacy and consent. Most caregivers are able to meet the care responsibilities during the early stages; however, as time passes they become more fatigued as stress increases. It is at this time that the risk for abuse increases. Home care staff should be alert for abuse and, whenever possible, prevent it from occurring. Risk factors include physical disability in the caregiver, a history of family violence, alcohol abuse by the caregiver or the dependent, decrease in family financial resources, or an emotional or psychiatric problem in the caregiver.[25] If abuse does occur, home care staff must take steps to protect the patient. State legal requirements must be followed. It is never a pleasant experience; however, the patient's needs must be considered at all times.

SUMMARY

The elderly home care patient has many needs. Interventions for physical problems are a priority; however, many of these interventions will affect the patient psychologically. The patient's illness also arouses many feelings in the patient and the patient's family/SOs. Some patients have a history of psychiatric problems that may influence the patient's responses to the illness and treatment. The elderly patient is a demanding patient, but knowledge of the aging process and its effects will help home care staff to provide the care appropriate to the patient's needs.

Exhibit 27–3 Guide to Selecting a Long-Term Care Facility

- Critical questions to ask before selection of a long-term care facility
  1. What kind of care is needed?
  2. What lifestyle would the patient like to lead in the facility?
  3. How close to the family should the patient be?
  4. What are the financial issues that need to be considered?
- Where to find information
  1. Local long-term care ombudsman; survey reports; complaints including number, type, and resolution
  2. Publications
  3. American Association of Retired Persons
  4. Health care providers
  5. State health department: report of latest survey of specific long-term care facilities
  6. Friends and family who have knowledge of long-term care facilities
- Initial telephone contact with long-term care facilities
  1. Is the facility certified for participation in Medicare or Medicaid programs?
  2. What are the facility's admission requirements?
  3. What is the "typical profile" of a resident in the facility?
  4. Does the facility require that a resident sign over personal property or real estate in exchange for care?
  5. Does the facility have vacancies or is there a waiting list?
- Visiting long-term care facilities
  1. Talk with residents and staff. What do they like about the facility? What do they do when they want something changed? What do the residents like about the staff? Ask some questions of visitors and volunteers.
  2. Visit, if possible, more than one time and at different times of days and different days of week. Are residents out of bed? Dressed appropriately? Eating? Participating in activities?
  3. Is a copy of the residents' bill of rights posted? Ask for a copy.
  4. What social services are provided?
  5. What treatment is offered and by whom?
  6. What is the physical condition of the residents?
  7. Assess the interactions between residents, between residents and staff, and among staff.
  8. How often do residents get a full bath?
  9. Are there opportunities to go outside?
  10. Do residents appear content? Some will not participate in activities, preferring to just watch.

continues

Exhibit 27–3 continued

11. Ask to speak with several family members of residents.
12. What medical services are provided? Can the resident have his or her own private physician? How often does the facility's physician visit? Do the physician and nurse develop the treatment plan together? Does the resident participate?
13. What is the staffing 24 hours a day?
14. When are restraints used? What is done to prevent their use? They should not be used for discipline or convenience of staff, and there should be no verbal, sexual, physical, or mental abuse, corporal punishment, or involuntary seclusion.
15. How much time is allowed for each meal? Is food delivered to residents who are unable or unwilling to eat in the dining room? Are snacks available? Are those residents in need of special equipment or assistance at meal time provided with such equipment or assistance? Ask to see menus for a month. Ask how special diets are handled. Ask to sample food. Are hot foods hot?
16. What are the plans for fire safety? Is there a smoking area?
17. Is the facility clean? Free of clutter? Bright? Good repair? Furniture appropriate? Can residents bring in personal belongings?

- Contract with the long-term care facility
  1. Components of the contract
     - resident rights and obligations including safeguards for resident's rights and grievance procedure
     - amount of money that must be paid each day or month
     - prices for items not included in daily or monthly charge
     - facility's policy on holding a bed if the resident temporarily leaves the facility for reasons such as hospitalization or vacation
     - statement regarding certification; Medicaid and/or Medicare
  2. Signing the contract
     - The admission contract is a legally binding contract.
     - Discrimination against Medicaid recipients is illegal.
     - Medicare payments must be accepted if the resident qualifies for Medicare.
     - Ask for a copy of the contract and review carefully at home; ask questions if needed.
     - If possible, review contract with lawyer.
     - Terms may be changed on the contract; however, the family member or resident as well as the long-term care facility representative must initial the changes.
     - Before signing, review for completeness, correctness; there should be no blank spaces.

Source: Reprinted from *Guide to Choosing a Nursing Home*, U.S. Department of Health and Human Services, Health Care Financing Administration.

NOTES

1. M. Trimbath and J. Brestensky, "The Role of the Mental Health Nurse in Home Health Care," *Journal of Home Health Care Practice* 2, no. 3 (1990): 1–8, at 1.

2. J. Kozlak and M. Thobaben, "Treating the Elderly Mentally Ill at Home," *Perspectives in Psychiatric Care* 28, no. 2 (1992): 31–36, at 31.

3. M. Harper, "Providing Mental Health Services in the Homes of the Elderly," *Caring* 8, no. 6 (1989): 5–9, 52–53, at 5.

4. K. Buckwalter and J. Stolley, "Managing Mentally Ill Elders at Home," *Geriatric Nursing* 12, no. 12 (1991): 136–139, at 139.

5. L. Bachrach, "The Challenge of Service Planning in Chronic Mental Patients," *Community Mental Health Journal* 22, no. 5 (1986): 170–174, at 171.

6. J. Kozlak and M. Thobaben, "Psychiatric Home Health Nursing of the Aged: A Selected Literature Review," *Geriatric Nursing* 15, no. 3 (1994): 148–150.

7. M. Harper, "Behavioral, Social, and Mental Health Aspects of Home Care for Older Americans," *Home Health Care Services Quarterly* 9, no. 4 (1988): 61–124, at 64.

8. K. Buckwalter and M. Smith, "Special Needs of the Elderly," in *Discharge Planning: A Manual for Psychiatric Nurses*, ed. K. Babick and L. Brown (Thorofare, NJ: SLACK, Inc., 1991), 146–158, at 149.

9. I. Abraham et al., "Outpatient Psychogeriatric Nursing Services: An Integrative Model," *Archives of Psychiatric Nursing* 5, no. 3: 151–164, at 157.

10. I. Abraham et al., "A Psychogeriatric Nursing Assessment Protocol for Use in Multidisciplinary Practice," *Archives of Psychiatric Nursing* 4, no. 4 (1990) 242–259.

11. J. Morley, "Physiological Aspects," in *Comprehensive Textbook of Psychiatry*, Vol. 2, ed. H. Kaplan and B. Sadock (Baltimore, MD: Williams & Wilkins, 1995), 2534–2539, at 2538.

12. J. Campbell, "Assessment," in *Geropsychiatric Nursing*, ed. M. Hogstel (St. Louis, MO: C.V. Mosby, 1990): 91–109, at 96–97.

13. North American Nursing Diagnosis Association, *Nursing Diagnoses: Definitions & Classification, 1995–1996* (Philadelphia: 1994), 13–14, 17–20, 29, 37, 60, 62–69, 75, 77, 79, 83, 86.

14. N. Keltner and D. Folks, "Pharmacokinetics and Psychopharmacology: Application to the Geropsychiatric Patient," *Perspectives in Psychiatric Care* 29, no. 1 (1993): 34–36.

15. R. Cosgay and V. Hanna, "Physiological Causes of Depression in the Elderly," *Perspectives in Psychiatric Care* 29, no. 1: 1993: 26–28.

16. M. Smith and K. Buckwalter, "Medication Management, Antidepressant Drugs, and the Elderly: An Overview," *Journal of Psychosocial Nursing* 30, no. 10 (1992): 30–36.

17. N. Keltner, "Tacrine: A Pharmacological Approach to Alzheimer's Disease," *Journal of Psychosocial Nursing* 32, no. 3 (1994): 37–39.

18. K. Brasfield, "Practical Psychopharmacologic Considerations in Depression," *Nursing Clinics of North America* 26, no. 3 (1991): 651–661, at 654.

19. B. Baldwin et al., "Geriatric Psychiatric Nursing," in *Principles and Practice of Psychiatric Nursing*, ed. G. Stuart and S. Sundeen (St. Louis, MO: Mosby–Year Book, 1995): 921–943, at 938–939.

20. A. Grieco, "A New Structured Database for Clinical Information," *Caring* 11, no. 5 (1992): 34–41, at 40.

21. J. Collins et al., "Uncovering and Managing Denial During the Research Process," *Archives of Psychiatric Nursing* 9, no. 2 (1995): 62–67, at 64.

22. Collins, "Uncovering and Managing Denial During the Research Process," 64.

23. M. Nelson, "Care of the Mentally Ill Older Person in the Home," in *Geropsychiatric Nursing*, ed. M. Hogstel (St. Louis, MO: C.V. Mosby, 1990), 283–302.

24. K. Weiler and K Buckwalter, "Geriatric Mental Health: Abuse among Rural Mentally Ill," *Journal of Psychosocial Nursing* 30, no. 9 (1992): 32–36, at 33.

25. Nelson, "Care of the Mentally Ill Older Person in the Home," 294.

SUGGESTED READING

Ashely, J., and T. Fulmer. 1988. No simple way to determine elder abuse. *Geriatric Nursing* 9, no. 5: 286–288.

Austin, A. 1989. Becoming immune to loneliness: Helping the elderly fill a void. *Journal of Gerontological Nursing* 15, no. 9: 25–28.

Bowlby, C. 1993. *Therapeutic activities with persons disabled by Alzheimer's disease and related disorders.* Gaithersburg, MD: Aspen Publishers, Inc.

Brown, H. 1989. The role of the home health care nurse in mental health assessment of the elderly. *Journal of Home Health Care Practice* 2, no. 1: 9–15.

Buckwalter, K., and M. Hardy, eds. 1991. *Nursing diagnoses and interventions for the elderly.* Redwood City, CA: Addison-Wesley Nursing.

Coffey, C., and J. Cummings. 1994. *Seven steps to effective parent care—A planning and action guide for adult children with aging parents.* New York: W.W. Norton & Company.

Craman, A. 1992. Community-based mental health services for the elderly. *Caring* 11, no. 1: 39–43.

Di Domenico, R., and W. Ziegler. 1994. *Practical rehabilitation techniques for geriatric aides.* 2nd ed. Gaithersburg, MD: Aspen Publishers, Inc.

Emlet, C. et al. 1995. *In-home assessment of older adults: An interdisciplinary approach.* Gaithersburg, MD: Aspen Publishers, Inc.

Ferran, C., and J. Popovich. 1990. Hope: A relevant concept in geriatric psychiatry. *Archives of Psychiatric Nursing* 4, no. 2: 123–130.

Folks, D. 1990. Clinical approaches to anxiety in the medically ill elderly. *Drug Therapy Supplement* 8, no. 1: 72–82.

Fopma-Loy, J. 1989. Geropsychiatric nursing: Focus and setting. *Archives of Psychiatric Nursing* 3, no. 3: 183–190.

Gallow, J. et al. 1995. *Handbook of geriatric assessment.* 2nd ed. Gaithersburg, MD: Aspen Publishers, Inc.

Geriatric patient education resource manual. 1996. Gaithersburg, MD: Aspen Publishers, Inc.

Hall, G. 1988. Alterations in thought processes. *Journal of Gerontological Nursing* 13, no. 3: 30–37.

Harper, M. 1988. Behavioral, social, and mental health aspects of home care for older Americans. *Home Health Care Services Quarterly* 9, no. 4: 61–124.

Harvey, S., and M. Seelman. 1991. Development of a mental health home care program. *Caring* 10, no. 3: 20–22.

Heim, K. 1986. Wandering behavior. *Journal of Gerontological Nursing* 12, no. 11: 4–7.

Hirst, S., and J. Miller. 1986. The abused elderly. *Journal of Psychosocial Nursing* 24, no. 10: 28–34.

Hogstel, M., ed. 1990. *Geropsychiatric nursing*. St. Louis, MO: C.V. Mosby.

Home care for people with Alzheimer's disease. 1995. Aspen Patient Education Video Series. Gaithersburg, MD: Aspen Publishers, Inc.

Lucas, M. et al. 1986. Recognition of psychiatric symptoms in dementia. *Journal of Gerontological Nursing* 12, no. 1: 11–15.

Shearer, R., and R. Davidhizar. 1994. It can never be the way it was: Helping elderly women adjust to change and loss. *Home Healthcare Nurse* 12, no. 4: 60–65.

Stroke rehabilitation patient education manual. 1995. Gaithersburg, MD: Aspen Publishers, Inc.

Strome, T., and T. Howell. 1991. How antipsychotics affect the elderly. *American Journal of Nursing* 91, no. 5: 45–49.

Strubel, L., and L. Silversten. 1987. Agitation behaviors in confused elderly patients. *Journal of Gerontological Nursing* 13, no. 11: 40–44.

28

Psychiatric Disorders and Neurological Diseases in the Elderly Patient

INTRODUCTION

The elderly patient in the home may have a psychiatric disorder or a neurological disease as well as a medical illness. This complex patient is a challenge to home care staff due to the additional problems associated with aging. The psychiatric disorders discussed in this chapter are mood disorders, late-life psychosis, delirium, sleep disorders, and substance abuse. The neurological diseases are nondegenerative dementing disorders, Alzheimer's disease, drug-induced neuropsychiatric syndromes, and neuropsychiatric aspects of a stroke.

PSYCHIATRIC DISORDERS IN THE ELDERLY PATIENT IN THE HOME

Mood Disorders

Mood disorders include depression, bipolar disorder, and anxiety disorders. Depression is the most common disorder in the elderly; however, many elderly also suffer from anxiety disorders. Anxiety is a normal emotion; however, if it becomes excessive and maladaptive, it interferes with functioning. Typical psychological and physiological symptoms in the elderly patient are[1]

- *psychological*: tension, nervousness, worry, irritability, difficulty concentrating, rumination, and dread
- *physiological*: palpitations, shortness of breath, dyspnea on exertion, choking sensation, heartburn, vomiting and nausea, insomnia, tremors, and restlessness

Phobias are the most common anxiety disorder in the elderly, and panic disorder is also common. Patients who experience these problems when they are younger may continue to have these problems as they age; however, these illnesses may also develop in old age. Patients who have late-onset panic attacks have less avoidance and report fewer symptoms during the panic attack than younger patients.[2] Phobias often focus on fear of crime and safety; however, in many cases the patient has real reasons to have these fears. The home care nurse should include these factors in the home assessment.

Because many elderly patients have medical problems, it is important to remember that anxiety is often associated with medical illness. If the patient has a high caffeine intake, this can cause anxiety or worsen it. Many patients are not aware of this dietary cause of anxiety. They will need education and support to decrease caffeine intake, and they may experience withdrawal symptoms such as headaches. Drugs such as over-the-counter medications for colds and allergies and prescription medications (e.g., amphetamines, bronchodilators, and some calcium channel blockers) can cause anxiety.[3] Assessment should include a medication history to identify medications that may be contributing to anxiety. Akathisia, a side effect of neuroleptics, may be mistaken as anxiety, because it causes a subjective sense of restlessness and agitation. Withdrawal from alcohol or sedative-hypnotic drugs can also cause anxiety. Elderly patients with endocrine disorders may exhibit symptoms of anxiety. This may be seen in hypo- and hyperparathyroidism, hypo- and hyperpituitarism, hypoglycemia, diabetes mellitus, and Cushing's syndrome. Parkinson's disease and stroke also increase the risk for anxiety. There is a high rate of alcohol abuse and sleep disturbances in patients with anxiety disorders. It is clear that any elderly patient who has symptoms of anxiety requires a thorough history and physical to rule out the various possible causes prior to determining treatment. The most common interventions include providing support; giving medications; and using interventions such as relaxation, identification of situations that cause stress, alternative methods of coping, and practice in the use of new coping strategies. Other interventions for anxiety are discussed in Chapter 20.

The psychiatric home care nurse sees more depression than any other problems in the elderly. Major depression is a significant problem in the elderly, especially in those with medical problems. Biological, psychological, and sociological changes increase the risk of depression in this age group; however, aging itself does not inevitably lead to depression. There are also physiological causes of depression that need to be assessed so that appropriate treatment can be provided. Some of these physiological causes include the following:[4]

- hypothyroidism
- neurological disorders (e.g., Alzheimer's disease, poststroke, multiple sclerosis, Parkinson's disease)

- cancer (e.g., breast, pancreas, prostate, lung, gastrointestinal)
- infections (e.g., tuberculosis, AIDS, meningitis, pernicious anemia)
- cardiovascular disease (e.g., cerebral arteriosclerosis, congestive heart failure, myocardial infarction)
- metabolic disorders (e.g., electrolyte imbalances, hepatic encephalopathy, uremia, alcoholism, collagen disorders)

Other factors that might cause depression are drug toxicity and sensory deprivation. Drug toxicity can occur when patients double dose, use over-the-counter medications, self-medicate, and make medication errors. Sensory deprivation can be extremely difficult for the elderly patient. If the patient is already confined to home due to illness, loss of hearing or sight means further isolation as well as limited ability to participate in recreational activities, such as reading, crafts, watching television, listening to music, and conversing with others.

Assessment of depression is not easy because many of the symptoms are similar to those for medical illnesses and are not the symptoms expected in depression found in younger patients. Typically the elderly patient experiences somatic complaints, anxiety, hypochondriasis, change in eating habits, inability to concentrate, difficulty making decisions, withdrawal, general irritability, suicidal feelings, decreased energy, and sleep disturbances. The nurse sees less of the usual symptoms of depression (e.g., guilt, sadness), as these are often masked by other symptoms. Exhibit 28–1 provides an example of a geriatric depression scale. According to Rossen and Buschmann, "Depression is often so insidious that neither the victim nor the healthcare provider recognizes its symptoms in the context of the multiple physical and social problems so many elderly people face."[5(p.131)]

Depression can affect physical and social functioning in elderly patients, affecting all aspects of life. Treatment focuses on antidepressant medications and supportive therapy for some elderly patients. The following interventions may be used:

- The assessment includes suicidal feelings and behavior with appropriate interventions taken.
- Because isolation is frequently a problem, the nurse and family/significant others (SOs) may identify others who might visit or call, agencies who provide visitors for elderly in the home, day treatment, or social groups. The home care nurse plans with the patient how the patient will increase contact with others.
- As nutrition is an important aspect of care for the elderly, assessment of nutritional status must be done. If the patient needs assistance (such as home-delivered meals, food stamps, grocery shopping), interventions to meet these needs should be clearly identified and implemented.
- An exercise plan appropriate for the patient is developed with the patient and implemented.

Exhibit 28–1 Geriatric Depression Scale (Short Version)

Answers indicating depression are boldfaced. Each answer counts 1 point; scores greater than 5 indicate probable depression. The scale can be used as a self-rating scale or observer-rater scale.

Question	Answer
1. Are you basically satisfied with your life?	Yes/**No**
2. Have you dropped many of your activities and interests?	**Yes**/No
3. Do you feel that your life is empty?	**Yes**/No
4. Do you often get bored?	**Yes**/No
5. Are you in good spirits most of the time?	Yes/**No**
6. Are you afraid that something bad is going to happen to you?	**Yes**/No
7. Do you feel happy most of the time?	Yes/**No**
8. Do you often feel helpless?	**Yes**/No
9. Do you prefer to stay at home, rather than going out and doing new things?	**Yes**/No
10. Do you feel you have more problems with memory than most?	**Yes**/No
11. Do you think it is wonderful to be alive now?	Yes/**No**
12. Do you feel pretty worthless the way you are now?	**Yes**/No
13. Do you feel full of energy?	Yes/**No**
14. Do you feel that your situation is hopeless?	**Yes**/No
15. Do you think that most people are better off than you are?	**Yes**/No

Source: Reprinted from J. Yesavage, "Geriatric Depression Scale," *Psychopharmacology Bulletin*, Vol. 24, No. 4, p. 715, © 1988, National Institute of Mental Health.

- Because depression and the medications used in treatment can lead to problems with constipation, it may be necessary to modify the patient's diet, increase fluid intake, exercise, and use stool softeners.
- Sleep disturbances should be addressed. (Interventions are discussed in the section of this chapter on sleep disturbances.)
- The patient's environment may be dark and depressing. Home care staff can encourage using lighting, opening drapes, increasing color, and listening to music. Too much silence is not helpful. Chapter 21 contains more interventions for depression. Exhibit 28–2 describes examples of other interventions.

Exhibit 28–2 Interventions for the Depressed Elderly Patient

Psychotherapeutic	*Psychosocial*
Convey hope	Establish a network if living alone
Present optimistic attitude	Arrange for transportation
Empathetic listening	Encourage family involvement
Cognitive therapy	Use the health care team
Behavioral therapy	Encourage positive coping patterns
Present alternatives and options	• Lower expectations of self
Use of expressive touch	• Compare self to cohort
Restoration of self-esteem	Discourage negative coping patterns
Reminiscence	• Somatization
	• Conversion symptoms

Source: Reprinted with permission from M. Buschmann et al., "Geriatric Depression," *Home Healthcare Nurse*, Vol. 13, No. 3, p. 50., © 1995, Pharmaceutical Media, Inc.

The elderly have the highest suicide rate, more than 50 percent higher than for young people or the nation as a whole.[6] It usually is not an impulsive act and is frequently associated with death of a loved one, physical illness, uncontrollable pain, fear of dying, a prolonged death that damages family members emotionally and economically, social isolation and loneliness, and major changes in social roles, such as retirement.[7] Chapter 29 discusses suicidal behavior and its treatment in more detail. Suicidal risk can be determined by considering the following questions:[8(pp.2–3)]

- Does the patient volunteer suicidal thoughts?
- Has the patient thought through plans for suicide?
- Does the patient have access to the means of suicide?
- Does the patient have an exaggerated concern about a real or imagined physical illness?
- Is there evidence of a sense of hopelessness?
- Is the patient extremely depressed and withdrawn?
- Is the patient an elderly white male?
- Is there alcohol involvement?
- Are there social contacts with whom to share emotional thoughts?
- Does the patient's cognitive status vary from day to day?
- Is there reason to suspect that the patient might not be taking prescribed medications?
- Is someone available at home for companionship until the depressed mood is controlled or resolved?

It is important to remember that most elderly suicides occur during the first episode of depression.[9]

Depression and anxiety in the elderly are sometimes difficult to distinguish. Treatment is different for each, and thus it is important to identify the problem clearly. The differences may be described in the following manner:[10]

- *depression*
  1. symptomatology: depressed mood, worse in the morning, lack of energy, terminal insomnia, feelings of guilt and anhedonia
  2. premorbid personality: usually had a better-adjusted premorbid personality, except in chronic depression
  3. clinical course: often has a history of regular cycles of depression with periods of remission
- *anxiety*
  1. symptomatology: anxious mood, worse in the evening, agitation, initial insomnia, panic attacks, phobias, symptoms of autonomic activation
  2. premorbid personality: usually poorly adjusted personality with dependent and avoidant traits
  3. clinical course: irregularly recurrent with somewhat incomplete periods of remission

Late-Life Psychosis

Late-life-onset psychosis is described as a syndrome that resembles early-onset schizophrenia and occurs after the age of 60. Late-life psychosis is found in up to 10 percent of elderly admissions to hospitals.[11] Common symptoms include persecutory delusions and auditory hallucinations. The content of the delusions are often influenced by the patient's isolation and homebound status. For instance, the elderly patient might think that people or gas are coming through the walls.[12] During assessment it is important to try to determine if symptoms of psychosis have been experienced in the past. The patient with early-onset schizophrenia never is cured. In this case, the patient would not have late-life-onset psychosis.

Risk factors for late-life-onset psychosis include genetics, female, sensory deficits (particularly auditory and visual), premorbid personality (particularly paranoid or schizoid), never married and no children, and lower social class.[13] The best treatment is antipsychotic or neuroleptic drugs. This is not always easy to accomplish because these patients usually do not seek treatment and frequently do not comply with the treatment plan. Depot medication may be required. It is important to remember that these patients are at risk for tardive dyskinesia, falls, anticholinergic side effects with low-potency neuroleptics (e.g., delirium, increased problems with glaucoma, cardiac abnormalities, and urinary obstructions). They may also experience problems with parkinsonian syndromes. The home care nurse must have good information about the patient's medical history and present problems in order to provide appropriate care in the home.

Delirium

According to the American Psychiatric Association (APA), delirium is "characterized by a disturbance of consciousness and a change in cognition that develop over a short period of time."[14(p.123)] It develops over a few hours or days and may change during the day. The delirium may be substance-induced or caused by medical conditions. Symptoms include the following:[15]

- disturbance in consciousness; reduced clarity of awareness of the environment; impairment of the ability to focus, sustain, or shift attention (This may require repetition of questions, and patient may answer previous questions as a result of inability to shift to present questions.)
- distractibility by irrelevant stimuli
- difficulty engaging in conversation
- memory impairment
- disorientation, particularly to time and place
- speech disturbance: rambling, irrelevant, pressured, incoherent, unpredictable changing of subjects
- perceptual disturbances: misinterpretations, illusions, hallucinations

Many medical illnesses and drugs can cause delirium. The common ones are[16]

- metabolic or endocrine: electrolyte abnormality (e.g., Na^+, K^+, Ca^{++}, and Mg^{++}), hyperglycemia or hypoglycemia, hypoxia or hypercarbia, liver or kidney failure, thyroid disorder, fever
- infection: sepsis, pneumonia, urinary tract infection, upper respiratory infection
- drug toxicity: anticholinergics, psychoactive medications (e.g., neuroleptics, tricyclic antidepressants, lithium, electroconvulsive therapy, steroids)
- alcohol or drug withdrawal
- central nervous system lesion: postictal state, raised intracranial pressure, head trauma, encephalitis, meningitis, vasculitis

Treatment for delirium depends on identifying the cause in order to focus treatment on that specific cause. Whenever possible, treatment for the symptoms of delirium should focus on psychosocial interventions rather than medications. If medications are prescribed, the neuroleptics and/or benzodiazepines should be given at the lowest possible dose. With some medications, such as haloperidol, the side effects mimic or worsen illness symptoms. Hospitalization may be required for patients who cannot be safely managed at home. The home environment needs to be predictable and provide orientation for the patient.[17] Stimulation should be minimized. The patient's room should be well lit to decrease illusions. Even at night, a night light should be used. Calendars and clocks should be visible, with family/SOs/caregivers and home care staff frequently reminding the patient of the day and date. If the patient usually wears eyeglasses and/or a hearing aid, these should be used. Family/SOs/caregivers should interact frequently with the patient. Delirium is reversible with care.

Sleep Disorders

Sleep disturbance and excessive sleep should be carefully assessed in the elderly patient to determine if the cause is medical or psychological. The elderly patient requires the same amount of sleep as a younger patient; however, the patient is less able to achieve and maintain stages 3 and 4 (deep sleep), so the elderly patient can awaken tired.[18] Part of the sleep assessment includes a sleep-wake log, which records the hours asleep and awake. Possible causes of a sleep disturbance include medical problems, psychological problems, neurological changes, drug-induced changes, breathing disorders, poor sleep habits, changes in sleep patterns such as sleeping more during the day, and the environment (e.g., too noisy, too light, uncomfortable, anxiety producing).[19] Elderly patients with sleep disturbances have a high risk of developing severe depression, so it is important to correct the sleep problem as quickly as possible. Sedative-hypnotic drugs should be used carefully and not just used when the patient says he or she is not sleeping well. Difficulty falling asleep is often caused by anxiety or physiological symptoms such as pain from arthritis. Middle or terminal insomnia is more common in depression, and antidepressant medication may alleviate this problem.

It may be necessary to teach the patient about sleep. This is preferable to using or overusing sedative-hypnotic drugs. Suggestions that may be given include the following:[20,21]

- Explain sleep cycle and changes with aging.
- Use bed only for sleep.
- Exercise.
- Take warm bath two hours before bedtime.
- Eat a light snack before bedtime (particularly milk and some high-protein snacks such as cheese and nuts, which contain L-tryptophan, a sleep promoter).
- Use relaxation exercises.
- Decrease intake of caffeine, preferably eliminating it.
- Decrease daytime napping.
- Wake up at a routine time.

- Remember that withdrawal from sedative-hypnotic drugs may increase sleep disturbance for two to eight weeks.
- Sleep disturbances decrease as depression decreases.
- Have patient rest in a recliner or have a quiet time in his or her room once in the morning and once in the afternoon; however if patient awakens during night, decrease this time.
- Drink warm milk before bedtime.
- Avoid turning on light when patient awakens during night.
- Read boring book before sleep.

Substance Abuse

Substance abuse does occur in elderly patients. Some have had a long history of abuse; a smaller group has had a more recent abuse history. Alcohol is the most abused substance; however, elderly patients also have problems with prescription drugs and over-the-counter drugs. Substance abuse may be a response to the many losses the elderly experience, loneliness, or physical illness. The elderly patient may try to self-medicate to relieve his or her symptoms.

Alcohol abuse leads to psychological and physiological problems. Exhibit 28–3 provides examples of complications of chemical dependence. These problems are complicated due to the physiological changes of aging. Because many elderly patients live in isolated situations with minimum social interactions and are no longer working, it is easy to cover up substance abuse. Patients who have a life-long alcohol abuse history usually have problems interpersonally and have a limited social support network. The latter occurs because they have abused their social support network too much in the past. Assessment and treatment guidelines for the elderly patient who abuses alcohol include the following:[22,23]

- Due to fears of stigma and denial, family/SOs may cover up or protect the patient.
- Job and family problems often are not motivating factors for treatment.
- The quantity of consumed alcohol is not always an important indicator; elderly persons experience reverse tolerance, requiring less alcohol to produce the same effect as the first drink did.
- Health problems make alcohol abuse more difficult to diagnose (e.g., general physical deterioration, malnutrition, mental deterioration, and social isolation).
- Intentional distortions and blackouts may make it more difficult to get information from the patient.
- Depression is very common in the elderly alcoholic. It may or may not disappear after abstinence.
- Antabuse should not be used for treatment with the elderly due to a decreased ability to cope physiologically with the adverse reactions.

- Treatment with thiamine, folic acid, vitamins, magnesium sulfate, electrolytes, and antianxiety medications to decrease withdrawal seizures may be used.
- The following should be cues to investigate further for a possible alcohol abuse problem (however, there may be other possible causes for these cues):
    1. confusion, staggering gait, and drowsiness
    2. frequent accidents and falls
    3. falling asleep while smoking
    4. tremulousness
    5. free-floating anxiety
    6. intermittent difficulty processing information
    7. fluctuating attention span
    8. overactivity
    9. overt, unprovoked anger
    10. lack of spontaneous thought
    11. selective attention and memory
    12. pessimism
    13. thought disturbances (e.g., racing, blocking, rigidity, paranoia)
    14. frequent hospitalizations and major illnesses
    15. organic mental impairment
    16. alcoholic hepatitis, pancreatitis with cholelithiasis, anemia, clotting disorders, cardiovascular disease, infections (particularly pneumonia), hypertension, diabetes, gastrointestinal problems (e.g., gastritis, esophagitis, chronic diarrhea)
    17. physical findings of peripheral neuropathy, enlarged liver, gynecomastia, cardiomyopathy, arrhythmia, tachycardia, elevated blood pressure
- A comprehensive assessment should include specific questions about drinking:
    1. How often do you drink?
    2. How do you drink?
    3. How much do you drink?
    4. What are your reasons for drinking?

After determining that there is an alcohol problem, staff should share information about alcoholism with the patient. Written material about alcoholism is given to the patient, and it should be discussed with the patient. When appropriate, Alcoholics Anonymous (AA) is identified as a resource for the patient. An AA visitor may also be used. All home care staff should encourage the elderly patient to discuss feelings, particularly those that might be related to alcohol abuse (e.g., loss, loneliness, hopelessness). Staff should help the patient identify opportunities to increase socialization and reinforce the patient's strengths.

Exhibit 28–3 Complications of Chemical Dependence

Exacerbation of preexisting chronic illnesses	Increased feelings of hopelessness
Stress-related physical problems	Decreased ability to make decisions
Lowered pain threshold	Feelings of selflessness
Increased signs and symptoms of depression	Feelings of worthlessness
Decreased appetite with potential for malnutrition	Feelings of helplessness
Accident proneness	Persistent irrational thoughts and fears
Sleep disturbances	Avoidant behavior
Physical collapse	Withering desire to survive
Increased isolation from family and peer group	Suicidal ideas
Escalation of anxiety	Psychosis or significant other psychiatric crisis
Increased feelings of insecurity	Fear of abandonment or rejection
Despair	Fear of losing control over all aspects of life
Fear of being punished by a supreme being	Fear of being denied a spiritual afterlife

Source: Reprinted with permission from J. Seibert, "Understanding Chemical Abuse and Dependence in the Elderly," *Journal of Home Health Care Practice*, Vol. 2, No. 3, p. 28, © 1990, Aspen Publishers, Inc.

Other substances abused by the elderly are opiates, prescription and over-the-counter medications, nicotine, and caffeine. The assessment data help to describe the patient's use of these substances. Long-term opiate addiction does not cause the physical problems that are found with alcohol abuse. Most elderly patients do not consider caffeine to be addictive, but it is. It may be necessary to educate patients and encourage them to stop or at least decrease caffeine use.

NEUROLOGICAL DISEASES IN THE ELDERLY PATIENT IN THE HOME

Description of Neurological Diseases

Dementia is one of the primary focuses of neurological disease in the elderly. Dementia is a broad category of organic mental disorders in which there is significant interference with activities of daily living, work, or social relationships. Dementia may be temporary or permanent. Symptoms include the following:[24]

- memory loss (usually the first symptom, which continues until memory is no longer testable; past memory is better than recent)
- loss of impulse control
- impaired abstract thinking (deceased capacity for generalization, differentiation, logical reasoning, and concept formation)
- decreased control of aggressive and sexual impulses
- personality changes
- mood disturbances
- emotional lability (sadness, irritability, combativeness, or inappropriate elation)
- delusions, hallucinations, and illusions

Dementia can have reversible causes or irreversible causes. Reversible causes include drug intoxication; some metabolic, infectious, cardiovascular causes; some brain disorders; pain; sensory deprivation; hospitalization; alcohol toxic reactions; anemia; turmoil; chronic lung disease; and nutrient deficiencies. If these are treated quickly, permanent damage can be prevented. This requires a careful assessment and history and physical. Irreversible causes are those for which there is no treatment, and they are diagnosed after other causes are ruled out. There are two important categories of the irreversible dementias: primary degenerative and multi-infarct dementia.

Alzheimer's disease is defined by Nelson as "a progressive disorder of the central nervous system with an average duration of 5 to 8 years from onset to death. It is an irreversible, insidious, life-threatening disorder that involves a progressive loss in cognitive ability, self-care skills, and adaptation that ultimately leads to the premature death of the afflicted individual.[25(p.185)] The disease course usually begins after the age of 70. It is thought that between 50 to 70 percent of all patients with dementia have Alzheimer's disease.[26] It is difficult to diagnose in its early stages. Williams has identified three stages by their symptoms:[27]

1. Symptoms of stage 1
   - memory loss
   - spatial disorientation
   - mistakes in judgment
   - decreased concentration abilities
   - perceptual disturbances
   - transitory delusions of persecution
   - muscular twitchings
   - time disorientation
   - affect changes
   - absent-mindness
   - lack of spontaneity
   - epileptiform seizures

2. Symptoms of stage 2
   - forgetfulness of recent and remote events
   - complete disorientation
   - increased aphasia
   - astereognosis
   - perseveration phenomena
   - insatiable appetite without weight gain
   - auditory agnosia
   - hypertonia
   - agraphia
   - increased inability to comprehend
   - agnosia
   - apraxia
   - hyperorality
   - alexia
   - socially acceptable behavior forgotten
   - unsteady gait
3. Symptoms of stage 3
   - marked irritability
   - seizures
   - loss or diminution of emotions
   - visual agnosia
   - apraxia
   - bedridden
   - helplessness
   - paraphasia
   - hyperorality
   - bulimia
   - hypermetamorphosis
   - decreased appetite
   - emaciation
   - unresponsive or coma

Multi-infarct dementia is a vascular disorder characterized by multiple large and small cerebral infarctions. Its progression is variable, and some of its symptoms are pseudobulbar palsy with emotional lability; dysarthria; dysphasia; convulsive seizures; fluctuation in level of cognition; states of confusion or delirium; explosive or unstable emotions; disturbances in memory, abstract thinking, judgment, and impulse control. There is no major change in personality.[28]

Assessment for dementias includes obtaining the following information:[29]

- What is the onset of the behavior? Sudden onset over several hours or days differentiates between delirium and dementia. (Dementia takes longer.)

- What is the time of the behavior? Time of day or night when the behavior is present and when it becomes worse is important.
- Is the behavior related to any precipitating factors? What makes it worse? Better?
- How have the patient's and the caregiver's activities of daily living been affected by the behavioral symptoms?
- What do the behavioral symptoms mean to the patient and to the caregiver?

In addition, the assessment should include a complete history and physical, mental status exam, and assessment of the patient's sensory status.

Interventions for the patient with dementia, particularly Alzheimer's disease, are never easy to identify or to implement. When the patient experiences stress, anxious behavior will be the result. Five groups of stressors are important for the patient to avoid.[30]

1. fatigue
2. change of environment, caregiver, or routine
3. misleading, overwhelming, or competing stimuli
4. demands to achieve that exceed functional capacity
5. physical stressors: pain, discomfort, acute illness, caffeine

Typical Problems and Their Interventions[31]

Wandering

Wandering is the tendency to move about aimlessly. It can be frustrating for family/SOs/caregivers and for home care staff. Possible reasons for this behavior are boredom; stress; or inability to express hunger, thirst, pain, or the need to use the toilet.

Suspiciousness

The patient believes that someone is trying to harm him or her or steal personal belongings. The following are suggested interventions to help the patient who feels someone wants to harm him or her:

- Maintain a daily routine.
- Keep rooms well lit, with no shadows.
- If possible, lock closets and drawers.
- Identify the places where the patient usually hides things.
- Avoid arguing with the patient.
- Approach the patient calmly and unhurriedly so that the patient will not feel he or she is being attacked.

Communication

Communication problems are very common. It is important to follow guidelines for good communication as discussed in Chapter 4. In addition, consider the following interventions:

- Do not give the patient a choice, as this can confuse the patient.
- If asking the patient to do something, break it down into simple steps.
- Do not discuss the patient's condition in front of the patient as if he or she does not understand.

Agitation

When the patient experiences the loss of cognitive abilities, coping strategies are also reduced and the stress threshold is lowered. The patient's response to these changes is often agitation. Medication may be required; however, other interventions should also be used. Consistency and a low-stress environment are important. As inadequate sleep and rest decrease the ability to cope, effort should be made to ensure that the patient gets enough sleep and rest. Exercise also helps to decrease anxiety. Limiting choices is important, because the patient feels stress with decision making.

Memory Loss

Memory loss and disorientation affect all areas of the patient's life, and these cause additional problems for everyone. Providing a clock and calendar may help the patient during the early stages of dementia. Efforts to decrease confusion should always be a goal. Keep pictures of family and friends with labels of their names where the patient can easily see them. Turning off the television and the radio when they are not being used will decrease background noise that might lead to delusions or hallucinations. There is disagreement about the use of reality orientation with dementia. Some authorities feel that if the patient no longer has the ability to remember, reality orientation expects too much from the patient.

Weight Loss and Incontinence

Patients may experience weight loss or incontinence. Home care staff should attempt to prevent these problems and to provide care to prevent complications (such as skin breakdown) from them.

SUMMARY

It may not be possible to provide home care for elderly patients with neurological illnesses as well as psychiatric illnesses in the home. The home care staff should carefully assess and reassess the patient and the family/SOs/caregivers' abilities to care for the patient in the home. Any time the patient can spend in the home is more beneficial for the patient; however, the nurse should be realistic about the patient's care needs, particularly safety. The family/SOs/caregivers need to rely on the nurse's ability to provide realistic advice.

NOTES

1. S. Smith et al., "Assessing and Treating Anxiety in Elderly Persons," *Psychiatric Services* 46, no. 1 (1995): 36–42, at 39.

2. J. Sheikh, "Anxiety," in *Textbook of Geriatric Neuropsychiatry,* ed. C. Coffey and J. Cummings (Washington, DC: American Psychiatric Press, Inc., 1994), 279–296, at 282.

3. Sheikh, "Anxiety," 285.

4. D. Steiner and B. Marcopulos, "Depression in the Elderly: Characteristics and Clinical Management," *Nursing Clinics of North America* 26, no. 3 (1991): 585–596.

5. E. Rossen and M. Buschmann, "Mental Illness in Late Life: The Neurobiology of Depression," *Archives of Psychiatric Nursing* 9, no. 3 (1995): 130–136, at 131.

6. J. McIntosh, *The Suicide of Older Men and Women* (Washington, DC: American Association of Retired Persons, 1993), 2.

7. McIntosh, *The Suicide of Older Men and Women,* 3.

8. R. Ham and B. Meyers, *Late Life Depression and Suicide Potential* (Washington, DC: American Association of Retired Persons, 1993), 2–3.

9. Y. Conwell, "Suicide Among Elderly Persons," *Psychiatric Services* 46, no. 6 (1995): 563–564.

10. J. Sheikh, "Clinical Features of Anxiety Disorders," in *The Psychiatry of Old Age,* ed. J. Copeland et al. (Chichester, England: Wiley, 1993), 107.1–107.5, at 107.4.

11. G. Pearlson and R. Petty. "Late-Life-Onset Psychoses," in *Textbook of Geriatric Neuropsychiatry,* ed. C. Coffey and J. Cummings (Washington, DC: American Psychiatric Press, Inc., 1994), 261–277, at 262.

12. Pearlson and Petty, "Late-Life-Onset Psychoses," 264.

13. Pearlson and Petty. "Late-Life-Onset Psychoses," 266.

14. American Psychiatric Association, *Diagnostic and Statistical Manual of Mental Disorders,* 4th ed. (Washington, DC: 1994), 123.

15. American Psychiatric Association, *Diagnostic and Statistical Manual of Mental Disorders,* 124–125.

16. L. Tune and C. Ross, "Delirium," in *Textbook of Geriatric Neuropsychiatry,* ed. C. Coffey and J. Cummings (Washington, DC: American Psychiatric Press, Inc., 1994), 351–365, at 359.

17. Tune and Ross, "Delirium," 362.

18. J. Campbell, "Assessment," in *Geropsychiatric Nursing,* ed. M. Hogstel (St. Louis, MO: C.V. Mosby, 1990), 91–109, at 106.

19. Campbell, "Assessment," 107.

20. E. Luke, "Psychotropic Drugs," in *Geropsychiatric Nursing,* ed. M. Hogstel (St. Louis, MO: C.V. Mosby, 1990), 110–129, at 126.

21. M. Nelson, "Organic Mental Disorders," in *Geropsychiatric Nursing,* ed. M. Hogstel (St. Louis, MO: C.V. Mosby, 1990), 177–212, at 201.

22. M. Kashka and S. Tweed, "Substance Abuse," in *Geropsychiatric Nursing,* ed. M. Hogstel (St. Louis, MO: C.V. Mosby, 1990), 227–259, at 239–245.

23. J. Seibert, "Understanding Chemical Abuse and Dependence in the Elderly," *Journal of Home Health Care Practice* 2, no. 3 (1990): 27–31, at 29.

24. Nelson, "Organic Mental Disorders," 178–180.

25. Nelson, "Organic Mental Disorders," 185.

26. Nelson, "Organic Mental Disorders," 185.

27. L. Williams, "Alzheimer's: The Need for Caring," *Journal of Gerontological Nursing* 12, no. 2 (1986): 21–28, at 23.

28. Nelson, "Organic Mental Disorders," 192.

29. Nelson, "Organic Mental Disorders," 196.

30. G. Hall, "Alterations in Thought Process," *Journal of Gerontological Nursing* 14, no. 3 (1988): 30–37.

31. A. Curl, "The Nursing Care of the Dementia Patient," in *Geriatric Mental Health Nursing: Current and Future Changes,* ed. K. Buckwalter (Thorofare, NJ: SLACK, Inc., 1992), 27–43.

SUGGESTED READING

Blazer, D. 1990. *Emotional problems in later life.* New York: Springer Publishing Co.

Blazer, D. 1993. *Depression in late life.* 2nd ed. St. Louis, MO: C.V. Mosby.

Buckwalter, K., and M. Hardy, eds. 1991. *Nursing diagnoses and interventions for the elderly.* Redwood City, CA: Addison-Wesley Nursing.

Burney-Puckett, M. 1996. Sundown syndrome: Etiology and management. *Journal of Psychosocial Nursing* 34, no. 5: 40–43.

Buschmann, M. et al. 1995. Geriatric depression. *Home Healthcare Nurse* 13, no. 3: 47–56.

Cohen, C. 1995. Studies of the course and outcome of schizophrenia in later life. *Psychiatric Services* 46, no. 9: 877–879, 889.

Cohen, D., and C. Eisdorfer. 1993. *Seven steps to effective parent care—A planning and action guide for adult children with aging parents.* New York: G.P. Putnam's Sons.

Curl, A. 1989. Agitation and the older adult. *Journal of Psychosocial Nursing* 27, no. 12: 12–14.

Dellasega, C. 1990. Coping with caregiving: Stress management for caregivers of the elderly. *Journal of Psychosocial Nursing* 28, no. 1: 15–22.

Dreyfus, J. 1988. Depression assessment and interventions in the medically frail elderly. *Journal of Gerontological Nursing* 14, no. 9: 27–36.

Grossberg, G., and J. Manepalli. 1995. The older patient with psychotic symptoms. *Psychiatric Services* 46, no. 1: 55–59.

Hall, G., and K. Buckwalter. 1987. Progressively lowered stress threshold: A conceptual model for care of adults with Alzheimer's disease. *Archives of Psychiatric Nursing* 1, no. 6: 399–406.

Horvath, T. et al. 1995. Dementia-related behaviors in Alzheimer's disease. *Journal of Psychosocial Nursing* 33, no. 1: 35–39.

Johnson, L. 1989. How to diagnose and treat chemical dependency among the elderly. *Journal of Gerontological Nursing* 15, no. 12: 22–26.

Kapp, M. 1995. Restraining impaired elders in the home environment: Legal, practical, and policy implications. *Journal of Case Management* 4, no. 2: 54–59.

Kennedy, G. 1995. The geriatric syndrome of late-life depression. *Psychiatric Services* 46, no. 1: 43–48.

Kimball, M., and C. Williams-Burgess. 1995. Failure to thrive: The silent epidemic of the elderly. *Archives of Psychiatric Nursing* 9, no. 2: 99–105.

Klozlak, J., and M. Thobaben. 1992. Treating the elderly mentally ill at home. *Perspective in Psychiatric Care* 28, no. 2: 31–35.

Krach, P. 1995. Assessment of depressed older persons living in a home setting. *Home Healthcare Nurse* 13, no. 3: 61–64.

Kurlowicz, L. 1993. Social factors and depression in late life. *Archives of Psychiatric Nursing* 7, no. 1: 30–36.

Kurlowicz, L. 1994. Depression in hospitalized medically ill elders: Evolution of the concept. *Archives of Psychiatric Nursing* 7, no. 2: 124–136.

Mace, N., and P. Rabins. 1991. *The 36-hour day.* Baltimore, MD: The Johns Hopkins University Press.

Matthis, E. 1994. Care of frail elders with relinquishing dispositions. *Home Healthcare Nurse* 12, no. 5: 30–35.

McCall, W. 1995. Management of primary sleep disorders among elderly persons. *Psychiatric Services* 46, no. 1: 49–55.

Smith, S. et al. 1995. Assessing and treating anxiety in elderly persons. *Psychiatric Services* 46, no. 1: 36–42.

PART VII

Psychiatric Emergencies
in the Home

29

Crisis Resolution
in the Home

INTRODUCTION

The seriously mentally ill encounter many crises in daily living, and many of these crises may lead to relapse and require more intensive treatment such as hospitalization. Crises that occur may be very frightening to the patient, family/ significant others (SOs), and to home care staff. Prevention of crises and emergencies is the preferred choice; however, there are times when prevention is not successful.

DEFINITION OF CRISIS

A crisis is caused by a stressful event. Benter defines crisis as "a disturbance caused by a stressful event or a perceived threat to self."[1(p.278)] The way the person usually copes is ineffective. Usually the precipitating event can be identified; however, sometimes it cannot be identified or it did not occur immediately prior to the person's responses. Aguilera has published extensively in the area of crises and states that "we all exist in a state of emotional equilibrium, a state of balance, or homeostasis. When something that is different (either positive or negative), a change, or a loss that creates a state of disequilibrium occurs, we strive to regain and maintain our previous level of equilibrium."[2(p.1)]

There are three types of crises: maturational, situational, and adventitious. *Maturational crises* are ongoing processes related to maturation (e.g., birth, adolescence, old age, and death). *Situational crises* can occur at any time and are related to daily living (e.g., loss of job, unwanted pregnancy, medical illness, divorce, or problems with children). *Adventitious crises* are accidental, uncommon, and unexpected events and do not occur in everyone's life (e.g., earthquake, tornado, flood, fire, major car accident). A patient may experience any of these types of crises during home care treatment or afterward. Staff will be available to help the patient and family/SOs cope with crises that occur during home care treatment and teach the patient and family/SOs coping skills to use after staff are no longer available.

CRISIS INTERVENTION VERSUS RESOLUTION

Crisis intervention is probably a familiar term to most nurses; however, emphasizing crisis resolution may be a different approach. Too often, the focus is on "limited assessment, triage, and disposition"; however, the focus should be on crisis resolution.[3(p.111)] When staff approach crisis from the point of view of resolution, outcome becomes more important. Are the patient/family/SOs able to cope and move on? Has the patient learned skills that can be used during future crises? Does the patient need more long-term help? What is the patient's view of the crisis and the outcome? Crisis resolution focuses on restoration of functional equilibrium as soon as possible to prevent further damage for the patient and the family/SOs.

PRECIPITANTS OF CRISIS

Patients with serious mental illness and their families/SOs live on the edge of crises that may happen at any time, similar to living on the edge of a volcano.[4] Common situations that can lead to a crisis for these patients include the following:

- *Medication noncompliance.* Medication noncompliance can be a very difficult problem for the patient, family/SOs, and staff. Steps that might be used to increase compliance include the following:[5]
  1. Staff and family/SOs should view the medication in the context of the patient's life. How can the medication help change the patient's life? What are concrete benefits from taking the medication (e.g., increased sleep, better concentration, decreased anxiety when with others)?
  2. Staff should always be concerned about compliance and discuss it openly with the patient and family/SOs. Identification of the reason for noncompliance can help specify interventions (e.g., if the patient forgets to take medications, develop methods to remind the patient).
  3. The patient and family/SOs need information about the medication. All health care workers who interact with the patient should know what medications the patient is taking.
  4. The patient should be involved in decisions about medications and allowed to express concerns. If the patient stops taking the medication, it is

important to maintain contact with the patient. Denial of illness may affect compliance. The patient needs to learn how to manage symptoms with medications. It is, however, important to recognize that the family/SOs cannot guarantee that the patient will be compliant with treatment. Blaming them for the patient's noncompliance is destructive.

- *Use and abuse of alcohol and drugs.* Patients who use and abuse alcohol and drugs may experience many crises. Staff should not be moralistic about this behavior but rather discuss the facts and the effects of alcohol or drugs on the patient. Family/SOs should not focus on the alcohol or drugs but rather the behavior that is objectionable (e.g., apathy, violence, noncompliance with treatment, excessive spending). Staff and family/SOs should hold the patient accountable for his or her behavior. In some cases to prevent abuse, it may be necessary for the family/SOs to control the patient's money. This may not be successful. As this action puts the patient in a more dependent position, caregivers should consider it carefully before carrying it out.
- *Violence and destruction of property*
- *Suicidal feelings and behavior*
- *Self-mutilation*
- *Running away from the home*

THE CRISIS PROCESS

Precipitating Event

The goal of crisis resolution is to return to precrisis functioning. It is easier to reach this goal if staff or family/SOs intervene quickly to prevent further problems. The first step is assessment. It is important to focus on the immediate problem remembering that the crisis usually has occurred within 10 to 14 days of the precipitating event. Feelings and behaviors commonly experienced during a crisis are anger, apathy, backaches, boredom, crying spells, diminished sexual drive, disbelief, fatigue, flashbacks, forgetfulness, headaches, helplessness, hopelessness, insomnia, intrusive thoughts, irritability, lability, nightmares, numbness, overeating or undereating, poor concentration, sadness, school problems, self-doubt, shock, social withdrawal, substance abuse, suicidal thoughts, survivor guilt, or work difficulties.[6] A patient may exhibit a pattern of behavior whenever a crisis is experienced. During the initial home care assessment, the nurse asks the patient how he or she responds when a crisis occurs. This may give clues to use in future assessments. The patient's family/SOs may also have important information to share. Staff should assess the following areas:

- What are the patient's needs?
- What are the events that threaten those needs?

- When did the symptoms appear or when did coping mechanisms stop working and symptoms begin?

The goal is to have the patient connect the precipitating event to his or her responses. The patient's perception of the event is more important than the perception of staff or family/SO. It is very easy to forget this, particularly if the crisis relates to something that is important to the staff member or family/SOs. It is, however, important that the patient has a realistic perception of the crisis. Staff need to help the patient assess the perception. Some patients may minimize, others may maximize, and some may even have difficulty recognizing a potential crisis situation or the early signs due to their chronic anxiety. Typical signs and symptoms of deteriorating mental status should be noted. These include the following:[7]

- signs of paranoia
- inability to listen
- increased anxiety
- decreased attention span
- decreased ability to make decisions
- asking for help (e.g., multiple telephone calls from the patient)
- irrational behavior
- increased safety risk (e.g., smoking accidents, nutrition, personal hygiene, suicidal feelings, self-mutilation, homicidal feelings)
- noncompliance with medications

Adequate Situational Support

Support systems may be professional or nonprofessional. To assess the patient's support system, ask the following questions: Who can the patient turn to for support? Is the person available when needed? Has there been a change in the support system? Does the patient need to develop new ones? Has the support system burned out? Can the support system be improved so that it is more available? What is the support system's view of the crisis and the patient?

Adequate Coping Mechanisms

Everyone uses coping mechanisms; however, some work better than others. A person may need to learn new coping mechanisms. It is important to assess the patient's strengths and previous coping mechanisms, experience with crisis in the past and results, and whether these coping mechanisms decreased the patient's anxiety in the past. In addition, assessment of the patient's suicidal and homicidal feelings should always be included.

Problem Resolution

Interventions are categorized in four ways, and staff and family/SOs may use all or some of them.[8]

1. *Environmental:* interventions focused directly on changing the patient's physical or interpersonal situation
2. *General support:* interventions that communicate staff support to the patient, empathy, caring, etc.
3. *Generic approach:* interventions focused on high-risk groups and with specific interventions (e.g., grief counseling, debriefing after a traumatic event, counseling after a disaster, rape groups, learning coping skills for the chronically ill)
4. *Individual approach:* interventions focused on the patient's individual needs

The outcomes for crisis resolution for the patient should state that the patient will do the following: [9]

- Describe the crisis event.
- Explore feelings and emotions related to the event.
- Discuss ways in which stressful events have been handled in the past.
- Identify alternative solutions or coping methods for the crisis situation.
- Implement possible solutions.
- Report satisfaction with coping abilities and level of functioning.

As interventions are planned, staff determine how much the crisis has disrupted the patient's life and how the patient's disequilibrium is affecting others in his or her life. The answers will help staff plan what must be done to support the patient and others in the home. If the crisis is not resolved, disequilibrium will continue; this will lead to further deterioration in the patient's clinical status.

SUICIDAL FEELINGS AND BEHAVIOR

What is the struggle that brings a person to the point of taking his or her own life? Generally, the person is experiencing extreme hopelessness, anger, and loss. This loss may be real or imagined. The person feels as if he or she has lost some part of himself or herself and feels a pervasive sense of worthlessness or depletion. There is a rejection of self. Suicidal feelings is a difficult topic for most health care professionals, whose focus is on curing patients. With a suicidal patient, staff and patient seem to be fighting against each other, with different goals. This frustration is communicated to patients, and it should be identified and discussed with the home care team. It is easy to be judgmental, but no situation is black or white. It is the patient's view that is important. Care is directed toward helping the patient cope with feelings and behavior.

The cognitive functioning of suicidal patients can be disturbed.[10] They often view themselves, others, and situations as either all good or all bad. In addition, they can have a rigid style of perceiving and reacting that makes it difficult for them to formulate alternatives to problems. These two deficits make it difficult for home care staff to discuss suicidal feelings and behavior realistically with the patient and to problem solve. Discussion and problem solving must take place; however, staff must consider how difficult it is for the patient.

The Dynamics of Suicide

When a patient is suicidal, the patient may experience any of the following:

- signals of severe distress
- feelings of inner disintegration
- anger at another person that is internalized in the form of guilt and depression
- attempts to manipulate another person to gain love and affection or to punish another person (This does not make the suicidal ideas and/or attempt any less serious. It is easy to be judgmental with this patient.)
- thought disorder, particularly with command hallucinations
- a desire to join a dead relative or significant other, such as seen with the elderly patient who has a deceased spouse
- substance abuse

The suicidal process can be described with the following steps. It is important to remember that the process is not as simple as it may appear; however, the steps provide a better understanding of the patient's experience.

1. The individual feels a frustration of personal needs.
2. Anger results.
3. The individual turns the anger inward. This leads to feelings of guilt, inadequacy, despair, depression, and hopelessness.
4. A stressful situation develops.
5. The individual perceives this situation as unbearable.
6. The individual tries to communicate his or her hopelessness to others.
7. The individual is not able to mobilize hope by himself or herself or through others.
8. The individual decides to terminate his or her life.
9. A plan is developed.
10. The plan is carried out.

A patient is at greater risk as a depression is improving than when severely depressed. Developing and implementing a plan require energy that is not available when severely depressed.

Whenever suicidal behavior is discussed, it is critical to discuss the issue of accidental death. Some patients never consider accidental death as a possibility, particularly those who threaten suicide but do not really want to die (e.g., the calculation of a "safe" dose is not correct, or the person who was expected home at a specific time does not come).

Risk Factors

According to Hillard, "Predicting suicide remains one of the greatest clinical challenges for mental health providers."[11(p.223)] The following are risk factors that have been identified:[12]

- presence of psychiatric illness
- presence of suicide plan
- presence and/or history of suicide attempt, particularly lethality and intention
- presence of a medical illness associated with pain and/or disability
- presence of alcohol/drug intoxication/abuse
- lack of adequate social supports
- elderly with medical illness
- presence of a family history of suicide
- command hallucinations to harm self

Assessment

The assessment of suicidal feelings and behavior should be done for every admission to home care, regardless of diagnosis. For patients who have increased risk, this assessment is repeated at each visit. For others, the assessment is done when staff observe changes that arouse concern or family/SOs are concerned about the patient's status. The areas that are assessed include verbal communication of intent, actual plan, actual attempt, signs of depression, past history related to self-destructive behavior, auditory hallucinations related to self-destructive behavior, any recent loss experienced (such as separation/divorce), illness in the family, change of therapist, or conflict with family resulting in increased anxiety. The home care staff might use any of the following questions to assess suicidal feelings:[13]

- Are you thinking of suicide?
- Do you wish you could end it all?
- Do you feel you would be better off dead?
- You've been feeling so miserable, I wonder whether you've considered suicide?

If home care staff believe that the patient might have suicidal feelings or the patient admits to these feelings, staff should ask the patient additional critical questions:

- Do you have a plan?
- What is the plan?
- Is it possible to implement the plan?
- When do you plan to do it?

Asking direct questions will not make the patient try suicide, and it is very important to be direct and communicate that the patient will be cared for rather than ignored. Exhibit 29–1 provides a more detailed list of signs and symptoms of suicidal feelings and behavior.

Interventions

Examples of desired outcomes for a patient who is suicidal include the following:

- The patient will discuss suicidal feelings.
- The patient will not act on suicidal feelings.
- The patient will participate in developing a treatment contract and follow the contract.
- The patient will participate in his or her treatment planning, assessment of progress, and discharge planning.

Examples of interventions for the suicidal patient in the home include the following:

- When a staff member makes an individual alliance with a patient who promises that he or she will be safe, this can be dangerous. All home care staff who work with the patient need to know about the patient's clinical status and the treatment plan to better ensure the patient's safety.
- Threats should not be dismissed as attention seeking; instead, the patient's condition must be carefully assessed and plans made for appropriate interventions.
- Information about suicidal feelings and behavior is communicated to the patient's physician on admission and whenever change occurs.
- All guns, sharp instruments, hanging devices, poisons, and hypnotic or sedative drugs are removed from the patient. However, it is important to remember that no place can be completely safe, particularly the home. Acknowledging this will prevent undue guilt.

Exhibit 29–1 Signs and Symptoms of Suicidal Feelings and Behavior

- Indicates decreased willingness to communicate with staff.
- Provides inadequate information for staff to feel comfortable with the patient's safety.
- Makes statements about suicidal feelings.
- Experienced a recent loss.
- Feels he or she is dying or is dead.
- Experiences increased physical complaints.
- Experiences signs and symptoms of depression.
- Expresses loneliness.
- Expresses hopelessness about the future.
- Expresses being tired and the wish to sleep and never wake up.
- Experiences increased anxiety.
- Expresses anger toward self.
- Experiences exaggerated or extended inactivity, apathy.
- Indicates lack of future plans.
- Experiences delusions and/or hallucinations, especially commands.
- Experiences change in health status (gets worse or better).
- Changes eating habits, sleep, dress.
- Experiences increased isolation.
- Displays sudden change in routine behavior.
- Gives away or sells personal articles.
- Plans or implements acts of self-mutilation.

- If there is serious concern about the patient's safety, the home care staff or family/SOs should not leave the patient alone for any reason. Arrangements must be made immediately to take the patient to the physician or hospital for further evaluation and, if needed, more intensive treatment.
- At all times the patient is treated respectfully; it is important to recognize that the patient feels humiliation about the loss of control and may believe that he or she is being punished.
- The patient should be told that he or she will be protected. The patient may be very angry about staff/family/SO observation; however, staff/family/SOs cannot take this personally and must consider the patient's safety as the first priority.
- If the patient is responding to command hallucinations, immediate treatment is required.
- The home care nurse provides time for the patient to discuss stressors leading to self-destructive feelings or behavior, or both. A treatment contract is

developed with the patient that focuses on "no harm" and what the patient will do if suicidal feelings are experienced.

- The home care nurse provides teaching related to depression, loss, anxiety, coping skills, and medications. This is paced according to patient's tolerance and ability to concentrate.
- If the patient must be taken to the emergency department, the home care nurse communicates with emergency department staff. Gaining access to the mental health system today is not easy due to cutbacks in reimbursement and services. The nurse provides data about the patient that will help emergency room staff in their decision making.
- If the patient must be hospitalized, the home care agency's policy regarding documentation and discharge is followed. The family/SOs need support and information about the hospitalization decision, even if the patient is discharged from home care. This is important for their well-being and their reactions to the home care agency, and may be important for continuity if the patient is readmitted to home care after discharge from the hospital. If there is patient consent, information is shared with the hospital.

Documentation is a very important part of the care of the suicidal patient. When the assessment indicates potential of self-destructive feelings or behavior, this is documented carefully by describing the patient's feelings and behavior. The notes should indicate when the patient's physician was notified, by whom, and the physician's response. All interventions and their results must be described. If the patient remains at home, the record and treatment plan should indicate the plan that will be followed until the nurse's next visit. Family/SOs and the patient must be an integral part of that plan. A treatment contract with the patient should be written and signed by the patient and the staff member. This plan is reviewed on each visit and amended as required; a copy is kept by the patient and in the patient's record.

If a home care agency has a patient who makes a suicide attempt or dies as a result of one, this is a crisis. The staff and the family/SOs will need support. Staff and families/SOs will have many feelings and questions, and these need to be addressed. Staff should review the incident carefully, without being judgmental. They should review the facts: who, what, where, when, and how? Staff then need opportunity to discuss feelings openly with one another. Some staff may feel guilt, anger toward the patient, frustration and hopelessness, or burnout from the incident.

Families/SOs may have negative feelings toward the staff and the home care agency. They may feel that staff failed, did not care enough, were not available, or were incompetent. Home care staff should provide support to the family/SOs immediately after the incident and refer them for further help as needed. If the family/SOs threaten legal action, the home care agency must consult the agency's legal counsel. (In fact, the agency should seek legal counsel any time a death of this type occurs.) Records are reviewed and staff are counseled regarding actions to be taken with the family/SOs.

ANGER AND AGGRESSION

There is no doubt that the topic of escalating behavior is troubling for staff, patients, and families/SOs. The first step in decreasing concern is to understand anger and aggression better. Anger begins with perceived anxiety, and it is a complex process. All people experience it, some more than others. Anger can serve a useful purpose, as it can promote a powerful feeling that is the opposite of powerlessness. A person expresses anger directly or indirectly. Direct expression is verbal expression against others or self or physical aggression. Indirect expression is aggression directed toward self such as self-derogation, suicidal wishes, somatic complaints such as headaches, sarcastic remarks, inconsistency, forgetfulness, and boredom.

When a person experiences anger, he or she has expectations, is frustrated when expectations are not met, and sees this as a threat to self. Feeling a high level of anxiety, powerlessness, and insecurity, the person copes by using anger unconsciously, changing anxiety to aggression, and reaching for the feeling of power rather than powerlessness. Violence is not an isolated act but rather part of a process. When the person responds with anger, it is expressed directly or indirectly; however, there are other directions the person may take. The experience may be seen as an opportunity to learn. Another possibility is that the person may be completely overwhelmed, and the anxiety escalates.

Anger may cause the person and those around the person to have a variety of responses. Many variables can affect the direction that the anger will take, such as: the anxiety level, amount of stress the person has been experiencing, the importance of the situation, possible consequences of the situation, the people involved, time of day, health status, medications, alcohol/drug abuse, support from others, reinforcement from others who say that the anger is appropriate, and financial issues.

It is important to recognize that anger does not equal physical violence. If home care staff become afraid that expression of anger will always lead to violence or is too much of a risk, they communicate to the patient that anger is bad and that it needs to be covered over. Appropriate expression of anger is something most patients need to learn how to do. Denial of anger will only increase the patient's stress.

Home care staff have a variety of reactions to aggressive behavior. Typical staff responses are fear, anxiety, aggression, withdrawal, inability to do the job, punitive actions toward patients, and attempts to make the home completely safe. The latter is never possible. Staff must first accept that if a patient really wants to do harm, it is possible. The goal is for staff to assess the patient prior to an incident and make every effort, without putting self at extreme risk, to prevent an incident. If staff become overly anxious about safety and fear the patient's behavior, the patient will feel this anxiety too, as anxiety can be contagious. It will affect the patient's behavior and the home environment. It is very important to work directly with the family/SOs about responses to the patient whose anger is escalating.

Risk Factors[14,15]

It is difficult to predict violence in any patient. Psychiatric patients do not have a greater risk for violence; however, most people think that they do. Risk factors for escalating behavior and violence for psychiatric patients include the following:

- past history of assaultive behavior
- diagnosis (e.g., drug/alcohol intoxication, organic brain disorder, paranoid schizophrenia)
- severity of illness
- denial by the ill person, staff, and families/SOs
- noncompliance with medications

Assessment

Prior to the first home visit, the nurse should review information from other sources (e.g., emergency department, referral source, hospital), particularly noting indications of escalation. When there is concern about the patient's anger during the admission assessment, home care staff should select the place for the assessment carefully. Privacy is important, but not at the expense of staff safety. If the nurse chooses to do the assessment in a room alone, the door should be kept open and the nurse should have easy access to the door. Family/SOs should be in the home and, if the patient's behavior deteriorates, the nurse should be willing to discontinue the assessment. The patient's mental status is assessed and possible problems identified. Throughout home care, the patient's affect and behavior are assessed as needed. The following assessment areas are particularly important: level of anxiety; noncompliance with medications; history of suicidal behavior; history of violent and/or destructive behavior; psychosis, especially with paranoid delusions or auditory hallucinations; substance use and abuse; and inappropriate interactions with other people, staff, and family/SOs. Behaviors that are associated with aggression include the following:[16]

- motor agitation: pacing, inability to sit still, clenching or pounding fists, jaw tightening, increased respirations, sudden cessation of motor activity

- verbalizations: verbal threats toward real and imagined objects; intrusive demands for attention; loud, pressured speech; evidence of delusional or paranoid thought content
- affect: anger, hostility, extreme anxiety, irritability, inappropriate or excessive euphoria, affect lability
- level of consciousness: confusion, sudden change in mental status, disorientation, memory impairment, inability to be redirected

Other indicators that the patient might be angry are forgetting appointments, refusing to see home care staff, maintaining silence, avoiding eye contact, turning away, and speaking with sarcasm.

If a patient is at risk for escalation, anticipatory planning is important. Home care staff plan how they will assess the patient and intervene prior to escalation. The assessment for anger includes the following components:[17]

- recent losses
- past history, particularly head trauma or seizures; childhood violence, fire setting, or truancy; sexual, physical, or psychological abuse; previous incidents of violence; legal history
- mental status exam
- appearance (e.g., tense, angry facial expression, clinched fists, angry stance)
- speech (e.g., loud, profanity, threatening)
- affect (e.g., labile)
- mood (e.g., angry, hostile, agitated)
- psychotic symptoms (e.g., paranoid or grandiose delusions, hallucinations)
- cognitive factors (e.g., disorientation, impaired judgment and insight)
- possession or availability of a weapon
- intoxication or withdrawal

Interventions

Therapeutic and Nontherapeutic Interventions

Interventions for anger and aggression may be nontherapeutic or therapeutic. The home care staff should be aware of these interventions as they work with patients who are angry. The most common nontherapeutic interventions, which reinforce anger, include the following:

- reacting with hostility
- intervening inconsistently
- setting limits in an overbearing manner
- failing to set limits
- displaying inflexibility

- intruding on the patient's personal space
- focusing on the patient rather than on the unacceptable behavior
- communicating that feeling anger is wrong or bad
- avoiding the angry patient
- showing little warmth toward the patient
- defending staff errors
- fearing the patient
- reinforcing behaviors to meet staff needs
- ignoring the behavior

The following therapeutic interventions are important to use with patients who are angry:

- Recognize the patient's feelings.
- Use a low, calm voice and speak slowly and clearly. Open-ended questions increase communication and allow the patient some flexibility.
- Listen to the patient and respond to the patient's issues.
- Give the patient time to clarify feelings.
- Give the patient the opportunity to maintain dignity.
- Avoid sarcasm or arguing with patient.
- Be honest and consistent.
- Help the patient accept that all people feel anger, and teach appropriate coping mechanisms.
- Help the patient assess his or her anger. (What happened before the feeling? What were the expectations? Were they met? If not, why not? Were the expectations realistic? What are possible responses of others and actual responses of others to anger? What are other methods for coping with anger?)
- Give the patient choices to avoid a power struggle.
- Do not push the patient into situations that will stimulate anger until the patient can cope.
- Use physical activity to decrease the energy that results from anger.
- Remain calm.
- Posture and body language are important. Avoid crossing arms across chest. A relaxed posture should be taken.
- Verbal intervention is very important, but only during escalation when the patient is becoming agitated, not when the patient is out of control. Recommendations for verbal intervention include suggestions that focus on the staff-patient interaction.[18] To encourage the patient to refocus on the situation or problem rather than acting out, it is helpful to ask the patient details about the reasons for the anger. Questions that begin with "how" or "when" are helpful. Instructions given to the patient should be brief and assertive. Staff should negotiate options with the patient. Using words such as "we" or "us" emphasizes cooperation. Staff should show concern as the patient speaks,

such as by nodding the head or saying "Go on." Questions that begin with "why" are not helpful. Telling the patient to calm down or belittling the patient's problem will only make the patient angrier.

Expected Outcomes

Examples of expected outcomes for the angry or escalating patient include the following:

- The patient will not injure self, others, or be destructive to property.
- The patient will identify behaviors and feelings that lead to escalation.
- The patient will ask staff or family/SOs for help when he or she feels a situation is escalating and cannot handle it.
- The patient will develop a treatment contract related to escalating behavior and follow it.

Home Care Interventions

Examples of interventions for the angry patient in the home include the following:

- The patient, family/SOs, and home care staff may develop a treatment contract that describes when the patient will take a quiet time in a specific room to decrease escalation. The contract must address criteria for use, the room, requirements such as open door, time period, and criteria to determine when the quiet period will be over. The patient and family/SOs must understand that this is not to be used as punishment but to provide the patient some time to gain control. On each visit, home care staff should ask if quiet times have been taken and the results. Quiet times may be used only when escalation becomes a problem or may be used routinely, such as daily, in order to ensure that the patient maintains control over behavior.
- The patient should take prescribed medications as ordered. If noncompliance occurs, staff assess the patient carefully for signs of escalating behavior. Some patients may have orders for medications when there are increased problems with anger and aggression. The patient and family/SOs should understand when these medications are to be used and the importance of using them.
- Home care staff and family/SOs should set limits with firm, clear direction using a soft, calm voice. The patient should be told that staff and family/SOs will help to keep the patient safe. Behavioral expectations must be simple and clear.
- Personal space can be an important issue with an angry patient. If the patient is sitting, the nurse should sit, because this position is less intimidating. There should be space between staff and the patient. If the patient is unable to sit or

stand still, pacing or walking with the patient may be helpful. It is best not to talk to the patient while standing behind the patient. The space between staff and the patient should not be so large that voices must be raised.

- Whenever there is a verbal altercation or inappropriate physical contact, immediate intervention is required. Communicate verbally and nonverbally that everyone must remain calm. At this time, follow-through and consistency are very important. Staff/family/SOs ask the patient to go to a quieter area in the home to gain control. Moveable furniture and other such objects are removed from the area.

- Home care staff and family/SOs should never put themselves at risk. If a situation cannot be handled, appropriate help is called. If the aggressive behavior is the result of psychotic thought (e.g., delusions or hallucinations), then the escalating behavior may not be easy to control. The telephone number for the local police; ambulance; and, if available, psychiatric emergency response team should always be accessible.

- The patient's physician should be contacted when there is a pattern that indicates escalating behavior that cannot be controlled or when the patient's behavior becomes disruptive and unmanageable.

- Home care staff should document the patient's clinical status related to anger and aggression and any incidents. Home care agency guidelines and standards should be followed. Documentation should continue after an incident, in order to assess changes and the results of interventions. Home care staff who visit the patient should communicate verbally with one another about the patient.

HOSPITALIZATION

The decision to hospitalize a patient is not an easy one to make—not because it is difficult to determine when the patient requires hospitalization but because of the feelings and reactions to the decision. The patient, family/SOs, and staff may feel guilt, anger, depression, frustration, and hopelessness. It is important to be clear about the reasons for the hospitalization and to recognize that the patient has a chronic illness and that there will be relapses and need for more intensive treatment. The home care nurse talks with the patient and the family/SO about their past experiences with hospitalization. Appropriate information and opportunity to discuss feelings may alleviate some anxiety. The patient may or may not return to home care, and staff must recognize this at the time of discharge from home care. Promises should not be made regarding future home care treatment unless specific information is known.

The home care staff should know about the community hospitals, their services, the quality of those services, and their admission procedures. Many patients are admitted to the hospital via emergency services and, thus, staff should know about these services and how to access them. The home care agency develops a procedure regarding admission to the hospitals and a reference manual that includes information about hospitals and other resources. During times of crisis home care staff should not have to hunt for information. The patient's insurance coverage is also an important factor in determining the type of service, length of stay, and availability of hospitalization for the individual patient.

FAMILY AND SIGNIFICANT OTHERS

Psychiatric crises and emergencies in the home are very traumatic for families/ SOs. Complex interpersonal and intrafamilial dynamics are important, along with the patient's symptoms. Clearly, the safety of family members/SOs is of concern; however, the experience of having violence erupt in the home disturbs its equilibrium. Families/SOs may walk around trying to be overly careful in order to avoid future problems. This will only increase the stress. Suicidal behavior arouses feelings of guilt, inadequacy, and fear. Again, the family/SOs feels that they must be very careful and supervise the patient. Home care staff must provide support to the family/SOs during and after these crises. Family/SOs will need practical information and someone to talk with about their feelings. Ideally, the home care staff will develop a plan with the patient and the family/SOs to be used in times of crisis. Questions that home care staff and family/SOs should consider as escalation occurs and when developing interventions include the following:[19]

- Is this a real confrontation?
- Is the violence or threat of violence an expression of psychotic thought?
- Does the ill family member use aggression deliberately as a threatening tactic to get what he or she wants?
- Does aggression occur because of the patient's tenuous control under stress?
- What type of situations have brought on violence in the past?
- Who tends to be present?
- Are there particular topics that set things off?
- Are there particular times of the day that are stressful?
- Have particular medications worked in the past?

Answers to these questions will provide guidance as to the best approach to take. As is true in most cases, the home care staff need to listen to the family/SOs. They have the long-term experience with the patient.

LEGAL ISSUES[20]

Understanding basic legal and ethical principles and their impact upon administrative and clinical decisions in crisis situations is an important part of home care. This understanding will reduce liability exposure for the home care agency and the staff. Legal issues are subject to constant change, depending on court decisions and changes in local, state, and federal laws. The home care agency must maintain current knowledge of these changes. See Chapter 6 for a detailed discussion of legal issues and the administration of psychiatric home care services.

SUMMARY

Crises and emergencies occur in the home when there is an ill family member. The major responsibilities of home care staff are to communicate to the patient and family/SOs that crises and emergencies will occur, to establish assessment and monitoring to identify potential crises, and to develop interventions with the patient and the family/SOs to be taken at appropriate times. Following a crisis or emergency, the home care nurse provides support; at the appropriate time, the nurse assesses with the patient and family/SOs the crisis situation to determine if other steps could have been taken and applies this new information to future planning and interventions. The focus is not blame but rather improvement.

NOTES

1. S. Benter, "Crisis Intervention," in *Principles and Practice of Psychiatric Nursing*, ed. G. Stuart and S. Sundeen (St. Louis, MO: Mosby–Year Book, 1995), 277–299, at 278.
2. D. Aguilera, *Crisis Intervention: Theory and Methodology* (St. Louis, MO: Mosby–Year Book, 1994), 1.
3. L. Mosher and L. Burti, *Community Mental Health: Principles and Practice* (New York: W.W. Norton & Company, 1989), 111.
4. A. Hatfield, *Family Education in Mental Illness* (New York: Guilford Press, 1990), 120.
5. Hatfield, *Family Education in Mental Illness*, 120–122.
6. Benter, "Crisis Intervention," 282.
7. A. Guarini, "The Challenge of Gaining Access to the Mental Health Care System: One Nurse's Perspective," *Journal of Home Health Care Practice* 2, no. 3: 17–25, at 19–20.
8. Benter, "Crisis Intervention," 287–288.
9. Benter, "Crisis Intervention," 287.
10. B. Rickelman and J. Houfek, "Toward an Interactional Model of Suicidal Behaviors: Cognitive Rigidity, Attributional Style, Stress, Hopelessness, and Depression," *Archives of Psychiatric Nursing* 9, no. 3: 158–168, at 159–160.

11. J. Hillard, "Predicting Suicide," *Psychiatric Services* 46, no. 3: 223–225.

12. S. Hogarity and C. Rodaitis, "A Suicide Precautions Policy for the General Hospital," *Journal of Nursing Administration* 17, no. 10: 36–42, at 41.

13. E. Kruse and G. Jones, "Development of a Comprehensive Suicide Protocol in a Home Health Care and Social Services Agency," *Journal of Home Health Care Practice* 3, no. 2: 59–63, at 52.

14. D. Blair and S. New, "Assaultive Behavior: Know the Risks," *Journal of Psychosocial Nursing* 29, no. 11 (1991): 25–30, at 26–27.

15. E. Torrey, "Violent Behavior by Individuals with Serious Mental Illness," *Hospital and Community Psychiatry* 45, no. 7 (1994): 653–662, at 652.

16. C. Hamolia, "Managing Aggressive Behavior," in *Principles and Practice of Psychiatric Nursing*, ed. G. Stuart and S. Sundeen (St. Louis, MO: Mosby–Year Book, 1995), 719–745, at 727.

17. P. Blumenreich, "Assessment," in *Managing the Violent Patient: A Clinician's Guide*, ed. P. Blumenreich (New York: Brunner/Mazel Publishers, 1993), 35–40, at 37–38.

18. J. Turnbull et al., "Turn It Around: Short-Term Management for Aggression and Anger," *Journal of Psychosocial Nursing* 28, no. 6 (1990): 7–10, 13.

19. Hatfield, *Family Education in Mental Illness*, 124–126.

20. A. Finkelman, *Psychiatric Nursing Administration Manual* (Gaithersburg, MD: Aspen Publishers, Inc., 1995), 5–1:1–5–1:8.

SUGGESTED READING

Blair, D., and S. New. 1991. Assaultive behavior: Know the risks. *Journal of Psychosocial Nursing* 29, no. 11: 25–30.

Blumenreich, P. 1993. *Managing the violent patient: A clinician's guide.* New York: Brunner/Mazel Publishers.

Cardell, R., and S. Horton-Deutsch. A model for assessment of inpatient suicide potential. *Archives of Psychiatric Nursing* 8, no. 6: 366–372.

Estroff, S. et al. 1994. The influence of social networks and social support on violence by persons with serious mental illness. *Hospital and Community Psychiatry* 45, no. 7: 669–678.

Finkelman, A. 1990. *Quality assurance for psychiatric nursing.* Rockville, MD: Aspen Publishers, Inc.

Forester, P., and J. King. 1994. Definitive treatment of patients with serious mental disorders in an emergency service, part I. *Hospital and Community Psychiatry* 45, no. 9: 867–869.

Forester, P., and J. King. 1994. Definitive treatment of patients with serious mental disorders in an emergency service, part II. *Hospital and Community Psychiatry* 45, no. 12: 1177–1178.

Guarini, A. The challenge of gaining access to the mental health care system: One nurse's perspective. *Journal of Home Health Care Practice* 2, no. 3 (1990): 17–25.

Harper-Jaques, S., and M. Reimer. 1992. Aggressive behavior and the brain: A different perspective for the mental health nurse. *Archives of Psychiatric Nursing* 6, no. 5: 312–320.

Harris, D., and E. Morrison. 1995. Managing violence without coercion. *Archives of Psychiatric Nursing* 9, no. 4: 203–210.

Hillard, J. 1995. Predicting suicide. *Psychiatric Services* 45, no. 3: 223–225.

Junginger, J. 1995. Command hallucinations and the prediction of dangerousness. *Psychiatric Services* 46, no. 9: 911–914.

Kruse, E., and G. Jones. 1990. Development of a comprehensive suicide protocol in a home health care and social service agency. *Journal of Home Health Care Practice* 3, no. 2: 47–56.

Merker, M. 1986. Psychiatric emergency evaluation. *Nursing Clinics of North America* 21, no. 3: 387–396.

Ragaisis, K. 1994. Critical incident stress debriefing: A family nursing intervention. *Archives of Psychiatric Nursing* 8, no. 1: 38–43.

Rickelman, B., and J. Houfek. 1995. Toward an interactional model of suicidal behaviors: Cognitive rigidity, attributional style, stress, hopelessness, and depression. *Archives of Psychiatric Nursing* 9, no. 3: 158–168.

Rozell, G. 1992. Is home care a dangerous occupation? *Caring* 11, no. 4: 50–53.

Segal, S. et al. 1995. Factors in the quality of patient evaluations in general hospital psychiatric emergency services. *Psychiatric Services* 46, no. 11: 1144–1148.

Stevenson, S. 1991. Heading off violence with verbal de-escalation. *Journal of Psychosocial Nursing* 29, no. 9: 6–10.

Tardiff, K. 1989. *Assessment and management of violent patients.* Washington, DC: American Psychiatric Press, Inc.

Torrey, E. 1994. Violent behavior by individuals with serious mental illness. *Hospital and Community Psychiatry* 45, no. 7: 653–662.

Turnbull, J. et al. 1990. Turn it around: Short term management and anger. *Journal of Psychosocial Nursing* 28, no. 6: 7–14.

Wilson-Nolan, B., and C. Toone. 1993. Responding to family violence. *Caring* 12, no. 4: 32–34.

Glossary

acrophobia—fear of heights

acting out—demonstrating behaviorally how one feels rather than verbalizing feelings

action—identifies how a drug is known to produce its desired therapeutic effect

actual diagnosis/problem—clinically validated diagnosis/problem

addiction—physical dependence on a substance

affect—outward manifestation of a patient's emotional feeling

agitation—chronic restlessness

agonist—a substance that acts to enhance or potentiate a substance or drug

agoraphobia—fear of being in an open, crowded space and being unable to escape

akathisia—a neuroleptic side effect in which the patient experiences motor restlessness

Al-Anon—self-help group for families and significant others of alcoholics

Alateen—self-help group for teenagers who are children or siblings of alcoholics

alexia—impairment in intellectual function characterized by the inability to comprehend the written word

ambivalence—simultaneous contradictory feelings

antagonist—a substance or drug that decreases or blocks the action of another substance or drug

anxiety—a form of tension; an emotional reaction to an object or experience that is felt to be a real or imagined danger or threat

aphasia—difficulty finding the right word

assessment—collecting and analyzing data about a patient

attention—the ability to focus on one activity

blocking—difficulty in recollection; interruption of a train of thought or speech due to emotional factors, usually unconscious

blood level—a laboratory test to determine the concentration of a drug in the plasma, serum, or blood; not accurate until a steady state is reached

blunting—a decrease or loss of emotional expression

body image—conscious and unconscious attitudes toward one's body

chemical dependency—pathological dependency on a chemical substance

chief complaint—the reason the patient comes for treatment, described in the patient's own words

circumstantiality—too many associated thoughts coming at one time with an inability to suppress them selectively

cognition—process of logical thoughts

compulsion—recurring impulse to perform a specific act

concrete thinking—logical and coherent thoughts; ability to sort, classify, order, and organize facts; with inability to generalize or deal with abstractions

condensation—process of reducing several ideas into one symbol

confabulation—unconsciously filling in memory gaps with material that is often complex; can be described in detail and appears logical

conflict—a situation in which a person experiences two opposite feelings or has two opposite reactions

defense mechanism—the means by which a person attempts to decrease anxiety, guilt, or shame

delirium tremens—diagnostic term that has been replaced with the term *alcohol withdrawal delirium*

delusion—a fixed, false belief contrary to evidence

dendrite—postsynaptic membrane of a neuron

denial—a defense mechanism; refusal to acknowledge what one sees, hears, or feels

depersonalization—feeling empty and unable to express feelings, and not feeling a part of self

diagnosis—making a judgment about a patient based on data collected

diurnal mood variation—changes in mood related to the time of day

drug interaction—the effect of two or more drugs taken at the same time, which changes the expected outcome and/or causes side effects

drug tolerance—requirement for increased doses of a drug to produce same physiological/psychological effect *dyskinesia*—inability to execute voluntary movements

dystonia—acute tonic muscle spasms due to use of a neuroleptic (e.g., muscles of tongue, jaw, eyes, neck)

echolalia—repetitive imitation of another person's speech

elation—high degree of confidence, boastfulness, uncritical optimism, and joy accompanied by increased motor activity

electroconvulsive therapy (ECT)— a treatment methodology in which electrical current is artificially placed on the temple(s) to produce a grand mal seizure

empathy—the emotional understanding of another person's experience; the ability to put oneself in another person's place and understand his or her feelings and behavior objectively

endorphins—naturally occurring peptides in the central nervous system that have a similar physiological effect to opiates

euphoria—exaggerated feeling of emotional and physical well-being inappropriate for actual environmental stimuli

extrapyramidal syndrome (EPS)—dysfunction of extrapyramidal system often due to side effects from drugs (e.g., tremors, drooling, shuffling gait, muscular rigidity, dystonia, akinesia)

flat affect—unchanging, extreme lack of emotional response

flight of ideas—verbally skipping from one idea to another before one is finished, with no connection between ideas

general appearance—patient's weight, coloring, skin condition, body build, odor, and physical impairments

half-life—the amount of time it takes a drug to reach a steady-state concentration; the amount of the drug in the body will increase and fluctuate with each dose until a steady state is reached; affects side effects and optimal dose for each patient; affects how frequently the drug needs to be taken

hallucination—a false sensory perception

health-promotion activities—patient teaching

human response pattern—functional health patterns used to organize the individual nursing diagnoses into categories; these are not mutually exclusive in that a diagnosis may relate to several patterns or just one pattern

hypomania—mild form of mania

inappropriate affect—emotion that is not appropriate for the situation

insight—ability to evaluate a problem accurately

intellectualization—a defense mechanism; control of feelings and impulses through thinking them instead of feeling them or acting on them

interpersonal—the relationship between people, behavior, and feelings *irritability*—a feeling characterized by impatience, annoyance, and easy provocation to anger

labile affect—rapidly changing emotion or mood

loose associations—a lack of relationship between ideas and emotions particularly related to similarities and continuity; changing topics rapidly

magical thinking—belief that merely thinking about an external event will make it occur

manipulation—influencing another person to meet one's needs and ignoring the needs of the other person

mutism—silent even though able to speak

Narcotics Anonymous (NA)—organization that is similar to Alcoholics Anonymous (AA) but for drug-dependent persons

neologisms—use of new expressions, phrases, or words or creation of new meaning for accepted expressions, phrases, or words

neuroscience—a branch of science that focuses on how the brain works in normal persons

neurotransmitter—a chemical compound that acts as a messenger for the nervous system

obsession—a persistent, unwanted, recurring thought

oculogyric crisis—side effect characterized by uncontrollable rolling upward of the eyes, caused by the effect of neuroleptic medication

paranoid ideation—an internal system of persecutory and/or grandiose delusions; internally appears logical to the person

perseveration—pathological repetition of a sentence, phrase, or word

pharmacokinetics—the process and rate of drug distribution, metabolism, and disposition

phobia—strong, persistent, abnormal fear of an object or situation

polypharmacy—concurrent use of several drugs; affects therapeutic efficacy, side effects, and leads to drug interaction problems

possible diagnosis/problem—the diagnosis/problem may be present but requires more data to confirm or to rule it out

potential diagnosis/problem—a diagnosis/problem with an increased risk if certain interventions are not initiated

pressured speech—sudden increase in the quantity of speech; appears loud and rushed

projection—a defense mechanism; a person perceives and treats unacceptable inner impulses as if they were outside one's self

psychosocial—patient's mental and social status and functioning *psychotropic drugs/medications*—the name for the group of drugs that includes neuroleptics/antipsychotics, antianxiety, antidepressants, hypnotics, sedatives, and stimulants

reality orientation—methods to ensure that a person is alert to the here and now

regression—a defense mechanism; when a person returns to a previous stage of functioning to avoid anxiety

self-esteem—a person's assessment of his or her own worth

splitting—viewing a person or a situation as all good or all bad

steady state—the amount of drug ingested equals the amount of drug excreted

synapse—the point at which the transmission of nerve impulses occurs; the gap between the membrane of one nerve cell and another nerve cell

synergistic—the reaction in the body between two or more substances that enhances each of the substances

tardive dyskinesia (TD)— a serious, chronic side effect from the use of neuroleptics (e.g., lip puckering; chewing; choreiform finger movements; tongue writhing or protrusion; movements of the neck, trunk, and pelvis)

target symptoms—symptoms of an illness that are most likely to respond to a specific drug or interaction

therapeutic relationship—the relationship between the patient and staff that helps the patient cope with problems

thought content—what a person thinks

thought process—how a person thinks

thought stopping—interrupting dysfunctional thoughts

tolerance—the decrease in the effect of a drug over time while taking the same dose; can lead to a decrease in side effects

treatment contract—a written agreement between a patient and staff or family/ SOs to do specific things in order to help the patient cope with a specific problem; time limited with specific evaluation times

word salad—combination of phrases, words, and sentences that are disconnected and incoherent

American Nurses Association Standards of Psychiatric-Mental Health Clinical Nursing Practice

Standard I. Assessment

The psychiatric-mental health nurse collects client health data.

Standard II. Diagnosis

The psychiatric-mental health nurse analyzes the assessment data in determining diagnoses.

Standard III. Outcome identification

The psychiatric-mental health nurse identifies expected outcomes individualized to the client.

Standard IV. Planning

The psychiatric-mental health nurse develops a plan of care that prescribes interventions to attain expected outcomes.

Standard V. Implementation

The psychiatric-mental health nurse implements the interventions identified in the plan of care.

Standard Va. Counseling

The psychiatric-mental health nurse uses counseling interventions to assist clients in improving or regaining their previous coping abilities, fostering mental health, and preventing mental illness and disability.

Standard Vb. Milieu therapy

The psychiatric-mental health nurse provides, structures, and maintains a therapeutic environment in collaboration with the client and other health care providers.

Standard Vc. Self-care activities

The psychiatric-mental health nurse structures interventions around the client's activities of daily living to foster self-care and mental and physical well-being.

Standard Vd. Psychobiological interventions

The psychiatric-mental health nurse uses knowledge of psychobiological interventions and applies clinical skills to restore the client's health and prevent further disability.

Standard Ve. Health teaching

The psychiatric-mental health nurse, through health teaching, assists clients in achieving satisfying, productive, and healthy patterns of living.

Standard Vf. Case management

The psychiatric-mental health nurse provides case management to coordinate comprehensive health services and ensure continuity of care.

Standard Vg. Health promotion and health maintenance

The psychiatric-mental health nurse employs strategies and interventions to promote and maintain mental health and prevent mental illness.

Standard VI. Evaluation

The psychiatric-mental health nurse evaluates the client's progress in attaining expected outcomes.

Source: Reprinted with permission from American Nurses Association, *Standards of Psychiatric-Mental Health Clinical Nursing Practice*, © 1994, American Nurses Association.

American Nurses Association Standards of Home Health Nursing Practice

Standard I. Organization of home health services
All home health services are planned, organized, and directed by a master's-prepared professional nurse with experience in community health and administration.

Standard II. Theory
The nurse applies theoretical concepts as a basis for decisions in practice.

Standard III. Data collection
The nurse continuously collects and records data that are comprehensive, accurate, and systematic.

Standard IV. Diagnosis
The nurse uses health assessment data to determine nursing diagnoses.

Standard V. Planning
The nurse develops care plans that establish goals. The care plan is based on nursing diagnoses and the medical treatment plan. The client and family participate in the planning process.

Standard VI. Intervention
The nurse, guided by the care plan, intervenes to provide comfort, to restore, improve, and promote health, to prevent complications and sequelae of illness, and to effect rehabilitation.

Standard VII. Evaluation
The nurse continually evaluates the client's and family's responses to interventions in order to determine progress toward goal attainment and to revise the database, nursing diagnoses, and plan of care.

Standard VIII. Continuity of care

The nurse is responsible for the client's appropriate and uninterrupted care along the health care continuum, and therefore uses discharge planning, case management, and coordination of community resources.

Standard IX. Interdisciplinary collaboration

The nurse initiates and maintains a liaison relationship with all appropriate health care providers to assure that all efforts effectively complement one another.

Standard X. Professional development

The nurse assumes responsibility for professional development and contributes to the professional growth of others.

Standard XI. Research

The nurse participates in research activities that contribute to the profession's continuing development of knowledge of home health care.

Standard XII. Ethics

The nurse uses the Code for Nurses established by the American Nurses Association as a guide for ethical decision making in practice.

Source: Reprinted with permission from American Nurses Association, *Standards of Home Health Nursing Practice,* © 1986, American Nurses Association.

Index

A

Abnormal involuntary movement scale, 346, 347
Abortion, 58
Acetylcholine, 280
Acquired immune deficiency syndrome. *See* AIDS
Acrophobia, defined, 577
Acting out
  anxiety disorder, 371–373
  defined, 577
Action, defined, 577
Active questioning, 216–218
Activities and support interventions log, 234
Activities of daily living, defined, 24
Actual diagnosis/problem, defined, 577
Addiction, defined, 577
Administrative commitment, 117
Admission
  admission criteria, 98–99
    reimbursement, 98
  informal admission, 116
  involuntary admission, 117
  types, 116–117
  voluntary admission, 117
Affect, defined, 577

Aggressive behavior
  crisis resolution, 567–572
    assessment, 568–569
    expected outcomes, 571
    interventions, 569–572
    risk factors, 568
  fear of aggression, 54
  schizophrenia, 449
Agitation
  defined, 577
  elderly patient, 551
Agonist, defined, 577
Agoraphobia, defined, 577
AIDS, 475–486
  assessment, 480–482
  behavioral disturbance, 485
  characteristics, 476
  cognitive dysfunction, 483–484
  crisis, 477–478
  depression, 478–479, 485
  family, 485–486
  illness phases, 477–478
  intellectual dysfunction, 483–484
  intervention, 482–485
  neuropsychiatric complications, 479–480
  personality disturbance, 485
  psychosocial aspects, 476

C